P9-DYA-186

Medicine
of the Earth

this book belongs to

Raymond E. Hirst Jr.

8/15/97   BS^s

401-949-0771

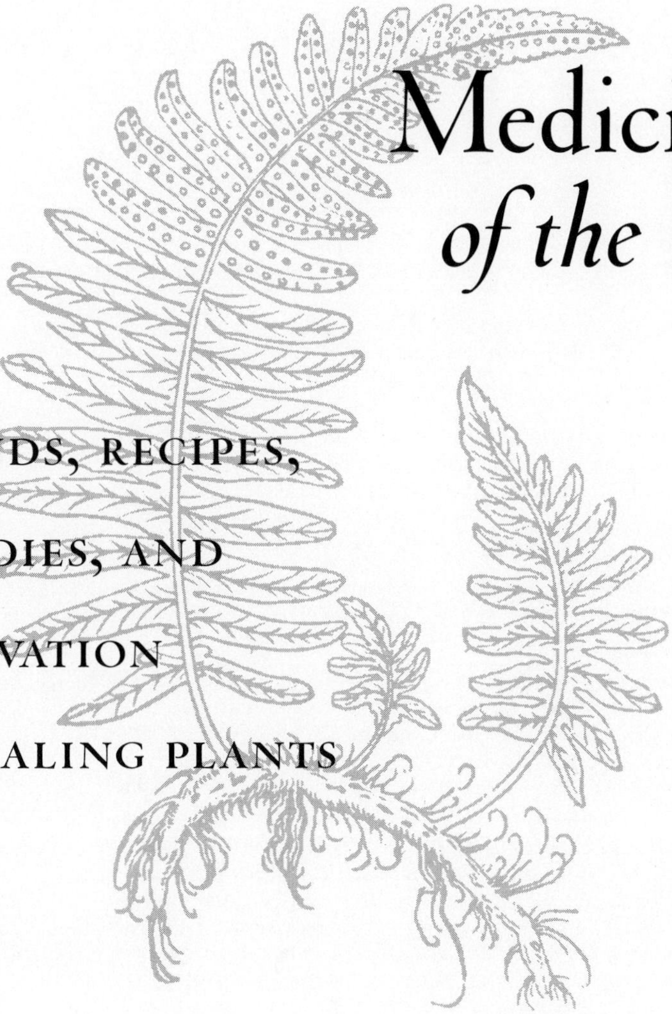

Medicine
of the Earth

LEGENDS, RECIPES,

REMEDIES, AND

CULTIVATION

OF HEALING PLANTS

SUSANNE FISCHER-RIZZI

Translated by Meret Liebenstein Bainbridge
Illustrations by Peter Ebenhoch

RUDRA PRESS   PORTLAND, OREGON

Rudra Press
PO Box 13390
Portland, Oregon   97213
Telephone: 503-235-0175
Telefax: 503-235-0909

© 1996 by Rudra Press

Originally published as *Medizin der Erde: Legenden, Mythen, Heilanwendung und Betrachtung unserer Heilpflanzen* © 1984 Heinrich Hugendubel Verlag, Munich, Germany

All rights reserved. No part of this publication may be used or reproduced in any manner whatsoever without written permission, except in the case of brief quotations embodied in critical articles and reviews.

Book and cover design by Bill Stanton
Cover photograph by Barry Kaplan
Edited by Julie Zinkus, Cheryl Rosen, and Ellen Hynson
Typography by Jeff Levin / Pendragon Graphics

The English edition of *Medicine of the Earth* sits before us in no small part because of the fastidious translation work of Meret Liebenstein Bainbridge, herself a student of naturopathy in the United States. Unless otherwise noted, translations into English of all poems, extracts from historical documents, etc., in this edition are by the translator.

This book is not intended to replace expert medical advice. The author and publisher urge you to verify the appropriateness of any herbal use with your qualified healthcare professional. Some herbs are potentially poisonous or can cause adverse reactions. Some herbs are regulated and / or restricted in their cultivation, collection, or usage. Always check with your qualified healthcare professional, local regulating agencies, and local herb societies or specialists regarding collecting, cultivating, or using any herb. The author and publisher disclaim any liability or loss, personal or otherwise, resulting from the information in this book.

Library of Congress Cataloguing-In-Publication Data
Fischer-Rizzi, Susanne
    [Medizin der Erde. English]
    Medicine of the Earth : legends, recipes, remedies, and cultivation
of healing plants / Susanne Fischer-Rizzi : translated
by Meret Liebenstein Bainbridge : illustrations by Peter Ebenhoch.
        p.   cm.
    Includes index.
    ISBN 0-915801-59-0 (alk. paper)
    1. Herbs—Therapeutic use. 2. Materia medica, vegetable.
3. Traditional medicine.   I. Title.
RM666.H33F5713   1996
615'.321—dc20   96-34014
                                                       CIP

00 99 98 97   10 9 8 7 6 5 4 3 2

CONTENTS

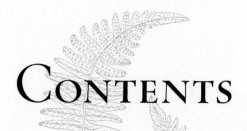

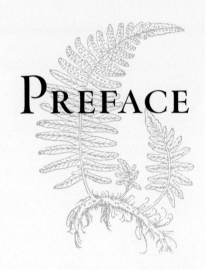

PREFACE

I ONCE ASKED a Native American medicine man if I could learn something about medicinal plants from him. He refused with the words: "First you must learn how to walk on the Earth." It was many years before I understood. I watched myself and my fellow human beings—how we walked on the earth; what relationship we had to her; how we perceived her, used her, consumed her. In truth, our taking is one-sided because we never consider giving back. In this way, we destroy the planet's harmony and health without noticing that we, too, fall into disharmony and alienate ourselves from nature's healing powers.

Two thousand years ago in Palestine, the Essenes wrote that people cannot live long or happily without honoring Mother Earth, without following her laws. I'm afraid this wisdom is almost forgotten.

Everything is connected. The earth vibrates in rhythm with the cosmos and in the smallest thing on earth we recognize the highest in heaven. And we are part of this cosmic web. For human beings, living in harmony with heaven and earth was once considered the fulfillment of life. In the fertility of the earth, in the growth of plants, in the maturation of fruits was recognized the unselfish giving of our earth. Plants, especially healing plants, were sacred. The ancients placed such plants under the command of gods, intoned prayers when gathering them, and processed them with care and gratitude. Today we have forgotten all of this. The Bible says that we have subjected the earth to our will. Unfortunately, we have lost sight of our responsibility and now suffer the consequences of our actions—dying forests and polluted water and air.

We have walked on the earth without respect. But it is not too late to re-learn her laws and live again in harmony. Indeed, in each healing herb we find some of the earth's vital energy. If we can receive it with awareness and gratitude, it will be strong medicine for us.

This is an attitude that is not learned from books. It comes from opening our hearts to it. Words cannot give you, the Reader, a true experience of a plant's essence, appearance, grace, or healing properties. To really connect to and understand their power, it is far better to observe these plants in nature.

As Author, my hope is to inspire you to learn from your own personal experience. I urge you to go outside, to pay attention, and, as I have, to ask questions: What energy does this plant have? What can I learn from it? What is its essence? What part of my body does it pertain to? Which plants do I find more appealing because of their remedies? How can I protect and propagate them?

Perhaps after experiencing a plant in nature we will recall some fairy tale once heard about it. This can give us some insight into understanding its essence. After all, myths and legends, plants associated with seasonal feast days, and old names are remnants of an older and deeper knowledge. I often feel nearer to understanding a plant through a story or name rather than through a scientific listing of its chemical make-up or a precise botanical description. For this reason, in *Medicine of the Earth* I have emphasized the old names and folklore.

As we rediscover the beauty and healing power of plants, we will become aware of our responsiblity and start thinking about how we can protect these healing gifts. For instance, we might pick only what we need and leave untouched those plants of which only a few still grow. On our walks we might gather seeds to plant in another location. And in our home gardens, we might cultivate plants to use for propagation. Lastly, we might find a way to contribute to organizations that hinder the further destruction of nature.

Medicine of the Earth describes only those plants that I have a personal relationship with—and whose healing powers I have observed and experienced firsthand on myself and others. Healing plants considered to be trees and shrubs are discussed in my book *Blätter von Bäumen* (in German).

I would like to thank all my teachers who have shared their knowledge and accompanied me on my path. Maria Keller, Kräutermutter ("Herb Mother") Flach, Fast Wolf, naturopath Josef Karl, and Veronica Andern. For helpful corrections, I am grateful to Dr. Probst and F. Wiedemann, Dipl. Hdl. My sincere thanks extends to my family who have supported me in many ways throughout my work on this book.

༄

SUSANNE FISCHER-RIZZI
Sulzberg im Allgäu

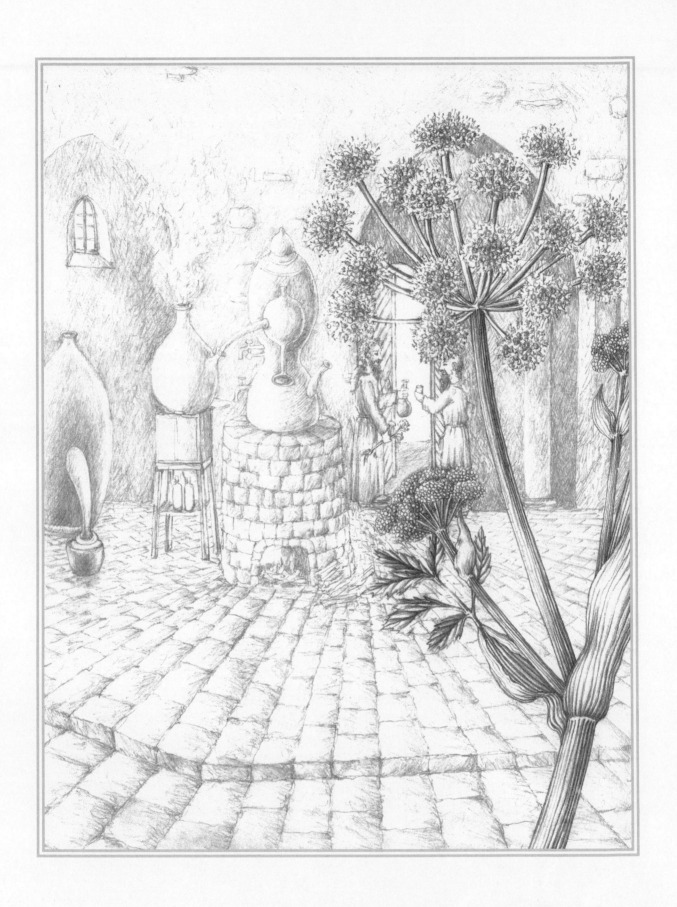

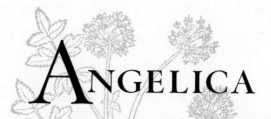

ANGELICA

Angelica archangelica / Angelica officinalis
Garden Angelica, European Angelica
Carrot family — Umbelliferae / Apiaceae

IN ALPINE FORESTS and wet meadows and along riverbanks there grows a Nordic giant— tall, of noble build and imposing stature, bursting with energy. Loving the moist cool air of the North, this plant was known through myths and legends in faraway Greenland, Iceland, and Norway long before the ancient Greek and Roman herbalists mention it.

Angelica is the plant's name—although a normal angel could never compete with her healing power. It would have to be an archangel; thus, *Angelica archangelica* or, in German, *Archangel-wort*. She is one of the best-known medicinal plants of our Nordic ancestors' medicine chest. Old herbalists sang her praises and famous physicians prepared valuable remedies from her root.

Nicholas Culpeper, the early seventeenth century physician and astrologer, felt it unnecessary to describe Angelica in detail to the readers of his herbal because "to write a description of that which is so well-known to be growing almost in every garden I suppose is altogether needles[s]."

Today it would be futile to seek Angelica in our home gardens. She has lost her inherited place and, undisturbed, now grows as a garden plant running wild over open fields. Early on, she was cultivated in Iceland, Greenland, and Norway where gardens grew with her alone. Preserved legal texts of the twelfth century state that a tenant farmer who had an Angelica garden must be allowed to take the plants when he moved. In Iceland, Angelica was even protected by a special law: it was forbidden to dig out Angelica plants on foreign land. In those days, Angelica root was an important commodity exported to countries where the plant was not native. Only in the fourteenth century did monks bring the roots from the North to plant in monastery gardens further south. Angelica made her way from there into rural gardens and then, in our time, to the wild.

Beginners in wild-crafting, however, should look closely because not every plant with an umbel like Angelica's is one. The Carrot family, to which Angelica belongs, offers one of the rare opportunities to get poisoned from gathering herbs. The Latin family name Umbelliferae derives from *umbella* (the umbel or "umbrella") and *ferre* (to bear); it describes the characteristic shape of the flower. In other words, Umbelliferae bear an umbrella-like flower. This large family comprises about 2,600 species, of which about 110 are native to Central Europe. Many members are well-known medicinal plants, vegetables, and spices; for instance, Carrot, Celery, Anise and Lovage, Caraway, and Salad Chervil. However, the black sheep in this family contain deadly toxins: Hemlock (*Conium maculatum*), a stupefying variety of wild Chervil (*Chaerophyllum temulum*), and Water Parsnip (*Sium* spp.). People familiar with Angelica rarely confuse her with these other plants. It is when gathering wild Parsley, wild Parsnip, or Chervil that a mix-up with a poisonous species is more likely.

We have to be especially careful of confusing Angelica with the deadly poisonous Water Hemlock (*Cicuta virosa*). Its roots are clearly divided into horizontal chambers with bipinnate or tripinnate leaves that are triangular in shape. And, in contrast to the aromatic celery-pineapple scent of Angelica, it has an unpleasant smell.

There are several "models" of our Angelica. There is Marsh Angelica (*Angelica palustris*), which we meet along swampy watercourses and in bogs and fens. She grows 20 to 40 inches tall, has pure white flowers, and is said to have less healing powers than her sisters.

In most instances, we encounter Woodland Angelica (*A. sylvestris*). We find her in forests as well as in wet meadows. She grows 30 to 60 inches tall and has white or slightly reddish flowers. Her leaf stalks are furrowed on the upper side and she has a thin taproot.

Finally, we stand before the giant Garden Angelica (*A. officinalis* or *A. archangelica*). We even have to look up to her because at the height of her development she is easily over eight feet tall. She is considered the strongest medicinally of these three native Angelica species.

When becoming familiar with plants we must utilize all our senses. After all, we are not in a museum. We are in a meadow or forest where we can touch the artwork. We cannot really know plants or establish relationships with them from reading books alone. Rather it is through sensory perception that we glean information about one plant that will protect us from confusing it with another. It is our senses that help us to understand its nature. How does the stem of a plant feel? Is it round, furrowed, smooth, hairy, cool, warm? Does the plant smell pleasant, aromatic, sweet, tart, acrid?

Let us examine the mighty Angelica stem. It is round and lightly furrowed and, when cut in half, hollow inside. The leaf stalks are round as well and, contrary to Woodland Angelica, without a furrow on the upper side. The leaflets of Angelica are two or more times pinnate with the terminal ones tripinnate; all are finely serrated. When we rub them together they emit the aromatic Angelica scent. (Hemlock would not meet this test of smell!) The giant primary stem has a purple tinge where it protrudes from the ground. The branching side stems originate from bulging, inflated sheaths and are the same color at their points of attachment. A gigantic flower thrones above it all, almost seeming to scatter itself. The entire globular umbel is dipped in a tender green. The individual rays, which we can clearly feel, are covered with downy hairs. Three years it has taken the plant to reach this height and now, toward the end of fall, she will die—but not before leaving many large seeds to begin a new generation.

Such a large plant, needing a proper anchorage, drills deeply into the soil. Anyone who has ever tried to pull up an Angelica root by hand surely will carry a sturdy spade into the forest the next time. As we dig, the scent attacks our noses. It smells strongly of celery and fresh pineapple with perhaps a hint of bitter almond. In fact, we can rely on our noses when gathering plants—a poisonous plant can often be ruled out because of its unpleasant odor.

During Europe's Middle Ages, the root of Angelica was considered a kind of panacea. As the plague spread across the land, physicians took Angelica along both to heal patients and to protect themselves. Muffled up tightly, they appeared at their patients' homes looking like giant black crows. Beneath their cowls, they wore a piece of Angelica tied around their necks to chew on.

Paracelsus, the early sixteenth century Swiss-born alchemist and physician, reports that he used Angelica successfully against the plague. At that time, Angelica was considered the remedy of choice against any type of contagion. Likewise Mattioli attests in his 1563 herbal that "Today we have again one of the noble and famous herbs, [one] that cannot be paid for because of its virtue against poison and especially against the plague, as various experiences bear witness of this."

During that difficult period, expensive "secret remedies" circulated that were supposed to guard against all diseases and contagion. Producers and vendors alike kept their ingredients a mystery. A number of these recipes became known and are still followed today. Most contain Angelica.

Much was rumored and written about one of these secret remedies, an electuary called Theriak. Considered a panacea, it was a thick paste prepared from different powdered plant substances, honey, and wine. Angelica was an important ingredient along with Gentian (*Gentiana lutea*), Valerian (*Valeriana officinalis*), Sweetflag (*Acorus calamus*), Ginger (*Zingiber officinale*) and others.

Elixirs of life were also highly prized in those times of high risk of infection. Healers, physicians, root diggers, alchemists, and barber-surgeons offered all-healing elixirs of life to their patients. In our time, many of these elixirs have been verified scientifically because ingredients such as Angelica, Cinnamom, Rosemary, and Thyme contain strong antiseptic chemicals.

One seventeenth century anti-contagion remedy still listed in many pharmacopeias of our time is the "Vinegar of the Four Brigands." The story

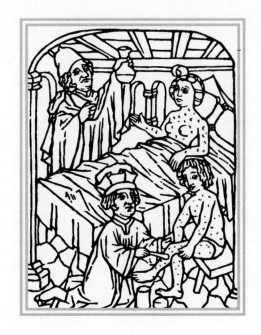

goes that while the plague raged in France, four brigands were plundering the houses of the stricken, miraculously without contracting the disease. When they were finally caught and sentenced to the gallows, they argued that rather than carry their secret to the grave, they would reveal all if their lives were spared. It was agreed and the brigands told. Henceforth, the secret concoction (herbs with strong antiseptic properties in an extract of vinegar) was called "Vinegar of the Four Brigands."

Other secret remedies and elixirs of life are still found in some form today, often as liqueurs. The monks who had introduced and cultivated Angelica in their cloister gardens processed her into elixirs. They usually steeped her in alcohol

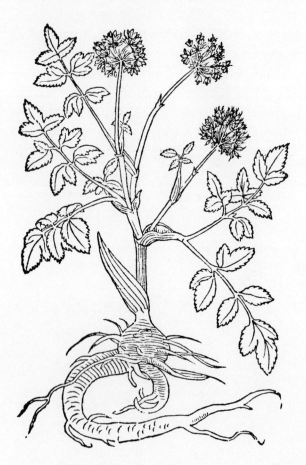

with other medicinal herbs and administered the herbal tincture to patients. For instance, the famous *Melissengeist* ("Balm Spirit") of the Carmelite nuns contains Angelica. It remains a proven remedy and is available in most drugstores in Germany today. The delicious Chartreuse liqueur originally was a very bitter Angelica tincture. Likewise, Swedish Bitters survived the Thirty Years War to be found today in natural food stores in America.

Let us return to the Angelica plant—an "Archangel" in plant form. Let it affect us. The old herbalists deduced a plant's mode of action from its appearance, relying on an invisible bond connecting them to Nature. Paracelsus urged his students not just to accumulate empty book knowledge but to comprehend in Nature the plants that they intended to use on patients. He taught them to recognize the *signatura plantarum*, the signs of a plant that express its healing powers. Students were told not to heed external attributes alone such as shape, color, and smell (as we have done with Angelica). They were also encouraged to understand the spirit and characteristic radiance of the plant.

German poet J. W. von Goethe, too, speaks of the deep secret of the Doctrine of Signatures in the following verse:

> You must, when contemplating Nature,
> consider one thing like all things.
> Nothing is inside, nothing is outside,
> for what is inside is outside.
> Thus seize without delay
> the sacred open secret.

Stand a few steps away from Angelica. See if we might be able to grasp something of her radiance. She has something erect, something strengthening, something generous about her. Her stature and refreshing aromatic scent give us courage. She could strengthen us when the body is weakened and in need of new energy, warmth, and fortitude. Culpeper expresses this attribute astrologically:

> [Angelica] is an herb of the Sun in Leo; let it be gathered when he is there, the Moon applying to his good aspect; let it be gathered either in his hour, or in the hour of Jupiter . . .

Angelica thus has the energy of the sun—vigor, heart energy, vitality. Leo gives her a generous nature; working on a wide level, she can strengthen the entire body. She resists Saturn and his diseases—epidemics, infirmity, chronic illnesses, hardenings, despondency, desperation, fear. Now we understand the old German name for Angelica: "Fearwort." She is an herb for the faint-hearted and disheartened, she brings joy into a dark mood. The Nordic bards of old knew this, crowning themselves with wreaths of Angelica flowers so that they would express rapture and gladness in their songs—and to take away their stage fright. Angelica was a symbol of enthusiasm and inspiration to them.

CULTIVATION

Why shouldn't we again set aside a small corner in our garden for Angelica? Then we will have these valuable plants on hand if we need a wild-growing specimen. Our ancestors, being experienced in cultivating Angelica, left us instructions. Here, in fact, is advice from the grand old man of herbology, Jacobus Theodorus Tabernaemontanus, who published his herbal in 1731:

> This herb is being grown off and on here in the gardens. The one especially being praised is that planted in large amounts near Freyburg im Breißgau by monks in the Carthausen. It is sold not only in Germany but in other foreign countries as well. From the seed, one grows young starts that are sown around St. Martin's Day (November 11) in the following way: One soaks the seed in fresh water overnight, and in the morning one throws it into good black soil. It comes out of the ground in spring like the seeds of Chervil, and the first leaflets that grow from it resemble those of Parsley. Plant these young starts in the new light in May, one and a half shoes [feet] apart. In the fourth year the stem thrusts forth, bringing flowers and seeds; when they fall off, the stem turns woody and rotten. When one sets Angelica into good firm soil, it will seed itself. From it, young plants will grow that one can transplant. They must, however, have well-tended soil kept free from weeds and watered often with tepid water.

Angelica is an impressive plant, growing up to six feet tall. In my herb garden grow an Angelica and a Chinese Rhubarb (*Rheum palmatum*) like two man-sized guardians standing above the smaller herbs.

Angelica enriches a garden, impressing visitors with its majestic appearance. Its leaves and especially the flower emit an aromatic, sweet scent. It loves deep, humus-rich, moist soil. We can grow it from seed or starts. Because the seeds lose their ability to germinate quickly, it is better to take the mature seeds from our first plant and thrust them right back into the soil. Sow the starts in late summer and thin them to grow about 6 inches apart. They winter over well. (As

we remember, this plant originated in the cold northern lands.) In spring, move your plants 30 to 60 inches apart. Water them well—Angelica tolerates neither long-lasting dry spells nor standing water. Also it prefers sunny places or semishade. Angelica is a biennial reaching its full height in the second or third year of growth. A solitary plant has great visual effect.

If you do not allow the plants to go to flower, the biennial Angelica will keep for several years, the stem becoming thicker and the root stronger. At the end of the first or during the second season, the roots can be harvested. The younger roots are smaller and thus better suited for making candy and tea; the older roots are often woody and wormy. Finally, Angelica will not thrive when cultivated every year in the same spot. I advise that you return to a particular location after five or six years.

HEALING PROPERTIES

Today we no longer need a remedy to protect us from contracting the plague. Nonetheless, we can rely on Angelica's antiseptic properties and ability to strengthen our resistance during the flu season or when traveling to foreign countries and the like. For this purpose, it is sufficient to chew a small piece of the root once in a while. During infectious diseases, consuming illness, or after surgery, Angelica can provide additional strength. It is a tonic for all debilitating conditions, be they of physical or psychological nature. It strengthens the nerves in times of weakness, despondency, agitation, and nervous palpitation. With its excellent combination of active ingredients, it can cleanse the body of toxins that strain both the organism and the psyche. It is recommended for heavy smokers and people who are exposed to toxins in their work environment (e.g., the paint and varnish industry, photo labs).

Anyone who has chewed on a piece of Angelica root knows its bitter taste. Angelica contains bitter compounds that stimulate the digestive system. Do not spit it out right away or sweeten its tea with sugar! A sweetened tea from a bitter herb is useless . . . The bitter compounds, or *amara* in Latin, take effect immediately by way of the gustatory nerves. They cause an increased secretion of saliva that stimulates the secretion of gastric juices in turn. Blood circulation improves and the blood-forming organs are stimulated. In short, bitter compounds are beneficial both to the stomach and intestines as well as to the entire organism. It is not without reason that "secret remedies for health and longevity" primarily contain bitter compounds. Today these compounds are also used in cancer therapy.

Therefore, chew the root slowly, drink the tea in small sips, and swallow the powder gradually. Angelica must have time to warm the stomach, stimulate digestion, and prompt one's appetite. An advantage over other stomach remedies is that it aids the nervous system. And since in most cases of gastro-intestinal conditions the nerves play a role, Angelica is an excellent remedy. It is helpful for digestive disorders—such as gastritis, gas, lack of appetite, an upset stomach after a fatty meal, and a lack of gastric acid. Only in cases of too much gastric acid is Angelica contraindicated—because it stimulates the production of gastric juice. Like all stomachics (remedies that stimulate stomach functions), Angelica

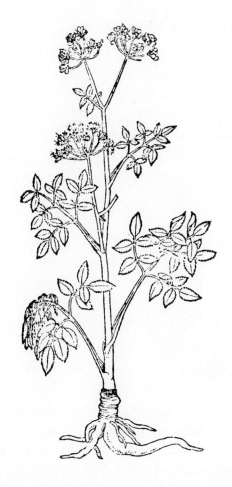

should be taken 15 to 30 minutes before eating to allow the stomach to "warm up" and digest even the heaviest of meals well.

In old herbals, Angelica is often found under the name "Chestwort." And it really is a healing plant for chest conditions due to its ability to promote the coughing up of phlegm. It dissolves the thick, sticky mucus that accompanies cough, bronchitis, and pneumonia, and it strengthens the local tissue and mucous membranes. It is a plant for long-standing chronic conditions of the respiratory pathways. In addition to ingesting Angelica tea or powder, one should rub a warming stimulating salve on the sufferer's chest and upper back.

Angelica also has an effect through the skin. It can be of aid for paralysis, neuralgias, rheumatism, and gout. Heinrich Pumpe says that for paralysis one should prepare a strong decoction of the seeds and bathe the affected limbs in it. A full body bath, however, should last no longer than 15 minutes. Follow this with a massage of Cowslip oil (*Primula elatior* or *P. veris*) or St. John's Wort oil (*Hypericum perforatum*) mixed with a few drops of essential oil of Angelica (*Oleum Angelicae aether*). For neuralgias or rheumatism, rub the oil or an Angelica salve into the affected parts and wrap them with a warm cloth.

Angelica salve is helpful in cases of chronic rhinitis and sinusitis because it dissolves mucus and warms. Apply it twice daily to the area of the paranasal sinuses, forehead, root of the nose, nose, cheeks, and angle of the jaw. Concurrently, inhale essential oils of Thyme (*Thymus vulgaris*), Eucalyptus (*Eucalyptus globulus* or *E. citriodora*), and Swiss Mountain Pine (*Pinus mugo*). It is also used for massage in cases of rheumatism, tense muscles, paralysis, and neuralgias.

On a cautionary note, one should avoid sunbathing or exposure to intense UV-radiation during any application of Angelica root preparations, whether internal or external. The furocoumarins contained in Angelica can make the skin more sensitive to light which, in turn, can lead to inflammation of the skin when combined with sun exposure or treatment with tanning devices.

As for digging up the Angelica root, it is best to proceed in late fall when the plant's energies have withdrawn back into the root. Wash it thoroughly and cut it into pieces or split the root lengthwise; hang it to dry in an airy and shady spot, laying out smaller pieces on a piece of cloth or wire rack. Once the root has dried out, store it in a closed container.

Although I talk about cultivating your own, Angelica can be found in herb stores or natural food stores as "Radix Angelicae." Likewise, if you prefer not to make your own, Angelica tincture is available in such stores.

Note: In this book I generally use the terms "tea" and "infusion" interchangeably. By them, I mean an herb steeped in boiling water—as when preparing a cup of tea. This is in contrast to a "decoction" in which the herb is boiled in water for a period of time.

❧ Angelica Tea

Take 1 teaspoon of the finely chopped angelica root and steep it overnight in 2 to 3 cups of cold water. The following day, bring it to a quick boil. This makes a daily dose to sip as you like.

❧ Angelica Root Powder

Prepare by grinding the dried angelica root to a fine powder with a mortar and pestle or in a coffee grinder. Store the powder in a tightly closed container. A daily dose is 2 to 3 pinches.

❧ Angelica Tincture

Fill a mason jar halfway with fresh, washed, and finely chopped angelica roots. Cover the roots with grain spirit or a fruit liqueur and close the jar tightly. Let the mixture steep for 3 weeks, shaking it occasionally. Strain the tincture into a dark bottle with a tight lid or stopper.

ᚠᚨ STOMACH BITTERS

a handful of each:

> angelica root (*Angelica archangelica*)
> gentian root (*Gentiana lutea*)
> wormwood herb (*Artemisia absinthium*)
> sweetflag root (*Acorus calamus*)
> 1 cinnamon stick
> grain spirit or fruit liqueur

Fill a mason jar halfway with the finely chopped herbs (fresh roots if possible). Add the cinnamon stick and pour in enough alcohol to fill the jar. Close it tightly and let the mixture steep for 2 to 3 weeks, shaking it occasionally. Strain the bitters into dropper bottles. Take 20 to 30 drops before meals.

ᚠᚨ WARMING STOMACH WINE

> 1 fresh angelica root (*Angelica archangelica*)
> 1 fresh sweetflag root (*Acorus calamus*)
> 1 liter red wine
> 1 teaspoon ground cinnamon

Chop the washed roots into small pieces. Put them in a jar with the cinnamon and red wine. Let the mixture steep for 2 weeks and then strain the wine into a bottle with a tight lid or stopper. Drink a small amount before meals.

ᚠᚨ VINEGAR OF THE FOUR BRIGANDS

2 ounces (about 60 grams) each:

> rosemary (*Rosmarinus officinalis*)
> sage (*Salvia officinalis*)
> peppermint (*Mentha piperita*)

½ ounce (about 15 grams) each:

> ground cloves (*Eugenia caryophyllata*)

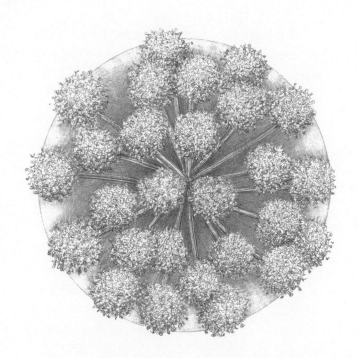

> zedoaria root (*Rhizoma Zedoariae*, from an herb store)
> angelica root (*Angelica archangelica*)
> a liter or so of good wine vinegar

Derived from an old pharmaceutical recipe from the Baden region of Germany:

Fill a large jar with dried or fresh herbs that have been finely chopped. Top it off with wine vinegar and close it tightly. Let the mixture steep for 2 weeks in a warm place, shaking it occasionally. Pressing the herbs well, strain the liquid into a bottle with a lid or stopper.

For internal use, take by the teaspoon during infectious disease or the risk of contagion. Use the vinegar externally to disinfect and cleanse.

ᚠᚨ ANGELICA SALVE

> 1¼ ounces lanolin
> 1 fluid ounce St. John's wort oil
> 2 grams beeswax, grated

15 drops essential oil of angelica

5 drops essential oil of marjoram

1 drop essential oil of thyme

While the lanolin and essential oils are available in herb stores, St. John's wort oil is best prepared at home. Pure beeswax can be obtained from a beekeeper or in a drugstore or crafts store. (Do not use bleached wax.) Because essential oil of angelica is expensive, buy the smallest bottle.

Slowly melt the lanolin in a pot or double boiler; add the St. John's wort oil and set it aside. In a separate pot, melt the beeswax while stirring constantly; add the essential oils and then the lanolin mixture. Remove from the heat and stir until the salve is nearly cool. Pour it into small salve jars with tight lids.

৪৯ CHARTREUSE

The original Chartreuse liqueur was made by Carthusian monks of "La grande Chartreuse" monastery near Grenoble, France. The historic recipe dates from 1605, its name protected under copyright law. The sweet and aromatic liqueur is also used in cakes, ice cream, and other desserts. The basic recipe follows.

herbal mixture:

50 grams lemon balm (*Melissa officinalis*)

40 grams angelica root

(*Angelica archangelica*)

8 grams thyme (*Thymus vulgaris*)

4 grams arnica flowers (*Arnica montana*)

50 grams peppermint (*Mentha piperita*)

5 grams hyssop (*Hyssopus officinalis*)

5 grams wormwood

(*Artemisia absinthum*)

4 grams whole mace

4 grams ground cinnamon

1 liter grain alcohol, wine spirits,

or brandy

Chop the herbs well, using fresh when possible. Place them in a jar with the mace that has been finely crushed in a mortar and pestle. Add the cinnamon and mix well. Pressing everything down tightly, pour in the alcohol to cover. Close the jar tightly and let it stand for 4 weeks, shaking it occasionally. Strain the liquid through a cloth, pressing the herbs well; store in a bottle with a lid or stopper. This herbal mixture makes excellent stomach bitters. Take 1 teaspoon before meals. While its taste is bitter (like any good stomachic), its aroma is very pleasant.

to complete the Chartreuse liqueur:

800 grams granulated sugar

(about ¾ pound)

1 liter water (about 1 quart)

250 millileters 90% alcohol

(about 8 fluid ounces)

Heat the water, stir in the sugar, bring it to a rolling boil, and let it bubble for 15 minutes. Skim the gray foam from the surface. A few drops of lemon juice ensures the success of the sugary syrup. While it is still hot, strain the mixture through a cloth, mix it with the herbal mixture and add the alcohol. Pour into bottles when it cools and let it rest for about 2 months to allow the full Chartreuse aroma to develop.

CULINARY USE

Historically, northern Europeans have long valued Angelica as a vegetable; they cook the stem and leaves. The Laplanders, according to Heinrich Marzell, gather the young flower umbels, chop them, and simmer them in reindeer milk until the mixture coagulates into a thick mass. This they stuff into reindeer stomachs, which they in turn hang up to dry for one year. The resultant cheese is touted as quite excellent. And in Iceland, for warmth, people still brew an alcoholic beverage from Angelica.

The young leaves with their aromatic scent are well suited as an herb for sauces, fish, and meat dishes. The juicy young stems are peeled and soft-cooked like rhubarb to be served topped with melted cheese or other sauce. Mixed with an equal amount of rhubarb, the young stems and leaf stalks can also be turned into a fruit butter or marmalade. They likewise go well with gooseberry or plum marmalade; cook them until they are very soft, peel them, and add them at the end of the cooking process. Candied like lemon peel, Angelica stems can garnish cakes, ice cream, and other desserts.

৪৯ Candied Angelica Stems

Gather the young Angelica stems before they flower, and let them be no thicker than your little finger. Peel, cut them into small pieces, and then boil them in water until they soften. Strain off the cooking water, reserving it as a bitter but health-promoting medicinal tea for the stomach, and set the stems aside. Prepare a sugar syrup by bringing 2 pounds of sugar and 1 quart of water to a rolling boil for 5 minutes. Pour the syrup over the Angelica stems, cover the pan with a cloth or lid, and let it sit overnight. The next day remove half of the syrup and save it to use in cakes, ice cream, frostings, or pudding. There should still be enough syrup to cover the stems. Add ½ cup of sugar to the pan and, once again, bring the mixture to a boil, spooning the mixture over

the stems. Repeat this procedure three more times without removing any syrup. Drain the stems, run them quickly under warm water, and spread them out on a baking sheet to dry.

Meanwhile, prepare a new sugar syrup: Bring 1 pound of sugar and 1 quart of water to a rolling boil, stirring vigorously until the syrup thickens. Stir the stems into this syrup for a few moments and then remove them with a slotted spoon. Spread them on a baking sheet, cover it with tin foil, and let them dry in the sun or in the oven with the door ajar,

Store the dried angelica stems in small boxes to use for decorating desserts. Similar in appearance to candied lemon peel (although frog green in color), they taste much better in my opinion.

Pour the remaining syrup into a bottle to keep in the refrigerator. Aside from its dessert value, it can be added to mineral water to make a refreshing angelica spritzer.

৪৯ Angelica Tea Cake

4 eggs, separated
½ cup angelica syrup (see "Candied Angelica Stems")
2¼ cups cake flour
½ cup melted butter
2 tablespoons rum
2 tablespoons rum-soaked raisins
¼ cup finely chopped candied angelica stems
the grated peel of ½ lemon

In a large mixing bowl, beat the egg whites until stiff; set aside. Whisk the egg yolks separately and fold them into the egg whites, add the angelica syrup, and beat for 15 minutes. Stir in the cake flour, melted butter, and remaining ingredients. Put the batter in a greased loaf pan and bake in a preheated 350° oven for 40 minutes or until done.

℘ CHARTREUSE CANDY

    2 cups sweet cream
    1 pound granulated sugar
    2 tablespoons honey
    2 tablespoons Chartreuse liqueur

Stirring the mixture constantly, boil the cream, sugar, and honey in a saucepan until it forms a sticky light brown mass (about 20 to 30 minutes). When a drop of this mass dropped into cold water does not disperse but forms a firm ball, the caramel is ready. Remove the pan from the heat and, when cooled slightly, stir in the Chartreuse—carefully so that it does not spatter. Spread the mixture on a greased baking sheet. Before the mass hardens, cut it into small cubes and wrap the candy in individual squares of wax paper.

BOTANICAL CHARACTERISTICS

Name: Angelica archangelica / A. Officinalis — Angelica

Distribution: Northern and central Europe, northern Asia, North America

Habitat: Meadows, forests, riverbanks, wetlands

Description: Plant can grow to 8½ feet; stems as thick as a person's arm are finely furrowed, hollow with a partial red tint; leaves are 2 or 3 times pinnate, originating from a bulging sheath. Globular, greenish flowers; aromatic scent in all parts; flowering from July to August.

Confusion with similar plants: With poisonous members of the Carrot family (Umbelliferae), such as Hemlock (*Conium maculatum*), Wild Parsley (*Petroselinum segetum*), Wild Chervil (*Chaerophyllum temulum*), and Water Parsnip (*Sium* spp.).

Collecting season:

    Root – Early spring or late fall

    Seeds – September to October

Active ingredients: Angelic acid, bitter compounds, essential oil, angelicin, coumarin

Astrological association: Sun / Jupiter

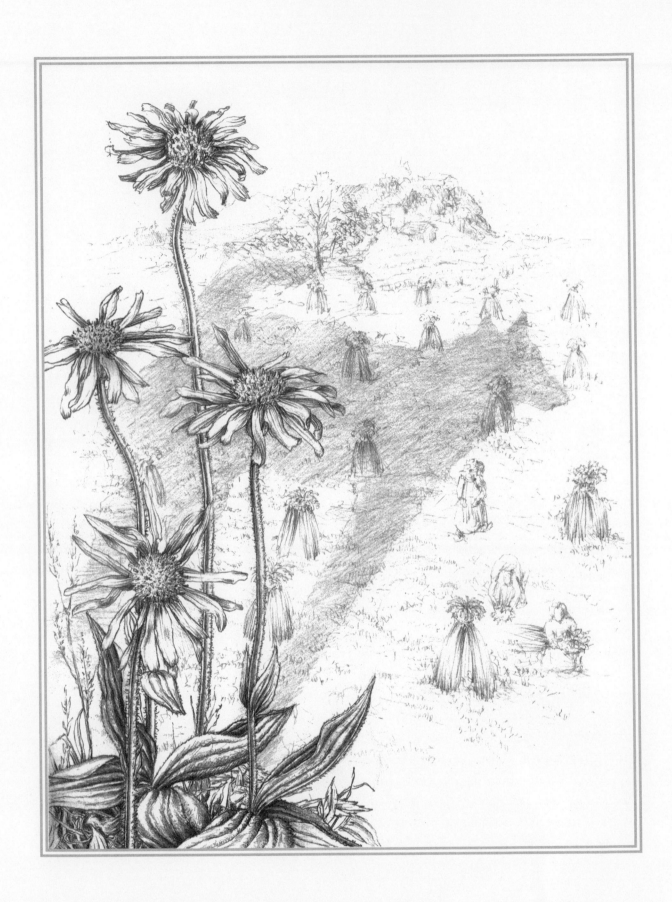

ARNICA

Arnica montana

Mountain Tobacco, Lambskin, Leopard's Bane, Wolf's Bane, Fallherb

Daisy family—Compositae / Asteraceae

ARNICA CARRIES THE WILD NATURE of the wolf after whom she is named. Her flowers are like yellow wolf's eyes in whom the captured mountain sun glistens. "Wolf's Eye," "Wolf's Yellow," *Wolfesgelega*—these old German names tell us about the wild, self-willed, even dangerous power of Arnica. Anybody who once sees her high up in the mountains will surely not forget her. We sense that she is both a strong medicinal plant and a strong poison. She opens up completely to the sun and radiates back in an orange yellow. And the scent! It is wild, aromatic, strengthening, heartening. The higher up into the mountains Arnica climbs to absorb solar energy, the more intense this aroma becomes.

She adores these heights and the intense radiation of the mountain sun. Up here I have discovered her radiant beauty in a fragrant alpine pasture. She shares the marshy lime-deficient soil with many other mountainous herbs—soft and tender white Cotton Grass, dark blue Scabiosa, tiny white Eyebrights, pale yellow Marsh Cinquefoils, erect Horsetails. The light green rosette of four to six basal leaves presses tightly to the ground as if to thrust itself into the air. The tall, gracious downy stem wastes little time with the formation of stem leaves. Usually once, or thrice at most, are smaller, opposite, and ovate pairs of leaves permitted to attach themselves to it; and maybe two opposite flowers on shorter stems below the main flower head. But then the stem flies upward to perhaps two feet above the ground, where finally the large bud bursts open to unfold a yolk yellow blossom. Around St. John's Day (Midsummer Day or June 24), when the sun has its strongest power, Arnica wants to suck itself full of sun energy. The old wolf names that she bears in German capture her unrestrained strength, her wildness, and her toxicity. And in the leopard names that she attracts in the English-speaking world lie her elegance and wild beauty.

Arnica is intimate with numerous multilegged guests—butterflies, bees, bumblebees, and a variety of other insects. These ensure pollination. However, when bad weather does not inspire insects to visit its flowers, Arnica fertilizes herself. The tube-shaped central florets unfurl little stalks or styles with sticky stigmata that probe adjacent florets for pollen. If they find none, these stalks will bend back far enough to reach their own pollen.

The flower really consists of 50 to 90 single tubular disk florets that crowd onto the receptacle. These short florets are framed by a ring of strap-shaped ray flowers. Both types sit in a cup of green bracts. The whole is called a compound flower head—hence the family name "Compositae." This family is varied and many of our well-known medicinal plants belong to it.

When picking apart Arnica's flower heads, we often discover other guests of the plant. The Arnica fly (*Tephritis arnicae*) especially likes to deposit its small black pupas here. These pupas and small insects must be plucked by hand from the flowers intended for medicinal use because they can increase Arnica's skin-irritating effects. In fact, significantly fewer allergic reactions occur in remedies produced from these "select" Arnica flowers than from carelessly processed plants. The German pharmacopeia, for instance, approves only select Arnica flowers.

A plant with such strong radiance has always attracted people and inspired different names. Most of them refer to Arnica's healing properties: Fallherb in English and, in German, "Wellbestow," "Prickherb," "Woundherb," "Snuffplant," the latter addressing the sneeze-provoking effect of the pulverized dried flowers. Used as a tobacco substitute, Arnica has been called Mountain Tobacco, "Smokeherb" in German, and *tabaco de montāna*. An old herbal tobacco recipe calls for a combination of Arnica flowers, Coltsfoot leaves, and Mullein flowers. Other names refer to the magical powers as-signed to Arnica—"Thunderwort," *Bilmes* herb, "Strengthwort," St. John's-Strength Flower.

Together with St. John's Wort and Male Fern, Arnica has been used in midsummer rituals since olden times. Her power is considered to be the strongest on St. John's Day. The peasants would set Arnica plants around their fields to protect them from the grainwolf. In the form of a horned devil with goat feet, this demon would stalk especially at this time of the year, riding his billy goat through the grain and turning it black. Or he might tie sickles to his legs and slash the blades in half. It was said that when the grain swayed in the wind, bending to one side and then the other, the grainwolf prowled the fields.

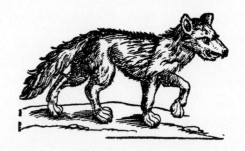

"He is back," the farmers would say, warning children to stay away. However, the grainwolf was beneficial as well as dangerous. He embodied the spirit and the power of the grain plants, bestowing energy for its maturation. If he left the fields, the grain would wither and the villagers would suffer from his raids. And, being a wolf's plant, Arnica hindered him. Only when the last patch of grain was cut would he slip away as a great sinister shadow. The women hesitated to bind the last sheaf of grain, fearing the wolf to be inside. Gathered around the last patch of un-mowed grain, the mowers would call out, "Now we catch the wolf!" Often the last sheath in the field was bound in the shape of a wolf and placed in the forest. Only then would the farmers remove the Arnica guardians and thank her for contributing to a successful harvest.

HEALING PROPERTIES

Arnica has many properties that bestow well-being. It has long been recognized as one of the best known remedies for healing wounds. According to the German clergyman and natural healer Parson Kneipp: "I consider Arnica tincture as the primary remedy for injuries and therefore cannot recommend it enough." I agree with him completely and recommend Arnica tincture for every first-aid kit.

Used externally, Arnica promotes the healing of wounds contracted through blows, punctures, falls, and cuts. It is anti-inflammatory and antiseptic, relieves pain from injuries, and promotes tissue regeneration. One can clean wounds, abscesses, boils, and ulcers with diluted Arnica tincture and dress them with a compress soaked in the same solution. For contusions, sprains, bruises, bursitis, arthritis, and inflammation of the lymphatic vessels, apply packs of diluted Arnica tincture. To relieve headaches and visual disturbances due to concussion, apply such compresses around the head and neck. Concurrently, homeopathic Arnica (4x) should be taken internally (ten drops three times daily). Gargling with diluted Arnica tincture will help tonsillitis, laryngitis, and hoarseness. For this purpose, add a few drops of Arnica tincture to a strong decoction of Burnet Saxifrage roots and swab mouth sores

and gingivitis with this diluted tincture. Finally, rub weary limbs and cold feet with Arnica oil.

Arnica is a powerful medicine that must be administered in proper dosage and form. If it is not diluted, the tincture or tea can cause skin irritations, eczema, and allergies. Special care must be taken with people who are prone to allergies, have red hair, and have fair skin. In such cases, Calendula or Comfrey would be preferable.

To prepare packs and washes, dilute one tablespoon of Arnica tincture in a cup of boiled water. (In cases where sensitivity is suspected, double the amount of water.)

Arnica tincture is available in herb stores, naturopathic pharmacies, and some health food stores. I personally recommend Wala brand Arnica essence and their Arnica towelettes for a home or traveller's first-aid kit.

℘ ARNICA TINCTURE

1 part fresh arnica flowers
5 parts grain spirits or vodka

Pick the flowers from the green flower head, removing any insects and other debris, and put them in a jar. Add the alcohol, close the jar tightly, and let it steep for about 2 weeks; shake it occasionally. Strain and store the tincture in a dark glass bottle.

℘ ARNICA OIL

fresh arnica flowers
cold-pressed olive oil or sunflower oil

Fill a jar halfway with arnica flowers picked free of insects and debris; fill to the top with oil. Close the jar tightly and place it in the sun for 3 weeks. Strain the oil from the flowers into a dark bottle.

Mixed with the oils of Calendula and Cowslip, it becomes an enervating massage oil for muscle fatigue and for skin care after bathing.

The German poet Goethe used Arnica to strengthen his heart. From his deathbed, he wrote:

With Life and Death fighting within me, I feel Life surge ahead with this flower on its standard as the hostile, stagnant, deadly depressing powers meet their Austerlitz. Rejuvenated, I sing her praises, and yet it is only she praising her own truly inexhaustible nature.

Arnica, bursting with health and strength, can restore the energies of a weary body. It has a stimulating effect, particularly on the heart and circulation, and can help prevent strokes. It strengthens the arterial and venous vascular system and is therefore helpful in arteriosclerosis, geriatric heart disease, coronary artery disease, and angina pectoris.

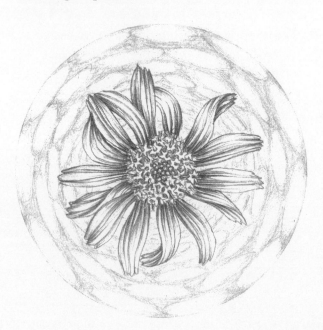

Its internal use, however, is not without risk. Overdoses of Arnica result in symptoms of poisoning (such as stomach cramps and damage to the mucous membranes, stomach, kidneys, and liver). To treat heart disease with Arnica, one should consult an experienced naturopath or physician. This is because reactions to the internal use of Arnica decoction or tincture vary greatly from person to person.

Arnica tincture has proved effective for circulatory problems and exhaustion from mountaineering especially in extreme altitudes. I can add that it was present in my own first-aid kit on a recent trek in the Himalayas. At 12,000 feet, a few drops of Arnica tincture restored me when my extremities felt heavy like lead and I wanted to give up.

✍ CIRCULATION DROPS

10 millileters arnica 3x
10 millileters cactus 1x
10 millileters crataegus 1x

For circulatory problems and states of exhaustion, take 3 to 10 drops in water. This mixture can be prepared for you in a naturopathic pharmacy.

In homeopathy, a mother tincture is the tincture base from which dilutions are made. Arnica tincture renders good service in concussions and strokes. A daily dose is five drops per tablespoon of water taken three to five times a day. As with all Arnica preparations, do not use it if sensitivity to Arnica is suspected.

In Germany, the Arnica plants used for preparations originate in Eastern Europe. In pharmacies and herbal stores, Arnica flowers are available as "Flores Arnicae" and the tincture as "Tinctura Arnicae."

Some commonly available products containing Arnica are: Arnica Sports Gel; Arnica-Kneipp; Arniflor for circulation problems, rheumatism, bruises, and strains; Arnica Wound Towelletes by Wala for wounds and as small compresses; Capillaron for weakness of the connective tissue; Arthrodynat Ointment for arthroses and diseases of the joints. This is only a sampling of German products that contain Arnica. As elsewhere in this book, I have chosen those that I can recommend from personal experience. Some are available in the United States.

VETERINARY MEDICINE

Arnica tincture and Arnica ointment are very useful in veterinary medicine for all kinds of injuries. For instance, an animal's wounds can be washed with diluted Arnica tincture. Sprains, arthritis, and bruises are aided by applying packs soaked with Arnica tincture.

CULTIVATION

Arnica loves lime-deficient, acidic soil (ideally with a pH of 4.5 – 5.5). My own garden has a peat bed where I cultivate plants that prefer this acidic soil. You can also plant Arnica in containers on a balcony or patio. However, when doing so, be sure to fill the bottom of the container with a layer of sand because Arnica does not like standing water. Peat moss is available at gardening supply stores or nurseries.

Arnica montana, which is not native to North America, can be difficult to germinate from seeds. After experiencing several failures, I finally ordered a few starts to plant in my bed so that I could watch them and make adjustments until I learned to rear my own plants. Sow the seeds in April or July. They germinate in 8 to 14 days. The transplants can stay outdoors throughout the winter protected with brush or mulch. They usually do not flower until their third season.

North American gardeners will find it much easier to cultivate their own native species. *A. chamissonis* thrives in regular garden soil and grows wild along the Pacific coast from Alaska to California. A species on the eastern seaboard, *A. lanceolata*, is found between Quebec and Maine, New Hampshire, and New York. Both can be used medicinally in the same way that *A. montana* is in Europe. Seeds and starts are commercially available.

BOTANICAL CHARACTERISTICS

Arnica is a protected plant in many countries.

Name: *Arnica montana* — Arnica

Distribution: Central and northern Europe

Habitat: Poor soil, unfertilized meadows; avoids limy composition, prefering acidic marshy soil up to 9,000 feet.

Description: Grows from 8 inches to 2 feet tall; ground rosette of 4 to 6 ovate to lanceolate basal leaves; stem holds 1 to 3 pairs of smaller opposite-facing leaves and occasionally 2 opposite-growing smaller flower heads. Flower is orange-yellow with an aromatic scent. Fruits are achenes with rough hairs and an acrid aromatic smell. Flowering time is May to July.

Confusion with similar plants: People who know Arnica only from pictures and descriptions are often at a loss confronting the vast number of look-alikes. However, anyone who has seen her and felt her effects will definitely not confuse Arnica with any other yellow flowering plant. Listed here are some plants commonly mistaken for Arnica. Note that none of them has Arnica's strong and aromatic scent, the strictly opposite-facing stem leaves, or 5 to 12 veins running through its ray flowers.

- Meadow Salsify (*Tragopogon pratensis*): Small, linear-lanceolate leaves; stem leaves have a wide base enclosing the stem; ligulate ray flowers only.

- Common Hawkweed (*Hieracium vulgatum*): The flowering head only contains ligulate ray flowers; the stem is umbellate and compound (branched); the basal leaves are dentate (toothed).

- Willowleaf Inula (*Inula salicina*): Inula flowers are often used in preparations to make Arnica flowers go farther. But they lack the typical aromatic scent and do not stimulate sneezing. The upper leaves enclose the stem and the leaves are linear lanceolate.

- Rough Hawksbeard (*Crepis biennis*): The flower cluster is an umbellate panicle with ligulate florets only. The lower leaves are pinnately lobed, the upper ones simple; the stem is often red at the base.

Collecting season: July to August

Active ingredients: Essential oils, resins, tannins, arnicaflavon, bitter compounds

Astrological association: Sun / Jupiter

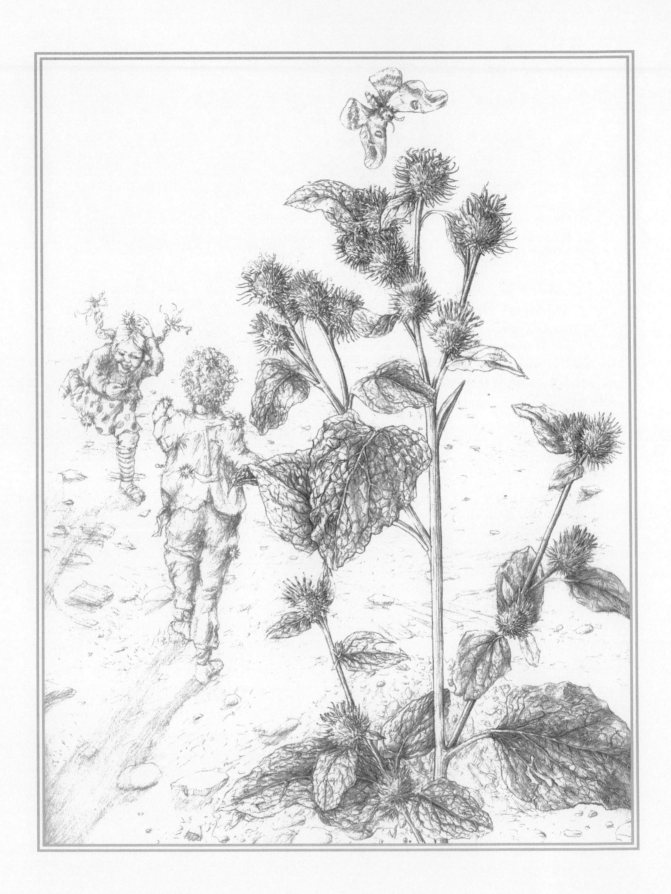

BURDOCK

Arctium lappa

Greater Burdock, Burs, Beggar's Buttons, Personata, Happy Major, Clotbur,
Cocklebur, Grass Burdock, Hardock, Harebur, Hurrbur, Turkey Burseed, Bardana

Daisy family — Compositae / Asteraceae

Great Burdock has a wretched long root, black on the outside and white within, and of a bitter taste. Its round stem is hollow and white mixed with crimson red, studded with many little side branches and small, narrow-pointed leaflets. The leaves being broad and long are blackish green with an ashen hue on the side facing the ground. Toward the hay month (July) appear her green round fruits or burs with their many crooked little hooks that help them stick to clothing. Green at first, after they flower these burs become quite beautiful, turning a light reddish brown as common thistles do. The seed is long and grey. Between leaves and branches grow the long prickly burs that resemble a hedgehog's head.

THIS CHARMING DESCRIPTION of Burdock comes from the 1731 herbal of Tabernaemontanus. We all know these prickly little burrs from our childhood. Their large, round flower heads attach themselves so readily to socks and pants, and once they get in the hair—what a mess. Yes, children know Burdock!

And I remember them, too. A few of the thick flower heads now lie on my table where I can study them in detail. I see why they stick so tenaciously to fabric and hair. The flowers sit within a stiff fur of hook-tipped prickles. In some, crimson pink flower petals blink shyly over the defensive bulwark of hooked spears. These rough, shaggy, hairy flower globes have given Burdock the botanical name *Arctium*, a derivative of the Greek word *arktos* for "bear"—no doubt a shaggy, furry bear.

Plants given bear names radiate a coarse but strong vitality. Our Burdock rises six to seven feet above the ground and is definitely somewhat bear-like in his appearance. Arranged around a robust stem are huge flabby leaves that I think are rather like elephant ears. The old name "Bardana" refers to these leaves and is said to come from the Italian word for "horse blanket" (*barda*). Burdock leaves are almost as big as a horse blanket—even resembling one in shape. They carry some darkness in their appearance; a hint of black seems mixed into the green of Burdock's leaves, inspiring a few wolf names for him ("Wolf's Herb" and "Wolfman"). To my German ancestors the wolf embodied dark powers, and so, astrologically, Burdock is under the dominion of Saturn and Pluto, the planet-rulers of such forces.

Burdock masters the dark powers, gaining great vitality from them and magically managing to produce red-violet flower petals. The old herbalists took this as a sign of Burdock's great healing powers. A plant that can master the darkness and transform it into new vitality can also control the dark juices and toxic substances in human beings. And since antiquity Burdock has been used to treat dyscrasia's imperfect mixture of blood and humors—excess toxins in the body.

In the prickly seed-vessels, small seeds ripen as fall approaches. The seeds are extremely oily and people used to extract this oil during times of hardship. They also used it as a tonic to strengthen the hair. Some people used the seeds as a plant oracle. Let us hear from Tabernaemontanus once again:

> Tragus reports that he usually finds two black oat kernels in every bur in the fall. And many naturalists observe that when the so-called burs open early in the fall they find in each bur two barley kernels enclosed. This indicates a fertile and perfect year. But when two pointed oat kernels are found, they take it for the opposite—namely, a future rise in price for all fruits.

At the opposite end of Burdock is the sturdy taproot. It drills itself into the ground to a depth of three feet, storing minerals, inulin, starch, and many other medicinal constituents in its tissue. Digging up Burdock roots requires a good spade. A small garden shovel is no match for the strength of this root. You can dig up the root of the two-year-old plant in the spring.

To develop such an imposing appearance both above and below the ground, Burdock needs nutrient-rich soil. He loves ammonia and you often will find him in the vicinity of dung hills. You can also look for him in dumps, along way-sides, and near fences. He seeks the company of people and likes to establish himself close to where we live. There he stands—a plump bear offering us his healing powers.

In the spring the first leaves rise from the root, purple near the root in beautiful contrast to the rest of the silvery young foliage. The fleshy root is a whitish color inside, greyish brown on the outside, and usually twisted and spindle-shaped. This is particularly evident in the dried root. After digging out the root, refill the hole with soil and a piece of the dug-up root.

HEALING PROPERTIES

The medical use of Burdock can be traced back to great and ancient physicians like Dioscurides, Galen, and Pliny, who described it in their writings. One of the herb's best-known successes was in France where it was said to have healed Henry III of syphilis. And the German doctor Hufeland, who counted the German poets Goethe, Schiller, and Herder among his patients, preferred Burdock for treating wounds and abscesses.

Burdock is a strong blood-cleansing remedy. Where the body accumulates too many toxins, where waste products fill the tissue and clog the skin, where the body attempts to cleanse itself through the skin (through ulcers, eczemas, boils, and skin eruptions), Burdock offers welcome support. It stimulates the organs of elimination: liver, gallbladder, spleen, kidneys, urinary bladder, and skin.

For skin diseases, I recommend a six-week course of treatment. The patient should either drink a cup of Burdock root tea or ingest a pinch of Burdock root powder three times a day. The external application of freshly mashed Burdock leaves enhances the effect. If fresh leaves are not available, use compresses saturated with the tea. However, because many of the root's active ingredients are lost in the heating process, it is more effective to chew the fresh root or ingest a powder prepared from the dried root.

To use remedially, it is best to dig up the root in the fall when the upper part of the plant is withering. Clean and cut the root into small pieces or thin slices and hang them up to dry. To prepare tea, briefly boil two teaspoons of the dried root in a cup of water. To prepare the root powder, finely pulverize the dried pieces in a mortar or clean coffee grinder for ingestion by the pinch. Do not store the root or powder for longer than a year.

Burdock root contains up to 45% inulin, which makes it especially useful for diabetics as well as for those suffering from liver and gall-bladder diseases. More about this in the culinary section.

During a cleansing fast, a course of treatment with Burdock aids metabolic stagnation and the elimination of waste products. I recommend it for any symptoms resulting from contact with toxic substances; for example, contact with chemicals such as varnishes and wood stain. These and other harmful substances tax the body immediately and long afterward affect the liver, kidneys, eyes, and lungs.

"Wood Tea" ("Spec. Lignorum"), of which Burdock is an ingredient, has long been recommended for all of the diseases mentioned. I include the recipe here.

Burdock root is available in herbal pharmacies and natural food stores as "Radix Bardanae." The homeopathic mother tincture "Arctium Lappa" is prepared from the fresh root. In Germany, commercially available Burdock oil does not have to contain Burdock root extract so I always advise my patients to make their own.

❧ "Wood Tea"

20 grams burdock root
    (*Arctium lappa*)
20 grams dandelion root
    (*Taraxacum officinale*)
20 grams lignumvitae
    (*Guajacum officinale*)
20 grams white sandalwood
    (*Santalum album*)

Steep 1 teaspoon of the tea mixture per cup of cold water and boil it for 10 minutes. A daily dose is 2 cups.

❧ Burdock Oil

Fill a mason jar with freshly crushed burdock roots and top it off with cold-pressed jojoba oil, sunflower oil, or wheat germ oil. Cover tightly and let it steep in a sunny, warm spot for 3 weeks. Strain the oil into dark bottles and keep them in a cool, dark place.

Use the oil as a liniment for diseases of the muscles, joints, and skin. Massage it into the scalp of a person suffering from dandruff and hair loss. And, if you have split ends, rub it into the ends of your hair.

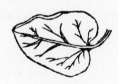

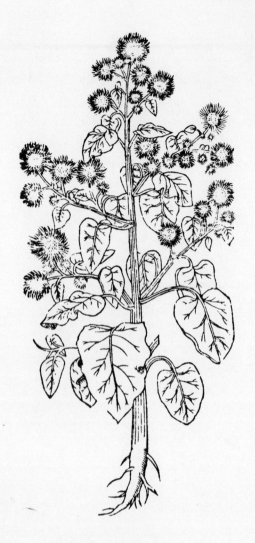

it, and sauté it in butter. Serve it warm or chilled with a lemon dressing or with yogurt, fresh herbs, and lemon juice.

The young leaves taste like spinach and can be steam-cooked and dressed with oil and vinegar. The young stems are also edible. You can steam-cook them in salted water before cutting them into small pieces for a salad. I then dress them with oil, lemon juice, mustard, oregano, and thyme.

VETERINARY MEDICINE

Burdock root is a good medicinal remedy for coughing, sickly sheep. To treat them, add freshly chopped root to their feed. For cattle and horses likewise suffering from cough, mix Burdock root, Coltsfoot (*Tussilago farfara*), Gentian (*Gentiana lutea*), and Oregano (*Origanum vulgare*) in equal parts to the fodder. Lastly, mixing the dried leaves into their food strengthens cattle.

CULINARY USE

All three Burdock components—roots, leaves, and stems—are used in the kitchen. In the past, a coffee substitute was made from the root (see the chapter on Chicory). And one old German name for Burdock, "Tobacco Leaf" (*Tubaksblad*), is still heard in the Eifel region, where the leaves are used as a tobacco substitute.

In Japan, the root is a popular vegetable. I think it tastes a little like an artichoke. Before its preparation, remove the thick root bark. Then cook the root in salted water until it is soft, slice

COSMETICS

Burdock is generally known as a tonic for hair growth. I clearly remember the bottles of Burdock hair oil on my grandfather's dressing table—and he had a very impressive bald head!

One recipe for "Burdock Hair Oil" that I found in a 1919 pharmaceutical manual contains olive oil, oil of benzoin, alkannin, chlorophyll, oil of bergamot, oil of lavender, rose oil, kumatrin—but no trace of Burdock root! Even today, many so-called Burdock hair oils that are available commercially do not contain Burdock root.

The following recipe for Burdock hair lotion, however, does include the named ingredient.

✧ Burdock Hair Lotion

> 40 grams burdock roots, freshly mashed
>   (*Arctium lappa*)
> 25 grams stinging nettle roots,
>   freshly mashed (*Urtica dioica*)
> 10 grams rosemary leaves
>   (*Rosmarinus officinalis*)
> 20 grams nasturtium leaves and flowers,
>   fresh or dried (*Tropaeolum majus*)
> 300 milliliters 70% alcohol
> 100 milliliters rose water

Fill a jar with the herbs and enough alcohol to cover. Replace the jar's lid and let the mixture steep for 3 weeks. Strain off the liquid, add the rose water, and store in a cool, dry place.

Cultivation

Burdock is a huge, imposing plant that can grow six or seven feet tall. With the addition of wide expansive leaves, it is best suited as a solitary plant at your garden's edge or near the house. It requires well-fertilized soil and a sunny habitat that is not too dry. An ideal place is near a compost pile where it will both receive needed nutrients and provide shade for the compost.

Seeds are available commercially. However, you can also propagate it with root pieces and root branches. Sown in March and April, seeds can take a month to germinate—so do not lose patience. Later, thin seedlings to a distance of two feet apart.

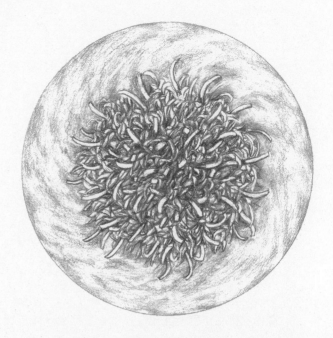

Burdock is a biennial plant that, in the first year, will form only a rosette with large leaves. In the second year, it will sprout a thick stem and purplish flowers. Harvest the root in the second year.

Seeds of the Japanese garden variety Burdock "Takinogawa" are not available in Germany. Once a friend, however, brought me a packet of seeds from Japan. They developed well and made a healthy and delicate vegetable. (As I mentioned earlier, the roots taste like artichokes.) The narrow roots can grow three feet long—and I never discovered the Japanese technique of pulling them out of the soil in one piece.

BOTANICAL CHARACTERISTICS

Name: Arctium lappa — Burdock

Distribution: Native to Europe and northern China, naturalized in North America

Habitat: Waysides, fences, dumps, near human dwellings

Description: In the first year: a large rosette of basal leaves; leaves are large, cordate, and stalked. In the second year: a stem up to 7 feet tall; rose-crimson flowers, stalked and globose, surrounded by prickly green bracts. Flowering time is July to September.

Confusion with similar plants: Possibly with Rhubarb (*Rheum* spp.)

Collecting season:
   Root – October
   Leaves and stem (for cooking) – in spring

Active ingredients: Inulin (27% to 45%), mucilage, tannins, bitter compounds, essential oil, phytosterols

Astrological association: Saturn / Pluto

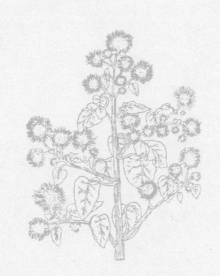

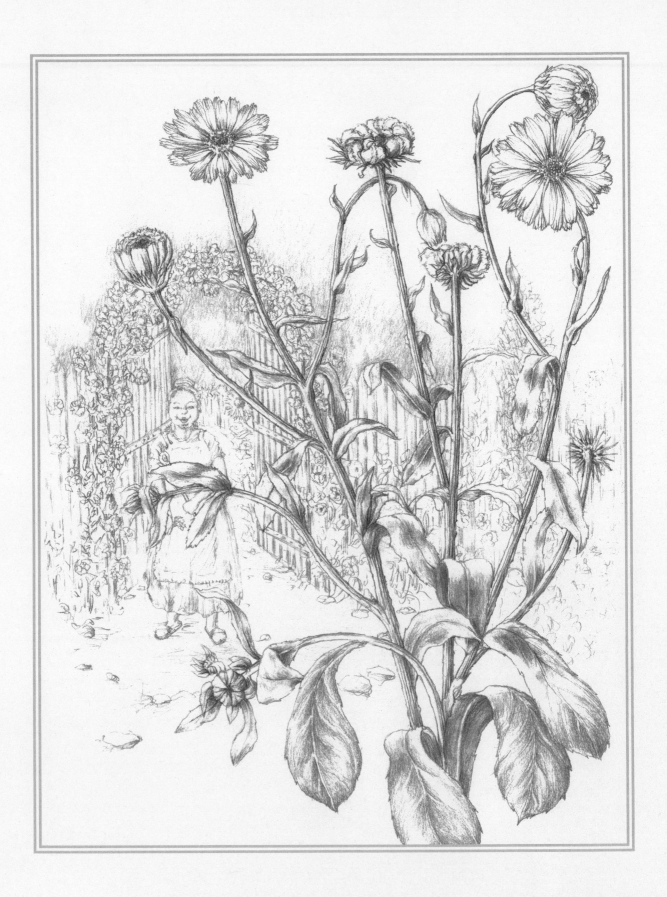

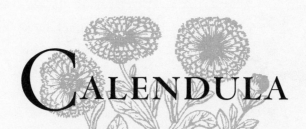

CALENDULA

Calendula officinalis
Pot Marigold
Garden Marigold, Marybud, Holigold, Bull's Eyes
Daisy family—Compositae / Asteraceae

IN MY HERB GARDEN is a bed with yellow medicinal plants where Wallflower and Golden Clover vie for radiance. Further back, the yellow becomes brighter and brighter until, reaching Calendula, it becomes pure orange. Next to the tender Wallflower and the delicately proportioned Golden Clover, Calendula looks stocky. She stands like a chubby, rosy-cheeked kitchen damsel in a white apron. Everything about her is round and placid, well-rooted, her light green leaf-skirts arranged neatly atop one another. Confident and warm-hearted, she gazes up into the sun. She has a place of honor in my garden because of her long tradition as both a medicinal and decorative plant. For many centuries the friendly Calendula appeared in every rural garden. A woman would make a salve from the herb as a helpful remedy for people and animals alike as well as toss her flowers into the cooking pot— hence, her common name Pot Marigold.

Calendula has many names that reveal her history and purpose. Observing her spreading nature in our garden, we certainly can understand the vernacular German names given to her

of "Rampant Flower" and "Curl Flower." Almost as soon as the strangely curled seeds are in the ground, the first leaf appears. Our little lady's leaves feel quite juicy and fleshy to the touch, and once one flower wilts, another rushes to greet the sun. Calendula blooms constantly in this manner from early June to the end of fall, even flowering into November or early December if the weather allows. Her name derives from the Latin *calendae*, meaning "the first day of the month," because she grows in so many months (*calendis*). A rampant bloomer, indeed!

Aside from peasant and herbal gardens, Calendula was regularly at home in burial grounds. Where Death exerted his irrevocable authority, people planted the "Flower of the Dead," her scent aromatic and strengthening and at the same time unpleasant and putrid. According to traditional wisdom, her inexhaustible botancal energy is a sign of eternal life. Even today Christian symbolism presents Calendula as an allegory for salvation after death.

It was several centuries before the Christian era that Albertus Magnus named her *sponsa*

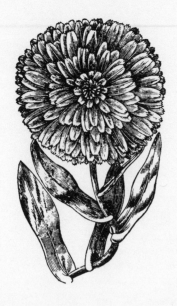

salis—"bride of the sun." Several other plants of the large Compositae family also bear this name: Daisy, Chamomile, Dandelion, and Chicory. This is because they each accompany the sun, turning toward the light, opening and closing their flowers according to the solar progression. Calendula, too, has her specific sun times and is a member of Linnaeus' "flower clock" that is described in the chapter on Chicory.

Who were these flower brides whose blooms resembling the radiant solar disk were dedicated to the sun? In recent decades, scholars have shed light on a forgotten world that existed before our current model of society. It was a matriarchal realm that survives in fairy tales, songs, images, and dreams. In my part of the world, countless folk tales and songs point to our inner connection to this time. The ancient ruler-priestesses, healers, and seers live on in stories of wise women and fairy godmothers. Today there are still hills in Germany called "Women's Mountain" (*Frauenberg*) where they once lived, healed, and pronounced judgment.

In those [ancient] societies, the sun was a sacred symbol of life and deliverance, its journey forming the secular and spiritual framework of the solar year. The priestesses—also brides of the sun—celebrated the solar holidays in sacred places. We know that modern Christian holidays like Easter, Whitsunday (Pentecost), St. Michael's Day (September 29), and Christmas are altered ancient solar feast days. Both Pagan and Christian feast days are meant to convey the same deep symbolism to their followers. Flowers who bloomed at these times and resembled the sun in shape were considered sacred—the Daisy during the vernal equinox, St. John's Wort at the summer solstice, Chicory and Calendula at the autumnal equinox, and for the winter solstice a plant that remained ever green—the Mistletoe that even today is present at Christmas in England and North America.

Some of these ancient sun brides are still dedicated to female goddesses such as the Germanic Freya or the Christian Mary. Calendula, always a plant of women and a plant of love, even bears the English name "Marigold." This flower-lady who blooms for such a long period is thought capable of producing undying love in one person for another—a magical love that forever puts forth new blossoms. An old folk song tells of a girl who planted our "Never-Wilt Flower" on the footprints of her beloved so that his love would never die.

In the evening I strolled down the lane
Where, under peach trees stood my
   sweetheart;
I obtained a peach from her by praying.
Quietly, my sweetheart reproached me:
Your mother has scolded me sharply
For bewitching you with my young blood;

But I never did! God is my witness that
Only your footprint I have chosen
To plant with Never-Wilt Flowers.
Don't wilt, beloved, you will have me, too.

HEALING PROPERTIES

The Daisy family has two prestigious wound herbs—Calendula and Arnica (*Arnica montana*). Although both have yellow flowers, they can easily be distinguished. Calendula arranges her yellow-orange petals in an orderly fashion around the disk while Arnica always looks slightly disheveled. And Calendula smells fainter while Arnica's scent is intensely aromatic. Lastly, Calendula is not a wildflower but only grows in cultivated gardens. In contrast, the wild Arnica grows high up in the mountains or in marshy meadows.

Both plants are primarily wound remedies. Arnica can dissolve bruises, affect tendons and ligaments, reduce inflammation of the joints, and help in cases of tendovaginitis. Calendula's different properties make it applicable when the skin is too sensitive and reacts allergically to the more caustic Arnica. Specifically, Calendula has vulnerary, disinfecting, and granulation-promoting qualities. It prevents the proliferation of scar tissue and is anti-inflammatory. It is a remedy for all wounds, especially for those that are purulent, inflamed, and healing poorly. It disperses ulcers and takes away pain during and after wound repair (for example, following amputations). It helps soothe inflamed nipples, diaper rash, leg ulcers, and eczema.

Classically, Calendula salve is prepared with lard. However, because lard is saturated with so many toxins from the environment, livestock feed, and "special additives," I no longer recommend it as a base for any remedy. The famous Calendula butter (*Ringelrosenbutter*) from the central European region of Silesia has long been used as a liniment for stomach problems. It was prepared with goat butter with the healing properties of the many herbs that goats eat. As an alternative to lard, I recommend its use if obtainable from biologically fed goats.

Another property of this sunny-faced herb is that it can stimulate the body's lymphatic system. I have had successful results with Calendula when administered internally as a tea and externally as a liniment. Specifically, I use Calendula salve or oil with Sweet Clover (*Melilotus officinalis*) and Figwort (*Scrophularia nodosa*) for lymphedemas, swollen lymph nodes, swollen tonsils with enlarged cervical lymph nodes, and lymph swellings after breast surgery. In addition,

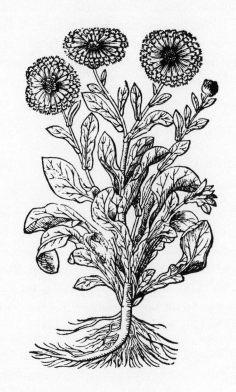

Calendula is an assisting remedy for painful or scanty menstruation.

For Calendula tea, salves, oils and so on, pluck the orange petals from the flower's green heads. And please review "Some Tips for Making Salves" in the chapter on Comfrey before making the following salve recipes. Calendula tea is available in herb stores as "Flores Calendulae sine Calycibus." The homeopathic mother tincture, which is especially useful for the treatment of allergic eczema, is prepared from the fresh flowering herb.

RINGELROSENBUTTER

500 grams goat butter (about 1 pound)
100 grams calendula flower petals
(about 3.5 ounces)

Slowly melt the goat butter in a double boiler; mix in the freshly plucked flower petals. Continue heating without boiling the mixture for 20 minutes, stirring constantly. Strain the butter through a clean cheese cloth; fill clean salve jars, cover tightly, and store in a cool, dark place.

CALENDULA OIL

fresh calendula flowers
cold-pressed olive oil (or sunflower oil)

Fill a clean wide-mouth mason jar with fresh calendula flowers that have been carefully washed and patted dry. Pour in enough olive oil to cover and screw the lid on tightly. Place the jar in the sun for 3 weeks, shaking it occasionally. Strain the oil through a clean cloth into bottles; store them in a cool place.

For a good massage oil, I mix this calendula oil with oils prepared in the same way from walnut leaves (*Juglans* spp.), rosemary (*Rosmarinus officinalis*), and lavender (*Lavandula* spp.). I also use Calendula oil as the base for making the following salves.

CALENDULA SALVE

220 grams lanolin (7.8 ounces)
270 grams calendula oil (9.6 ounces)
a handful of fresh-plucked calendula petals
55 grams beeswax, grated (2 ounces)
40 grams calendula tincture (1.4 ounces)

Melt the lanolin in a double boiler and slowly add the calendula oil, mixing thoroughly. Add the flower petals and heat for 15 minutes without boiling, stirring occasionally. Strain the mixture through a clean cheese cloth and return it to the pan. Add the grated beeswax and reheat enough to melt it. Now stir in the calendula tincture. Pour the salve into clean salve pots and let it cool before storing.

A "SPECIAL" CALENDULA SALVE

calendula salve [see the preceding recipe]
½ teaspoon Peruvian balm
castor oil
10 grams propolis tincture (0.4 ounces)

To make an especially potent medicinal salve, I add Peruvian balm (balmtree, *Myroxylon balsamum*) and propolis tincture to the preceding recipe for calendula salve. Both salves have strong vulnerary, germicidal, and disinfecting properties. Peruvian balm is a dark brown, tenacious, pleasant-smelling mass obtainable from herbal pharmacies. However, some people react allergically to it so be sure not to overdose or apply it in its pure form. Propolis tincture is available in herb stores or health food stores.

To prepare the "special" salve: Dissolve the Peruvian balm by stirring it into a little hot castor oil; set it aside. Reduce the quantity of calendula oil from the previous recipe by 10 grams (0.4 ounces). Likewise, reduce the amount of calendula tincture by 10 grams (0.4 ounces) and use only 30 grams (1 ounce). Follow the preceding recipe and at the end stir in the Peruvian balm and propolis tincture.

❦ Calendula Tincture

Fill a mason jar halfway with fresh, washed, and chopped calendula flowers. Cover the flowers with grain spirit or a fruit liqueur and close the jar tightly. Let the mixture steep for 3 or 4 weeks, shaking it occasionally. Strain the tincture into dark bottles.

This tincture is suitable for treating open wounds and as a rinse for gum inflammation. As a dressing, dilute 1 teaspoon calendula tincture in 1 cup of boiled water.

❦ Calendula Tea

Pour 1 cup of boiling water over 1 teaspoon of calendula flowers that have been washed and chopped. Let the mixture steep covered. A daily dose is 3 cups.

For a lymph remedy, prepare a tea of equal parts calendula flowers and sweet clover (*Melilotus officinalis*).

❦ A Women's Tea for Painful Menses

calendula (*Calendula officinalis*)
chamomile (*Matricaria chamomilla*)
lady's mantle (*Alchemilla vulgaris*)
yarrow (*Achillea millefolium*)

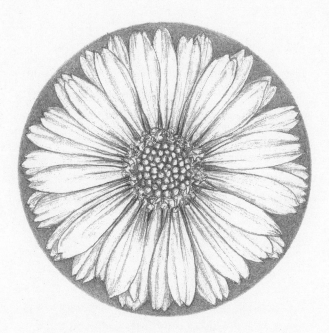

Mix these four herbs in equal parts and prepare a tea following the procedure used for calendula tea in the preceding recipe. A daily dose is 2 to 3 cups. (You may also refer to the chapters on Mugwort and Silverweed.)

Veterinary Medicine

St. Hildegard von Bingen praised Calendula as a remedy for animals, recommending it to treat flatulence in sheep caused by bad feed. For this purpose, give the sheep fresh Calendula juice. For cough in cattle or sheep, spray freshly pressed Calendula juice into the nostrils of the affected animal. I have had great success using Calendula salve on animals for wounds, injuries, and inflammation (for example, inflammation of the udder). For this, mix together equal amounts of Calendula and Comfrey salves. Calendula tea is also suitable for washing wounds.

COSMETICS

Because Calendula soothes reddened and inflamed skin, we can use the tea as a facial cleanser, for compresses, and as a hair rinse for a dry and brittle scalp. Calendula oil is also useful for dry, sensitive skin and cracked hands.

❧ CALENDULA ROSE CREAM

> 40 grams egg yolk (about 1.5 ounces)
> 60 grams calendula oil (about 2 ounces)
> 2 drops essential rose oil

Warm the egg yolk in a double boiler over hot water and whisk it until it is creamy. Add the calendula oil a drop at a time, whisking constantly until it thickens into the consistency of a salve. Finally, stir in the rose oil and pour into a salve jar with a tight lid.

Calendula rose cream is true nourishment for dry, irritated, and inflamed skin. It does not keep long, however, so make it in small batches and keep it in the refrigerator. Finally, always use the more expensive, pure rose oil and never a synthetic version.

CULTIVATION

Although a smaller, wild variety of Calendula is native to southern European regions, to obtain the fresh flowers needed for oils, tinctures, salves and so forth, it is necessary to cultivate it in our gardens. And, thankfully, this is not difficult—this cheery damsel is easy to cultivate. The plant thrives on any soil but prefers deep, loamy, nutrient-rich earth. Seeds are available from your local nursery or garden center.

If you plan to use Calendula for medicinal purposes, be sure to choose varieties with orange double flowers. Otherwise seeds of decorative varieties are available in shades ranging from cream to deep orange. In early April, you may seed directly into the open ground, later thinning the young plants to 8 inches apart. Water these sun lovers well but avoid standing water. Calendula grows well in containers and flower boxes.

A few hints: If you let a few plants mature and self-seed, you will see many small Calendula plants grow at that spot the following year. And, because the evaporation of its roots can kill nematodes, Calendula is a good companion for roses or carrots and will strengthen and protect them from pests.

CULINARY USE

Once used to color butter, dried Calendula petals impart a lovely yellow color to foods. I use them in sweets, puddings, desserts, rice, and egg dishes. To extract the pigment from the dried petals, steep them in a hot liquid.

BOTANICAL CHARACTERISTICS

Name: *Calendula officinalis* — Calendula

Distribution: Southern Europe, northern Africa, western Asia, elsewhere cultivated in gardens

Habitat: In gardens, although they occasionally run wild

Description: These annual plants can grow 1 to 2 feet high; ramified stem; leaves succulent green, hairy, spatulate at the base but smaller and narrower further up; bright orange-yellow flowers with green receptacles.

Confusion with similar plants: None

Collecting season: Flowering from June to October, and occasionally into November

Active ingredients: Essential oil (in the ray flowers up to 0.12%), flavonoids, bitter compounds, carotenes, tannins, saponins

Astrological association: Sun / Venus

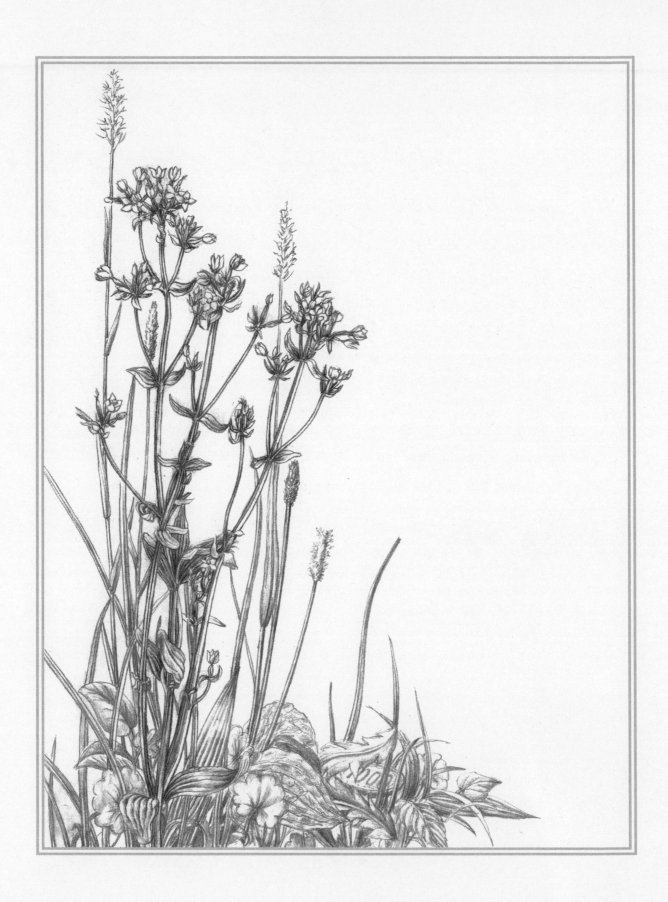

C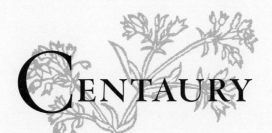ENTAURY

Centaurium erythraea (C. minus, C. umbellatum, Erythraea centaurium)
Common Centaury, European Centaury, Bitter Herb, Lesser Centaury
Gentian family—Gentianaceae

Tired of my debts, I will plant some
Thousand Guilder Herbs in my garden.
Thereafter I will guard my golden treasure,
Attend to arts and belles-lettres,
And, when I die, leave my heirs
This Croesus of plants.

from Karl-Heinz Waggerl's
Humorous Herbarium

ONE SIP OF A TEA made from this herb—whose German name means "Thousand Guilder Herb"—will make you question why this plant is worth a thousand pieces of gold. The mouth contracts, the taste buds react with dismay, and the courageous woman swallowing her first cup of Centaury tea will make a face and exclaim, "Ugh! How awful!" But the wise patient will reach again for her teacup, remembering that what is bitter in the mouth is healthy for the stomach.

Centaury is so bitter that the ancient Romans rightly called it "bile of the earth" (*fel terrae*), an epithet recognizing its power to stimulate the digestive system by increasing the secretion of gastric juices and the function of the gallbladder.

Its healing past records that it was also used to treat severe febrile diseases, bite wounds, and injuries. And surely, any herb that will restore one's health after such illnesses is worth a thousand guilders! The herbalist Parson Kneipp, too, highly valued Centaury and often prescribed it to his patients for fevers and stomach problems. Of it he writes:

Named for a large sum, help will this herb
give for free to anyone.

But first, to understand its botanical and English name we visit ancient Greece. There we meet Chiron the Centaur, half human and half horse, who purportedly taught the healing arts to Hercules, Achilles, Jason, and Aesculapius. With the help of this herb, Chiron healed purulent arrow wounds on his own horse legs. In remembrance, the plant was named *Centaurea*, or Centaury in English. This connection was lost in Germany. Instead, my ancestors translated the Latin name into what seemed more logical: *centum* for "hundred" and *aurum* for "gold." And indeed, until the fifteenth century, "Hundred Guilder Herb" was its name, that is, until its value later increased to one thousand guilders.

Chiron's herb was known early on as a powerful healing plant. In old herbals I sometimes find it under mysterious names like "Red Aurin," "Wild Laurin," or "Laurin's Herb." It makes me think that there was once a connection between Centaury and the Dwarf-King Laurin in Dietrich von Bern's legend. Do you suppose he included "Laurin's Herb" in his beautiful rose garden?

"Blessing the herbs" is long celebrated in Europe. Originally a Pagan custom, it asks for the blessing of the Goddess on the healing herbs of which Centaury is one. It is still practiced on August 15th, the Day of the Assumption of the Blessed Virgin, in the Catholic regions of southern Germany where I live. On that day women bring ritually arranged herbs in bundles of seven, nine, or another sacred number to the church for Mary's blessing. (See the illustration in the chapter on Mullein.) This bundle is later placed conspicuously in the living area of the home or above the stable door if used for animals. Traditionally, these sacred herbs are used in cases of serious family illness or thrown into the fireplace to guard against lightning.

Some old German names tell us of the high esteem in which Centaury was held. For instance, "Mad Dog's Herb" and "Dog Bite Herb" refer to one of the plant's medicinal uses. In the moors around the German town of Lüneburg, "mad dog butter" was administered to the bite victim of a rabid dog. And in Mecklenburg, people called the plant "Stand Up and Go Away" because, once administered to someone, the patient could do just that—stand up and be gone.

Whether used as a remedy for the stomach, wounds, or fever, Centaury was valued everywhere. A rider who encountered the valuable plant in his or her path was admonished not to pass by without picking it. Unfortunately, a rider traveling in the late afternoon or evening was unlikely to spot the plant from horseback. The bright rose-colored flowers are extremely sensitive, opening only in the warmest morning sun. By early afternoon, its five petals close—as they do in cool temperatures, in darkness, upon touch, or when rain approaches.

Centaury chooses to grow in wooded meadows and along grassy banks where it can seek protection from winter's cold and summer's heat. Early in the day when the sun shines, the small pink flowers emerge from the grass appearing tender, light, friendly—yet timid. And this is when special admirers come visiting to pollinate. Fluttering in many colors around the small flowers, they are butterflies sporting names like "Checkered Skipper" and "Chalkhill Blue."

Let's take a closer look at this shy young plant with pink veil and linden green leaf mantle. From the soft, pale yellow root a basal rosette originates clinging tightly to the earth. From the center a rather stiff stem rises 4 inches (and sometimes up to 20 inches) above the ground. Every pair of leaves along the stem is arranged crosswise to the one above it. The matte green leaves are of elongated ovate or lanceolate shape with five prominent parallel leaf veins. The stem branches out at the top to allow the flowers to sit in cyme-like arrangement on loosely forked flower stalks. And the pink hue of their small five-petaled flowers radiates as intensely as the light blue of the little spring Gentians. Both plants, along with Common Bogbean (*Meny-*

anthes trifoliata), belong to the Gentian family. All bitter herbs, these three cousins enjoy a reputation for healing bad stomachs.

Unfortunately, Centaury's popularity has contributed to its decimation in nature. Classified as "partially protected" under German law, we can pick the plant above the ground but may not damage its roots or move it from its location. Another species growing in Germany is used less frequently for medicinal purposes. "Branching Centaury" (*Centaurium pulchellum*) grows only six inches tall and has a stem that branches out from the ground. It prefers wet meadows and ditches and also enjoys partially protected status. *Note: Before gathering plants in the wild, always check with the local library, national and regional park authorities, or nature societies for regulations regarding protected plants in your area.*

HEALING PROPERTIES

Not all plants containing bitter compounds are considered to be medicinal bitters; for example, Yarrow (*Achillea millefolium*), Coltsfoot (*Tussilago farfara*), Arnica (*Arnica montana*), German Chamomille (*Matricaria chamomilla*), Lady's Mantle (*Alchemilla vulgaris*), and Hops (*Humulus lupulus*). The effect of the bitter compounds must be predominant before a plant is included in the bitter herbs group (or *amara*), which is then divided into three subgroups:

1. *Amara tonica*: Plants that contain only bitter compounds and no other chemical constituents of importance.

2. *Amara aromatica*: Plants that, besides bitter compounds, also have a substantial content of essential oils. The respective essential oil unfolds yet another zone of action in the body—for example, nerves, liver, gallbladder. This group includes Angelica (*Angelica archangelica*), Sweetflag (*Acorus calamus*), and Wood Avens (*Geum urbanum*).

3. *Amara acria*: Exotic plants like Ginger (*Zingiber officinale*), Lesser Galangal (*Alpinia officinarum*), and Pepper (*Piper nigrum*) belong to this group. Bitter and acrid at the same time, they are used mostly as spices.

The most important alpine natives of the first group are Common Centaury (*C. erythraea*), Yellow Gentian (*Gentiana lutea*), and Common Bogbean (*Menyanthes trifoliata*). All three have a very high content of bitter compounds. Struggling through a self-trial, I compared teas made from these plants in terms of bitterness—and Yellow Gentian definitely won the prize, its taste in the mouth being slow to subside. This oral sensation, by the way, is expressed scientifically as the plant's "bitter factor" by giving the dilution in which a compound still retains a bitter effect. For example, Centaury's bitter factor is 1 to 3,500 (meaning it still tastes bitter and has a bitter effect in a dilution of 1 part Centaury to 3,500 parts water). Common Bogbean's bitter factor is only 1 to 1,500. But neither hold a candle to big brother Yellow Gentian's bitter factor of 1 to 20,000! These values come from Dr. R.F. Weiss's *Lehrbuch der Phytotherapie* (Stuttgart, 1974).

Bitter compounds affect our body by stimulating our digestive system. This begins in the mouth when the taste prompts the salivary glands to secrete more saliva. This in turn signals the stomach to start working. This is precisely why bitter medicines should never be ingested in the form of capsules, tablets, or pills. For the same reason, a bitter tea used medicinally should not be sweetened because we want the bitterness to induce the secretion of saliva.

Bitter compounds stimulate the entire body and it is not surprising to discover that all great panaceas contain large quantities of bitter herbs. (Remember the sixteenth century plague remedy Theriak mentioned in the chapter on Angelica.)

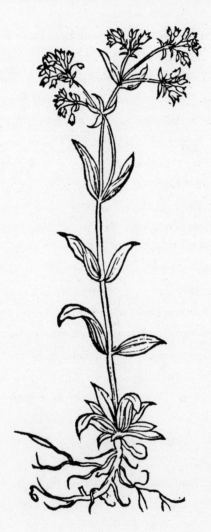

Bitter compounds can promote heart function, increase vessel tone, increase the production of red and white blood cells, and stimulate the entire metabolism.

Remedies containing bitter compounds should be ingested 15 to 30 minutes before meals—and in the proper dosage. This is because a small amount can stimulate digestion but too much can produce the opposite effect. It is therefore better to take small doses of bitter remedies regularly over an extended time period rather than larger doses occasionally.

Centaury helps in cases of poor appetite, weak stomach function, or general weakness of the digestive system. It restores strength to someone recuperating from illness and is a good remedy for anorexia nervosa as an adjunct to psychotherapeutic treatment. In addition, it is recommended as an adjunct remedy for liver-gallbladder dysfunctions and for diabetes. *Note: However, do not use it for an acid stomach (acidosis) or heartburn.*

From June to September, when Centaury is flowering, we can pick it for teas, tinctures, wine, and so on. The best time is at midday when the sun is shining and the flowers are fully open. Cut the plants off above the ground, tie them into thin bundles, and hang them upside down to dry. To store, cut the dried bunches into small pieces.

In my country, native plants cannot keep up with the demand. Therefore most of the Centaury tea available in German herbal stores and pharmacies comes from Morocco. If you prefer to take Centaury as drops, you can easily make your own tincture. (See the following recipe section.)

❧ CENTAURY TEA

2 teaspoons fresh or dried centaury herb

2 cups cold water

Pour the water over the herb and let it stand overnight. The next day, strain off the liquid and sip it throughout the day. Two cups is a daily dose.

❧ CENTAURY TINCTURE

Fill a dark mason jar halfway with finely chopped fresh centaury. Top it off with grain spirit or a fruit liqueur and close the jar tightly. Let the mixture steep for 2 weeks, shaking it occasionally. Strain the tincture into a bottle with a tight lid or stopper.

Take 20 drops before meals, 3 times a day.

❧ TINCTURA AMARUM

3 grams centaury herb, powdered
   (*Centaurium erythraea*)

3 grams yellow gentian root, powdered
   (*Gentiana lutea*)

2 grams bitter orange peel, mature,
   powdered (*Citrus aurantium matur.*)

1 gram bitter orange peel, immature,
   powdered (*Citrus aurantium immatur.*)

1 gram zedoary root, powdered
   (*Zedoaria* spp.)

50 grams wine spirits 68%

Because centaury can be mixed with other stomachics, I include this old and familiar recipe for stomach drops from the German Pharmacopeia. Prepare it as you do the centaury tincture in the preceding recipe.

❧ CENTAURY WINE

2 handfuls fresh centaury herb
   (*Centaurium erythraea*)

2 tablespoons bitter orange peel, mature
   (*Citrus aurantium matur.*)

1 bottle Málaga wine

Chop the centaury herb finely and add it, with the bitter orange peel, to the wine. Let this mixture steep for 2 weeks before straining the liquid into a bottle with a tight lid or stopper. As an aid to digestion, have a small glass before meals.

Málaga wine is a sweet fortified wine from Spain that in years past was very popular. Ask your local wine merchant for something comparable.

Centaury's bigger and more bitter brother, Yellow Gentian, is also used to improve stomach function. Only the root is used, and when

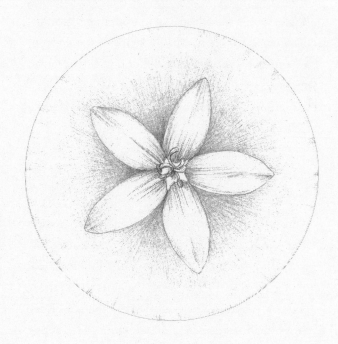

steeped in boiling water, it can be taken as a tea. From the root, you can also prepare a tincture or a liquor (commonly called "Gentian schnapps"). Its areas of application are weak stomach function, anorexia nervosa, and lack of appetite. It generates blood and is strengthening for exhaustion and after severe illnesses. As noted earlier, however, Yellow Gentian can irritate a sensitive or overly acidic stomach. Centaury has a weaker effect on the stomach but also influences the liver, gallbladder, and pancreas. Before digging up a Yellow Gentian root (*Gentiana lutea*), check on its protected status in your area. In Germany, it is protected.

Common Bogbean loves boggy, wet habitats. Its three large leaves resemble those of the small Clover (*Trifolium repens* or *T. pratense*). The white or reddish white flowers are funnel-shaped with hairy fringes. For Bogbean tea and tincture, follow the aforementioned procedures—but use only the leaves. Besides bitter compounds, Bogbean (or Buckbean) also contains saponins, tannins, and resin and is helpful for loss of appetite, weak stomach function, bloatedness, and strengthening during febrile diseases.

Centaury is available in herb stores as "Herba Centaurii."

CULTIVATION

A biennial, Centaury loves soils rich in loam and lime—and sunny places like a grassy meadow where it can grow undisturbed. In June you can plant the tiny brown seeds in pots or manure beds by pressing them lightly into the soil. Keep them well moistened. Later, thin the young plants to a distance of 6 or 8 inches apart.

Centaury will flower the following year and self-propagate thereafter.

VETERINARY MEDICINE

In the past, farmers added Centaury to the fodder of horses and cattle showing blood in their urine (hematuria). They placed it in the drinking water of sick chickens. Even today fresh or dried Centaury is mixed into the fodder of horses, cows, and sheep suffering from emaciation and loss of appetite.

❧ A REMEDY FOR ANIMALS

2 parts centaury herb
  (*Centaurium erythraea*)
2 parts yellow gentian root
  (*Gentiana lutea*)
1 part wormwood herb
  (*Artemisia absinthium*)
1 part stinging nettle herb
  (*Urtica dioica*)
1 part fenugreek seed
  (*Trigonella foenum-graecum*)

Chop the herbs finely and grind them into a powder. Administer 2 to 4 tablespoons to the animal depending on its size.

This mixture has proved effective for loss of appetite, emaciation, and general weakness in animals.

BOTANICAL CHARACTERISTICS

Name: *Centaurium erythraea* — Centaury

Distribution: In almost all of Europe, North Africa, western Asia, and North America

Habitat: Woodlands; arid, warm grasslands

Description: Plants grow 4 to 20 inches tall; basal rosette with obovate leaves; square stem with elongated, ovate to lanceolate crosswise leaves, prominent parallel leaf veins, entire margins. Inflorescence is a cyme with rose red or (rarely) whitish flowers.

Confusion with similar plants: With "Branching Centaury" (*C. pulchellum*) that branches from the ground up and grows to only 6 inches.

Collecting season: Flowering time is July to September

Active ingredients: Bitter compounds with small quantities of the intensely bitter secoiridoidglycosides; flavones, flavonoids, and traces of an essential oil

Astrological association: Sun / Venus

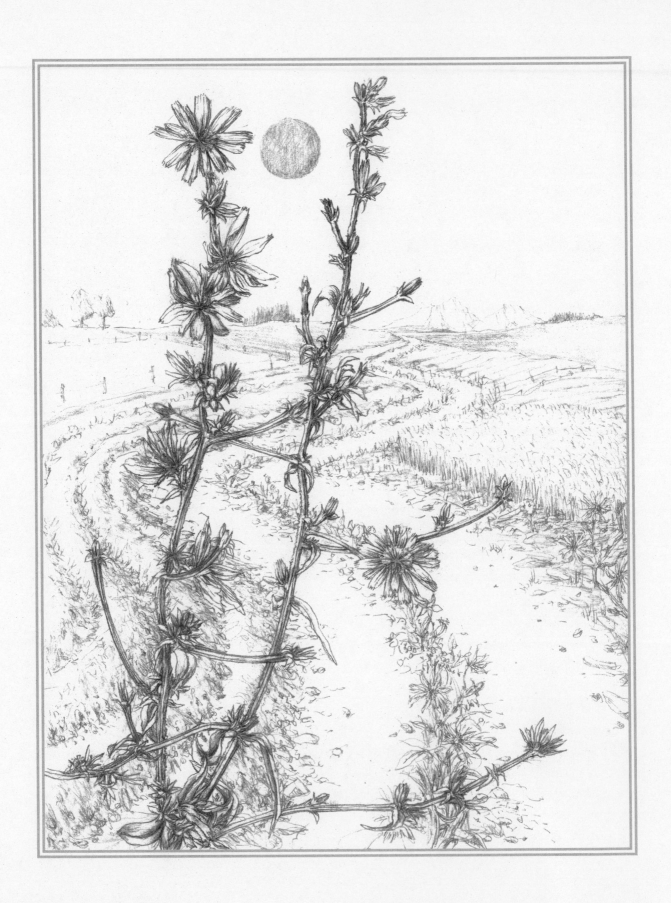

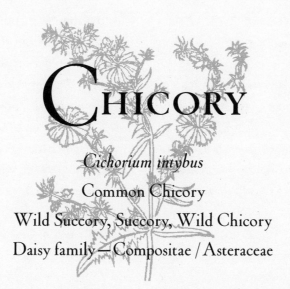

CHICORY

Cichorium intybus

Common Chicory

Wild Succory, Succory, Wild Chicory

Daisy family — Compositae / Asteraceae

ONCE UPON A TIME there was a princess who had a lover more handsome than any other. But one day her prince mounted his horse, rode to the east, and was seen no more. Saddened, the princess wanted to die but a glimmer of hope kept her going. Every morning she would arise and with her chambermaids await his return. Finally, God in His mercy transformed these sorrowful ladies into flowers along paths and roads where they might keep watch forever. The princess became the solitary white Chicory; the chambermaids, the more abundant blue ones. And there they remain to this day, facing east toward the rising sun. Their faces follow the golden orb as it moves and, and as it sets, they hang their heads in sorrow. Hope returns, however, by the next morning along with bright, new flowers to salute the sun.

Today we still see them along the wayside—the lovely blue Chicories and an occasional white one. They are the companions of travelers just like the small, dark broad-leaved Plantain and the proud, tall Mugwort who likewise prefer to live outside the confines of cultivated gardens.

All three tend to the physical ailments of those who wander near.

The beautiful Chicory is a flower for the soul. The sight of her alone gives joy and strength to travelers. But few take the time to stop and gaze into her blossom-eyes. Since the eighteenth century's Romantic period when her blue flowers received much attention, it has become lonely around Chicory. In fact, if not for her cousin, the cultivated Chicory and coffee substitute, she might be forgotten.

Our forebearers recognized the power of certain flowers—especially blue ones—to heal the human soul. The Native North Americans still know this. They say the path of the heart and of the soul is the color of a blue flower. Even in European healing traditions, blue flowers have long been used to heal depression and melancholy. They were also considered a remedy for the eyes because their power comes from our looking at them with our eyes—the deepest mirror of the soul. Along with Chicory, other blue flowers that appear in old herbals as remedies for the soul and eyes are Columbine,

Borage, Verbena, Cornflower, and Sweet Violet.

But how can we experience the relationship between flowers and the human soul today? How can we re-open our senses to the healing power of plants? With Chicory, it is not so difficult. To begin, we can simply go outside and sit down in front of a flowering Chicory. It is best to choose a clear day because traditional wisdom calls her power strongest in radiant sunshine. Gazing into her blue eyes, we now let them do their work. Afterward, we can look into the dark flowers of a Figwort or a poisonous Black Henbane and compare their energy.

The British physician Edward Bach (1886–1930) was one of the first people in our time to rekindle awareness of the soul energies of plants. He even captured them in remedies. From his long years of practice, he understood that disease originates largely from emotional disharmonies (such as fear, impatience, anger, and stress) that make the body susceptible to illness. Dr. Bach sought to heal his patients with remedies that could affect these relationships without producing harmful side effects. He developed 38 basic remedies prepared from fresh flowers that specifically addressed the energies of the human soul. Since then, his Bach flower remedies—the sky blue Chicory included—have helped countless people.

Stories and legends about this flower with its strong radiance would fill a book. The first written mention of Chicory appears on an Egyptian papyrus 4,000 years before the Christian era. And the Roman scholar Pliny informs us from first century A.D. Eygpt that she was still considered to be a magical plant. Indeed, since ancient times Chicory was coveted for magical purposes,

wisdom that later spread to German regions and lived on throughout the Middle Ages.

What could not be done with the magic of Chicory! We still know of spells and rituals dating from the seventeenth and eighteenth centuries. She was supposed to bring success in love. It was also believed that she could make one invulnerable. And when prepared in a certain complicated ritual, she could yield a cloak of invisibility. She was the famous herb (called "No More Pain" in German) that fairy godmothers from the forest gave to women threatened with bleeding to death in childbirth. Our old friend Paracelsus, the sixteenth century Swiss-born alchemist and physician, even claims that Chicory root turns into a bird every seven years. I venture that this means that a remedy made from her root may lift the heaviness of melancholy and allow the soul to be as light as a bird once more.

One can also accomplish ordinary tasks with Chicory and other plants. For instance, 200 years ago the great naturalist Carl von Linné (Linnaeus) noticed that certain plants, as if having an internal clock, opened and closed at specific times and, when planted in a circle according to their progression, gave him the time of day. Linnaeus planted the first flower clock in Uppsala, Sweden, using nine plants. And because her flowers opened early and closed again by midmorning, this living dial started with Chicory.

If you would like to plant this wondrous "flower clock" in your yard or garden, I have listed the flowers with their respective times. However, flower times vary by location, climate, and season. So, like Linnaeus, you will have to experiment in making your own version.

Flower-opening times:

- Chicory (*Cichorium intybus*)
    4 to 5 A.M.
- Dandelion (*Taraxacum officinale*)
    5 to 6 A.M.
- Common Hawkweed (*Hieracium vulgatum*)
    6 to 7 A.M.
- White Waterlily (*Nymphaea alba*)
    7 A.M.
- Pink Carnation (*Dianthus gratianopolitanus*)
    8 A.M.
- "Field Marigold" (*Calendula arvensis*)
    9 to 10 A.M.

Flower-closing times:

- Dandelion (*Taraxacum officinale*)
    8 to 10 A.M.
- Chicory (*Cichorium intybus*)
    10 A.M.
- Sow Thistle (*Sonchus oleraceus*)
    11 A.M. to NOON
- "Field Marigold" (*Calendula arvensis*)
    NOON
- Common Hawkweed (*Hieracium vulgatum*)
    2 P.M.
- White Waterlily (*Nymphaea alba*)
    5 P.M.
- St. Bernard Lily (*Anthericum liliago*)
    7 to 8 P.M.

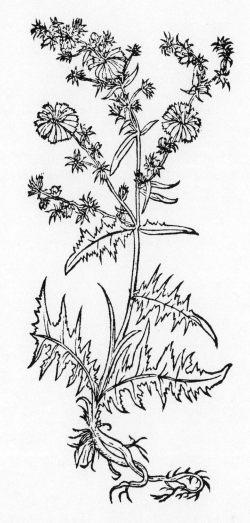

HEALING PROPERTIES

Ancient physicians viewed the spleen as the seat of the darkest of the four humors that circulate in the human body. They called this humor "black bile" or *melancholé*. Its predominance in a person was made evident through symptoms of melancholy, impure skin, and disturbed liver and gallbladder functions, evidence that toxins circulating in the body were slowly poisoning it. To purify the blood, medical practitioners stimulated the functions of the spleen, liver, and gallbladder. Chicory, a cleanser of both soul and body, was recommended for melancholy because it was one of the few spleen remedies found in nature's pharmacy. At the same time it tonified and healed the liver and gallbladder. This makes Chicory a remedy for all ailments of these three organs; for instance, stasis of the liver and gallbladder (cholestasis), stasis in the area of the

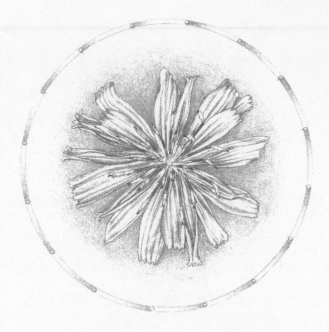

pressed juice from the whole Chicory plant ingested by the teaspoon.

Chicory root is available in herb stores as "Radix Cichorii." The homeopathic mother tincture "Cichorium" is prepared from the fresh roots.

❧ Chicory Root Tea

1 teaspoon chicory root (fresh or dried)
1 cup cold water

Steep the chicory root in cold water. Bring it to a boil; let it bubble for 5 minutes. A daily dose is 2 to 3 cups.

❧ Liver-Gallbladder-Spleen Tea

chicory root (*Cichorium intybus*)
dandelion root – Radix Taraxaci
    (*Taraxacum officinale*)
milkthistle seeds – Fructus Silybi mariani
    (*Silybum marianum, Carduus marianus*)

Mix the ingredients in equal parts and prepare them like the chicory root tea. A daily dose is 2 to 3 cups.

❧ Chicory Wine

1 liter good red wine
1 handful chicory roots
    (*Cichorium intybus*)
1 handful rhubarb roots
    (*Rheum palmatum* or *R. officinale*)
2 tablespoons buckthorn bark
    (Glossy Buckthorn, *Rhamnus frangula*)
1 teaspoon anise
1 cinnamon stick
2 tablespoons dried orange peel
    (pesticide-free)

portal vein, weak function of the spleen, hepatitis, and jaundice. And because Chicory also stimulates gastric and intestinal functions, I recommend Chicory wine for constipation.

It is used for the general cleansing of impure skin. For eczemas, Chicory is combined with Burdock root (*Arctium lappa*) and Fumitory (*Fumaria officinalis*). It even has a mild effect on a fourth organ of elimination and blood cleansing—the urinary bladder. A remedial tea uses Chicory root that is gathered in the spring or fall when the plant's strength is still held within the root. The root is then washed, cut it into small pieces, and dried carefully. (Another method is to cut the root open lengthwise and string the halves on a cord to dry.) The herb is also dried to use in tea mixtures.

But I am still not finished with Chicory's healing properties. All parts of the plant contain high quantities (up to 25%) of inulin, especially the root. This can lower the blood sugar level, making it a remedy for the pancreas. For a course of treatment for diabetics, I recommend fresh

After grinding all the ingredients in a mortar, pour them into a mason jar. Add the red wine and cover tightly. Let the jar stand in a warm spot for 3 weeks, shaking it occasionally. Strain the liquid into a dark bottle. Enjoy a snifter-full following meals.

Note: Use Chinese medicinal rhubarb found at an herb store—not your garden variety.

❧ Wine for Heart and Mind

chicory flowers (*Cichorium intybus*)
hyssop leaves and flowers
 (*Hyssopus officinalis*)
balm (*Melissa officinalis*)
raisins
1 vanilla bean
1 liter sweet red wine

The invigorating and heart-strengthening property of chicory is captured in this old wine recipe. To begin, combine equal amounts of the fresh herbs. Mash a handful of raisins in a mortar and add them to the herbs; place this mixture in a large jar. Add the vanilla bean and sweet red wine, close the jar tightly, and let it steep for 3 weeks. Strain the wine into a bottle and enjoy!

❧ Tea for Diabetics

chicory root – Radix Cichorii
 (*Cichorium intybus*)
dandelion root – Radix Taraxaci
 (*Taraxacum officinale*)
French bean pods – Fructus Phaseoli sine
 semine (*Phaseolus* spp.)
stinging nettle – Herba Urticae
 (*Urtica dioica* or *U. urens*)
goat's rue – Herba Galegae
 (*Galega officinalis*)

whortleberry leaves – Folia Myrtilli
 (*Vaccinium myrtillus*)

Combine equal amounts of the herbs. Steep 3 tablespoons of the herbs in 1 liter cold water; boil it for 5 minutes, remove from the heat, and let it steep for another 10 minutes. Drink 2 to 3 cups daily.

As a course of treatment, drink this tea for 3 weeks. Then alternate it with a tea mixture for the kidneys or the liver. Then return to the tea for diabetics for another 3 weeks.

❧ Preserved Chicory Flower Sugar

This recipe comes from Tabernaemontanus' herbal dated 1731. Because blue chicory flowers are not available year-round, we can strengthen ourselves with this confection on a cold winter day.

From the beautiful blue flowers of Chicory a beneficial and attractive sugar preserve is made in the following manner: Take 1 part plucked fresh flowers and cut them into small pieces on a board. Crush them afterward in a stone mortar and, during the crushing, gradually add 3 parts sugar. When it is mixed well and then shaped into an electuary, place it into a sugar bowl or a porcelain box. Place this in the sun for a while and keep it to use throughout the year.

This will strengthen the heart and revive the faint-hearted. It will serve against palpitations caused by heat as well as open, cleanse, and strengthen the liver. It will expel bile and mucus and serve against a burning stomach and chase away heartburn. It will arrest fevers and approaching dropsy and cool the heated liver and all internal members. In summa, this sugar serves all ailments and the same is said of the herb and syrup.

Culinary Use

In 1836, when Napoleon's colonial trade embargo brought a coffee shortage to the European continent, people turned to the cultivated variety of Chicory as a coffee substitute. Europeans grew it as a field crop and made "Chicory coffee" from the thick swollen roots, refining its taste by adding figs. While the beverage was fashionable at the time, its virtue may have derived only from need because, once the embargo was lifted, the consumption of real coffee returned.

Traditionally, Chicory coffee is prepared by cutting the roots into small pieces, which are then brushed with fat and roasted with sugar in tin drums. It is then immediately ground and packaged. To give it a dark color, the powder is exposed to damp air in a cellar for several weeks. You can make your own coffee substitute at home by drying small pieces of Chicory root in the oven and grinding them in a coffee grinder.

In Germany, when I was a child, we asked for "Hound Legs" at the corner pastry shop and got freshly candied Chicory roots. A popular and healthy form of sweets, its name derived from the notion that Chicory grew at the side of the road where dogs walked.

Chicory root has often been a lifesaver for people during times of famine. For a bitter-tasting vegetable substitute, the roots are sliced, soaked in water, and boiled to eliminate their acrid flavor before preparation. They can then be sautéed and served with a white sauce, a lemon-cheese sauce, or yogurt. The pale green leaves also make a fine salad. With its high inulin content, the roots and leaves are beneficial in the diet of diabetics.

Interestingly, Chicory has a sister long established in our vegetable gardens—endive (*Cichorium endivia*), who with a high tannin content retains some of the old healing power. Other cultivated relatives include coffee chicory, French or Belgium endive, iceberg lettuce, and radicchio.

Cosmetics

Applied internally or externally, Chicory is a cleanser. However, to treat impure skin always combine external cleansing with internal ingestion in the form of tea to cleanse the blood. (See the respective plants for this.) To prepare a compress or facial cleanser, put two teaspoons of the root in two cups of water and let it boil for 10 minutes. Then add a few Chicory flowers and let the mixture steep a while before straining it. Place the compress on the face and let it penetrate for 15 minutes. For inflamed skin, add a few Plantain leaves (*Plantago major*) with the Chicory flowers to soothe and disinfect the skin.

Cultivation

Chicory is a hardy, unpretentious plant that is particularly suited for sowing in a meadow. If you plan to harvest the roots, plant them deeply into nutrient-rich soil. If starting seeds (which have the ability to germinate for many years), do so only after all danger of frost, later thinning seedlings to 8 inches apart. In late fall, the roots can be dug up and stored in a cellar. When placed in a box of sand in the spring, they will sprout.

BOTANICAL CHARACTERISTICS

Name: *Cichorium intybus* — Chicory

Distribution: Throughout Europe, North America, northwest Africa, and western Asia

Habitat: Waysides, wasteland, dry soils

Description: Grows 1 to 3 feet tall; stiff, erect, angled stem; leaves deeply pinnately toothed, smaller toward the tip, hairy underneath; bright blue or white flowers, ligulate florets in flower heads. Root is a spindle-shaped taproot with a white milky juice. Flowering time is July to September.

Confusion with similar plants: None—although the young leaves may possibly be confused with Dandelion.

Collecting season:

    Roots – March to April; September to October

    Herb and flowers – July to September

Active ingredients: Bitter compounds, intybin, inulin, sugars, starch, mineral salts, and vitamins

Astrological association: Venus / Mercury

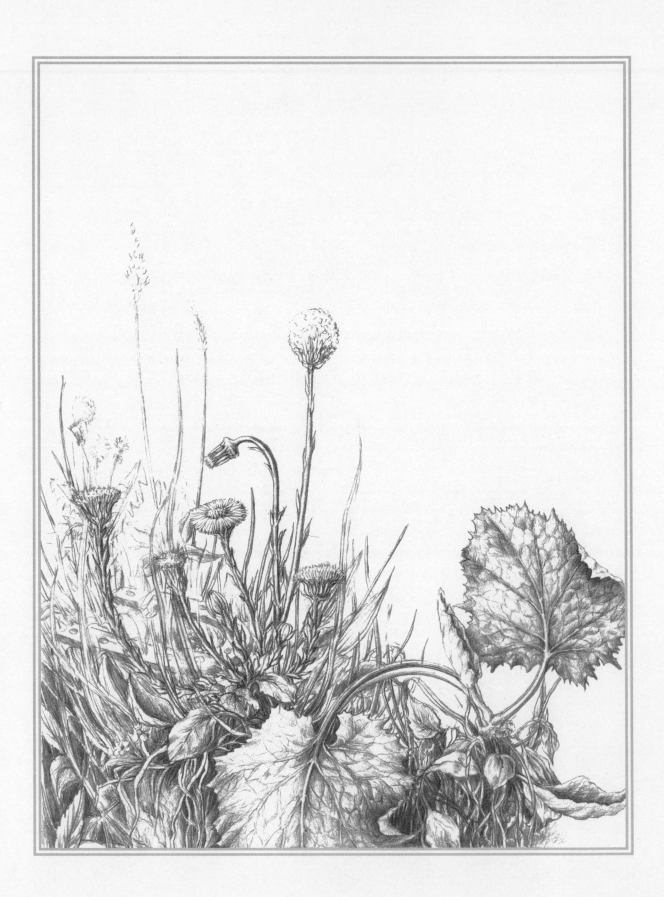

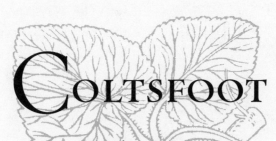

COLTSFOOT

Tussilago farfara

Common Coltsfoot, Coughwort, Foal's Foot, Horse Hoof, Bull's Foot,

British Tobacco, Butterbur, Flower Velure

Daisy family — Compositae / Asteraceae

EARLY ON, when winter gives up only a few patches of earth to the approaching spring, one small plant hurries to push his scaly neck from the soil and show his round yellow flowers. What wayfarer would not pause to acknowledge these cheerful faces! This year I discovered my first Coltsfoot in February and marked the day with a little sun on my calendar. Nevertheless I waited a long time before spring made headway into the mountains of the Allgäu region of the German Alps where I live. Not until late March did I find a cluster of these radiant flowers in a sun-filled quarry.

In rocky, sunny places, Coltsfoot unfolds his flowers in spring. He is one of the "indicator" species—a plant that indicates a particular type of soil. Coltsfoot is an indicator species for clayey, loamy, marly, and calcareous (or alkaline) soil. According to Madaus, Coltsfoot is the only plant that can grow on pure lignite, the brownish black coal that lies between peat and bituminous coal in evolution. Our sunny friend radiates so much light and optimism that he cannot help but succeed in such an environment.

Among plants that prefer alkaline soils are Coltsfoot (*Tussilago farfara*), Forking Larkspur (*Delphinium consolida*), Greater Burdock (*Arctium lappa*), Yellow Sweet Clover (*Melilotus officinalis*), Herb Robert (*Geranium robertianum*), Field Pennycress (*Thlaspi arvense*), and Euphorbia (*Euphorbia exigua*). Their acidic-soil counterparts include Alpine Dock (*Rumex alpinus*), Knotgrass (*Polygonum aviculare*), Common Horsetail (*Equisetum arvense*), Common Speedwell (*Veronica officinalis*), Corn Buttercup (*Ranunculus arvensis*), Common Hempnettle (*Galeopsis tetrahit*), Whortleberry (*Vaccinium myrtillus*), Cottonsedge (*Eriophorum scheuchzeri*), and Lily of the Valley (*Convallaria majalis*).

Just as Stinging Nettle growing in iron-rich soils exhibits a high iron content in its leaves, so Coltsfoot growing in zinc-rich soils absorbs a significant amount of zinc. And, in fact, it is the quantity of different minerals in Coltsfoot that is the source of his specific healing properties. The high content of potassium nitrate (saltpeter) in the ash of the burnt plant is striking. According to Straßer's ash analysis, Coltsfoot ash shows the

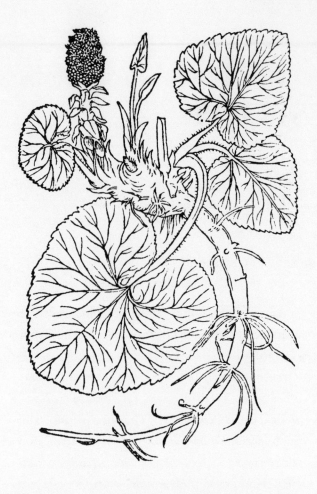

leaves for asthma and bronchitis. He experienced the same results: the mucus membrane of the hard palate became slippery and the expectoration of phlegm stuck in the bronchi was stimulated.

A high content of potassium nitrate has made Coltsfoot one of the best known medicinal plants for cough. Followers of Hippocrates were already using Coltsfoot as a cough remedy, naming it *bechion*. The first and second century A.D. Greek and Roman scholar-physicians Diosurides, Galen, and Pliny recommended the smoke from the burning leaves in cases of cough and difficulty in breathing. Pliny instructed that, for an inveterate cough, one should place Coltsfoot roots on glowing coals of cypress and inhale the resulting smoke through a funnel. Coltsfoot's Latin name, *Tussilago farfara* comes from the Latin *tussis* ("cough") and *agere* ("to expel").

Coltsfoot appears at just the right time of year to heal us from a late-winter cough. These sunny "cough banishers" with their honey-scented flowers crowd together in masses due to a vastly ramified creeping root system. From the basic axis, runners six or seven feet long branch out to hold the small, budding flower heads. In addition, Coltsfoot seeds germinate quickly and easily, the light they need controlled by a special pigment system. Clustered beneath the snow waiting for the liberating sun, the plump red-violet buds with their glistening scales that appear covered by cobwebs will soon open and extend into a flowering carpet six inches high.

The flower heads at the terminal end of the sprout open into beautiful flowers long before the plant's leaves develop. *Filius ante patrem* ("the son before the father") was Coltsfoot's

following composition: 28.23% potassium, 2.36% sodium, 21.10% calcium, 8.48% magnesium, 1.02% iron, 4.44% phosphorus, 26.55% sulfur, and 7.82% silicic acid.

In past times, pharmacies sold so-called "saltpeter paper" (*charta nitrata*), a filter paper saturated with potassium nitrate solution, to people suffering from asthma, bronchitis, or severe cough. They, in turn, would light this paper and inhale its fumes. Saltpeter fumes lower the susceptibility for respiratory spasms and help one cough up mucus by stimulating its excretion by the mucus membranes. The German pharmacologist Hugo Schulz experimented on himself by engaging in the old custom of smoking Coltsfoot

name in the Middle Ages in reference to this peculiarity. Once the small flowers finally lower their faces to the ground, the stems begin to grow and the tired flowers assume new robes, now resembling withered Dandelion flowers with a multitude of small white hairs. Only when the seeds in slow surrender to the wind are carried off to new places does life stir in the leaf buds. Rolled up into a point, the Coltsfoot leaves stretch out toward the light and unfurl at the ends of their stems. Now we see why the plant's German name is "Hoof's Lettuce"—the leaves are shaped like horseshoes. The reference to lettuce comes from *lapatica*, a medieval term indicating large-leafed plants like Burdock or Dock. But in spring they are soft with both sides covered in a thick, white felt (tomentum). Indeed the botanical name *farfara* comes from the Latin word for flour (*farina*). By summer the toothed, horseshoe-shaped leaves stiffen, the hairs on top disappear, and they can grow six inches long and eight inches wide. In late summer the underside darkens.

Butterbur (*Petasites hybridus*), a close relative, has similar leaves which can cause cases of mistaken identity. Like Coltsfoot, Butterbur even forms flowers before leaves. However, while both plants belong to the Daisy family, Butterbur's flowers are totally different. Sitting in a cylindrical cluster, its many flowers range in color from pink to pale violet. The later-forming leaves, like Coltsfoots', have cordate stalks with a serrated edge and whitish wool below (although Butterbur's leaves are not as sharply serrated and appear rounder). But once full grown, there is no doubt who they belong to— the largest in Germany, Butterbur's leaves can

reach a diameter of two feet! Fortunately, confusing Butterbur with Coltsfoot is relatively harmless because neither are poisonous and they enjoy similar medicinal properties.

HEALING PROPERTIES

As mentioned earlier, the cough banisher Coltsfoot is among our best known cough remedies. Like Mullein (*Verbascum thapsiforme*) and Ribwort Plantain (*Plantago lanceolata*), it has long been counted among the traditional antitussives. In teas for chest cold, which are often sold pre-mixed in Germany, each herbal plant addresses a particular aspect with its medicinal properties. Once you know these, you can prepare your own tea blend suited to individual symptoms of respiratory illness. (You will find additional information in the chapter on Mullein).

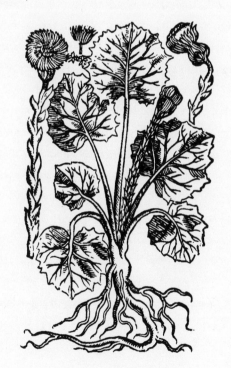

Coltsfoot belongs to the so-called mucilaginosa, "mucous drugs" with an enveloping and moistening effect around the throat opening. Used mostly in the areas of the mucous membranes, they soothe irritated or inflamed mucous membranes by forming a thin protective coat over them. This lowers the feeling of pain, reduces irritation, and promotes faster healing. Other members of this plant group are: Flax (*Linum* spp.), Iceland Moss (*Cetraria islandica*), Common Mallow (*Malva sylvestris*), Marshmallow (*Althaea officinalis*), Corn Poppy (*Papaver rhoeas*), and Licorice (*Glycyrrhiza glabra*).

Besides mucilage, Coltsfoot leaves contain 17% tannins as well as many minerals, a combination that allows mucous membranes to firm and strengthen. In addition, Coltsfoot can dilate the bronchi and loosen stagnation in the most delicate parts of the lungs, aiding the expectoration of viscous catarrh.

Usually, Coltsfoot is administered in cases of spasmodic chronic cough. When taken before breakfast, it helps to dissolve the sticky mucus that accumulates overnight. It is an excellent remedy for cough in older people, although we should not overlook Coltsfoot in the treatment of acute cough and bronchitis. Dr. W. Bohn recommends it even in the beginning stages of pulmonary tuberculosis. He also reports that, as an adjunct therapy, it has helped many patients with silicosis and emphysema.

To prepare Coltsfoot tea, I gather the flowers in March and April and dry them carefully. Later, from April until June, I collect the leaves to dry, crumble, and add to the dried flowers. Herbal teas that do not contain many essential oils—like this one—can be stored in boxes or linen sachets. Antitussive herbs are generally used in mixtures. You can make your own or buy them from your local herb or health food store. I include a few well-proved recipes here.

As with Ribwort Plantain (*Plantago lanceolata*), Coltsfoot leaves can be used in the preparation of "Earth Chamber Syrup," a remedy that is both potent and popular with children. (The recipe is in the chapter on Plantain.) But "flower honey" is another tasty remedy included here for cough, bronchitis, and colds.

Inhaling the smoke of dried Coltsfoot leaves placed on glowing coals is a treatment rarely seen these days. Smoked like tobacco, the dried leaves are crumbled finely and stuffed into a pipe or rolled into cigarettes. To impart a more pleasant flavor, connoisseurs even soak the fresh leaves in honey water or brandy before drying them quickly in the sun or oven. Smoked Coltsfoot has demulcent and antispasmodic properties and covers the mucous membranes with a filmy protective coat. I personally find sipping Coltsfoot tea to be more pleasant . . .

For treating cough or bronchitis, besides drinking tea or syrup made from Coltsfoot or other antitussive herbs, I recommend the inhalation of essential oils. Their properties help to dissolve phlegm and kill bacteria. *Note: Only use pure and natural essential oils. Adulterated or synthetic products can be harmful to the body.*

For inhalations I recommend White Thyme oil (*Thymus vulgaris*), Eucalyptus oil (*Eucalyptus globulus*), Hyssop oil (*Hyssopus decumbens*), and Myrtle oil (*Myrtus communis*). Hyssop oil is effective for treating cough and bronchitis as well as for stimulating mental functions. It is suggested for people who work in occupations requiring mental focus, alertness, and clarity of thought.

To treat cough and bronchitis, add one or several drops of the essential oils to a pot of boiling water. Remove the pot from the burner, carefully cover your head and the pot with a large towel or blanket, and inhale the fumes. The body also absorbs essential oils through the skin. Massaging the chest and back with a liniment containing these essential oils supports the inhalation treatment. We can further strengthen the body with Elderberry juice (*Sambucus* spp.) or Sea Buckthorn juice (*Hippophae ramnoides*).

Another remedial application of Coltsfoot is for scrofula. (Read the chapter on the medicinal properties of Figwort [*Scrophularia nodosa*].) Because scrofula is considered a precursor of tuberculosis, it should be recognized and treated as early as childhood. Even if someone never falls ill with tuberculosis, a scrofulous predisposition can have a negative effect throughout one's lifetime. A scrofulous predisposition can result from other childhood diseases, poor nutrition, lack of sunlight and fresh air, and living in damp quarters. There are two distinct types of scrofulous children: one is skinny, pale, and irritable; the other is large and flabby with a red face. Both types can exhibit characteristics such as difficult teething, swollen glands, cradle cap, skin rashes, chronic rhinitis, and sinusitis. Also, in most cases the mucous membranes are in poor condition—which is why scrofulous children are particularly susceptible to illness. Coltsfoot has long been used as a remedy for scrofula. Today's medical professionals explain that this is because of its high content of minerals and mucilage. For scrofula, especially in children, I recommend a

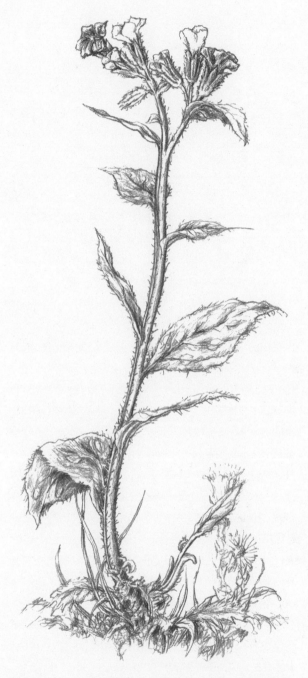

six-week course of treatment with Coltsfoot twice a year. In the spring, administer two tablespoons of freshly pressed or commercially available juice from the leaves daily. In the fall, administer a teaspoon of powder prepared from dried Coltsfoot leaves three times daily.

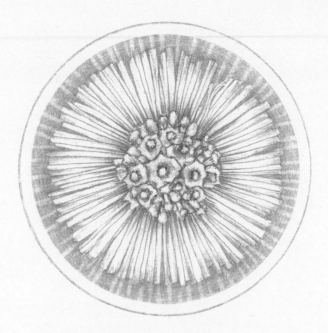

Other plants used for treating scrofula in children are Oak (*Quercus robur*) ingested in the form of acorn coffee; Walnut leaves (*Juglans regia*) added to healing baths; and Beccabunga Speedwell (*Veronica beccabunga*) given in the spring as a freshly pressed juice mixed with an equal part of Coltsfoot juice. Figwort (*Scrophularia nodosa*) is better suited for treating adult cases of scrofula.

Coltsfoot's astringent, disinfecting, and vulnerary qualities make it a good remedy for treating varicose veins and leg ulcers. For a compress (preferably applied overnight), I mash fresh leaves with a rolling pin, place them in two or three layers of cloth, and then wind it tightly around the leg. A more detailed description of treatments of circulatory problems of the legs and leg ulcers is given by Heinrich Pumpe in his pamphlet called *The Twelve Most Important Medicinal Herbs in Their Application in Folk Medicine* (Munich, 1957, in German only).

Coltsfoot is available in herb stores as "Folia Farfarae" (leaves), "Flores Farfarae" (flowers), or "Flores et Folia Farfarae" (flowers and leaves). The homeopathic tincture is made from the fresh leaves.

✌ Coltsfoot Tea

Pour 1 cup of boiling water over 2 teaspoons of coltsfoot tea (dried flowers and leaves). Let it steep and drink sweetened with honey if desired. A daily dose is 3 cups. For viscous mucus, drink a cupful when you first get up in the morning.

✌ "Species Pectorales"

the traditional recipe:

"Rad. Althaeae" conc. gross 16.0
"Rad. Liquiritiae" conc. gross 6.0
"Rhiz. Iridis" conc. gross 2.0
"Fol. Farfarae" conc. gross 8.0
"Flor. Verbasci" conc. gross 4.0
"Fruct. Anisi" cont 4.0

modern equivalents:

marshmallow root, cut (*Althaea officinalis*)
licorice root, cut (*Glycyrrhiza glabra*)
sweet violet root, cut (*Viola odorata*)
coltsfoot leaves, cut (*Tussilago farfara*)
mullein flowers, cut
   (*Verbascum thapsiforme*)
anise, crushed (*Pimpinella anisum*)

A traditional chest cold tea from the German Pharmacopeia followed by a list of the modern equivalents: Pour 2 cups of boiling water over 4 teaspoons of the mixture. Let it steep before drinking.

❧ Tea Blend for Chest Cold

coltsfoot flowers and leaves
    (*Tussilago farfara*)
mullein flowers (*Verbascum thapsiforme*)
linden flowers (*Tilia cordata*)
lungwort herb (*Pulmonaria officinalis*)

Mix the herbs in equal parts and make an infusion by boiling 2 teaspoons in 1 cup of water.

❧ Flower Honey

Tightly pack a large mason jar with an inch and a half of fresh coltsfoot flowers. Pour in enough honey to cover the flowers. Depending on the season, add a layer of any of the following flowers, again topping it off with honey: cowslip (*Primula veris*), sweet violet (*Viola odorata*), corn poppy (*Papaver rhoeas*), or mullein (*Verbascum thapsiforme*). Place the jar on a warm, sunny windowsill to steep for 2 weeks. Squeeze the honey from the flowers and mix in a few drops of essential fennel oil.

Cosmetics

Coltsfoot is tried and true in herbal cosmetics. A high sulfur content gives it antiseptic and cleansing properties that reduce excessive secretion of the sebaceous glands in oily skin and hair. Tannins are astringent, strengthening, and antiseptic. Finally, the mucilage in Coltsfoot protects the skin.

A strong tea from the flowers and leaves can be used as a facial cleanser, compress, or steam bath for the care of blemished, inflamed, oily skin and enlarged pores. Applications of mashed fresh Coltsfoot leaves can also soothe swollen eyes. Furthermore, if you suffer from a flaking scalp or have hair that easily becomes oily, try rinsing your hair after shampooing with a concentrated infusion of Coltsfoot leaves. Between washings, massage the scalp with Coltsfoot tea.

For dandruff, wash your hair with water that has been boiled with a handful of Coltsfoot flowers, then cooled and strained. Prepare a hair rinse from equal amounts of Coltsfoot flowers and Nasturtium (*Tropaeolum majus*).

❧ Coltsfoot Rose Astringent

fresh coltsfoot flowers
grain alcohol (as for a tincture)
rose water

Fill a mason jar halfway with coltsfoot flowers; add alcohol to cover. Let the mixture steep for 3 weeks, strain it, and add an equal amount of rose water. Use the astringent as a facial cleanser for oily skin.

❧ Facial Wash for Blemished Skin

coltsfoot flowers and leaves, fresh or dried
    (*Tussilago farfara*)
fumitory herb
    (*Fumaria officinalis*)

Mix together equal parts of these herbs; reserve. Pour 2 cups of boiling water over a handful of the herbs, let it steep covered for half an hour, and strain the liquid. Use as a facial wash.

CULINARY USE

Young Coltsfoot leaves, gathered from March until June, make a delicious vegetable. They can be steamed by themselves or added to casseroles or soups. (I love Coltsfoot and potatoes!) You can also stuff them like cabbage leaves after boiling them in salted water until they are limp (about five minutes).

For a tasty side dish, chop the leaves (minus their stems) into small pieces and sauté them in an oiled pan over low heat. Serve the greens with soy sauce and roasted sesame seeds or with nutritional yeast flakes and sour cream.

The taste of Coltsfoot flowers is both sweet and tart. I use them in spring to garnish desserts, salads, and cold cuts. I also add them with Sweet Woodruff (*Asperula odorata*) to make a white wine punch. And when simmered in the milk used to make vanilla pudding, the flowers impart a pleasant flavor.

❧ MASHED POTATOES WITH COLTSFOOT

1 pound potatoes
milk
butter
nutmeg, freshly ground
sea salt
1½ cups coltsfoot leaves, cut into strips

Boil the potatoes until soft and mash them with butter, milk, and seasonings to taste. Steam the coltsfoot leaves in a little water and mix them into the mashed potatoes.

❧ COLTSFOOT-POTATO HOT POT

1 pound potatoes, cut in cubes
2 onions, minced
1 cup coltsfoot leaves
light vegetable broth
salt
marjoram
sour cream
parsley

In a well-oiled pan, sauté the onions until soft; add the potatoes. Cut the coltsfoot leaves into strips and stir into the mixture. Add vegetable broth to cover and salt and marjoram to taste; cook until coltsfoot and potatoes are soft. Serve garnished with sour cream and fresh parsley.

CULTIVATION

The modest Coltsfoot is a hardy plant that prefers to grow in sunny places with moist, loamy, calcareous soil. As early as February it delights the world with bright yellow flowers. Later on, as leaves reach their full size, they may cover smaller adjacent plants—a point to consider when planting them. Coltsfoot is available as starter plants or seeds. Sow the latter in spring, later thinning seedlings to eight inches apart. Coltsfoot propagates easily by itself.

BOTANICAL CHARACTERISTICS

Name: Tussilago farfara — Coltsfoot

Distribution: Europe, North Africa, western Asia, and the Americas

Habitat: Stony fields, waysides, wastelands, quarries

Description: In spring whitish, woolly, violet-flowering stems are covered with leaf-like scales; flowers are terminal and golden yellow; leaves do not appear until the end of flowering time, they are basal, long-stalked, angular-cordate with rough indentations and a finely serrated edge, their underside is white-felted.

Confusion with similar plants: Similar to Dandelion flowers, Coltsfoot flowers are smaller and are leafless during flowering time (unlike Dandelion). In spring, Coltsfoot leaves may be confused with Butterbur leaves (although not as conspicuously angular and less deeply indented); later Butterbur leaves grow much larger.

Collecting season:
    Flowers – March to April
    Leaves – April to June

Active ingredients: Mucilage, bitter compounds, tannins, saltpeter, minerals, inulin

Astrological association: Sun / Mercury

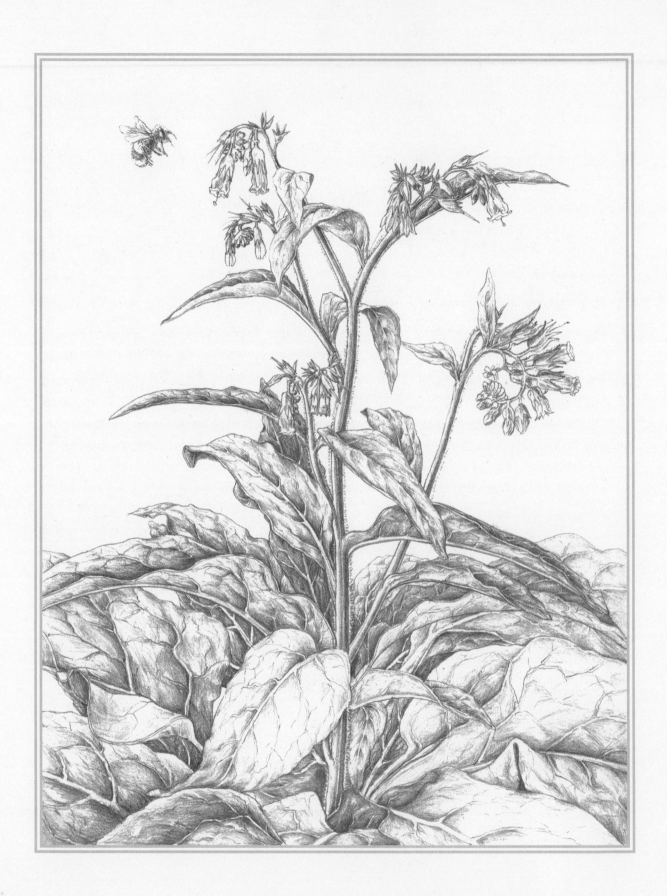

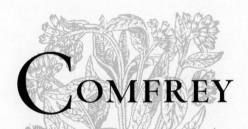

COMFREY

Symphytum officinale
Common Comfrey, Healing Herb, Knitbone, Woundwort,
Blackwort, Bruisewort, Wallwort
Borage family — Boraginaceae

AT THE OUTERMOST CORNER of my garden, I curiously watch the drama of two giants confronting each other. The pumpkin from the nearby compost pile has intruded into the Comfrey field. The Comfrey plants grow close together, their large, fleshy leaves spreading around the high stem as much as possible. They seem to have sucked up all of the soil's vitality in order to grow bigger and bigger. The pumpkin plant, fat and gluttonous, winds through the Comfrey forest like a giant snake, trying to create more space with its enormous umbrella-size leaves.

This little plot of Comfrey might very well be the most productive part of my plantation. It is a living medicine chest that presents me with wheelbarrows full of valuable remedies. I come here often in the summer months to enjoy the pale violet flowers of the Canadian Comfrey. And I am not alone—swarms of bumble-bees enjoy the bell-shaped flowers with their sweet nectar.

To avoid any mix-ups right from the beginning of our acquaintance, let me introduce the different plants in my Comfrey field. In the left-hand corner grows the native, old trusted Common Comfrey. His epithet "officinalis" modestly infers that we are dealing with a medicinal plant of rank and name. He was already being processed long ago in the *officin*, the workshop area of old pharmacies, and listed in the official pharmacopeia. He is an old and revered medicinal plant of stately appearance. Large, lanceolate leaves that appear somewhat plump and crudely fashioned are arranged around a thick, fleshy stem that can reach up to three feet in height. Leaves as well as stem do credit to the Borage family, of which Comfrey is a member, because they are covered with pointed, rough hairs. The leaves are fused to the stem, running down alongside it as if they could not let go.

This was a sign to the old botanists of Comfrey's great determination, a gesture expressing its cohesive power. To the human body, this means that Comfrey can join back together what has come apart. And indeed Comfrey has long been used with great success as a remedy for broken bones and tissue damage. The plant was

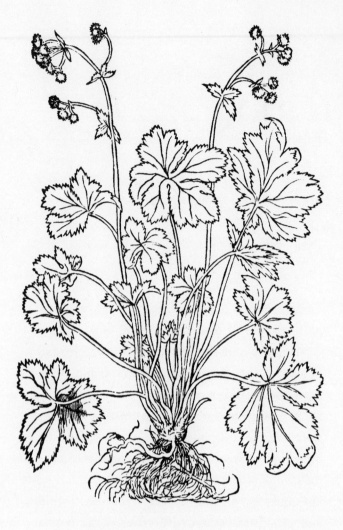

tury herbal that Comfrey's character "is an herb of Saturn and, I suppose, under the sign of Capricorn—cold, dry, and earthy in quality."

Comfrey flowers are either pale yellow or purplish blue. Long ago, plants with purple flowers were called "Comfrey Men" and those with yellow flowers "Comfrey Women." The flowers sit on overhanging terminal stems that are rolled up like spirals.

Further to the right in my garden grows "the wandering Comfrey" (*Symphytum peregrinum*). He is not a European native but comes from distant Siberia and the Ukraine, a hybrid crossbred from *S. officinale* and Caucasian Comfrey (*S. caucasium*). In the second half of the eighteenth century, this wanderer (also known as *S. asperum* or Prickly Comfrey) was brought to England from St. Petersburg by an English gardener in the service of Catherine II. By way of Canada, this species spread to the United States, New Zealand, and Australia. Today he is generally called Canadian Comfrey.

Canadian Comfrey grows taller than Common Comfrey. And with leaves and stems that are hairy but far less bristly, he makes a valuable feed crop. Despite his size, he appears softer and lighter overall. Even the green of Canadian Comfrey's leaves is friendlier, seeming to soften his Saturn nature. Hovering above the weight of his appearance—again on spiraling stems—are pale violet flowers. They, too, appear lighter than those of his smaller brother. The leaves of the European native contain the chemical symphytocynoglossin, which has a mildly paralyzing effect on the central nervous system. While only found in very small quantities, this ingredient produces an analgesic effect when Comfrey leaves are

recognized to bear the sign of the planet Saturn and to stand for the joining, fixing, hardening energies. In truth, when a Comfrey root in the ground has been cut into, it will grow together again—another sign of the plant's joining force. Plants of Saturn often have hard, rough surfaces (Horsetail, for example) and the green of their leaves (like Comfrey's) appears darkened with a tinge of black. Also, plants bearing Saturn's imprint do not open their blossoms to the light— they bend down. Comfrey's flowers, too, open toward the ground. The physician and astrologer Nicholas Culpeper wrote in his seventeenth cen-

applied to wounds. However, Canadian Comfrey lacks this chemical and makes an excellent fodder for domestic animals. The leaves can be harvested up to six times a year and are high in protein, minerals, and vitamins B_{12}, A, and C.

Both Common Comfrey and Canadian Comfrey are sometimes listed under Black Salsify ("Blackroot" in German). However, while the garden species of Black Salsify (*Scorzonera hispanica*) has black roots, it is not a Comfrey species but a member of the Asteraceae family. Common Comfrey and Canadian Comfrey both belong to the Borage family, Boraginaceae, which contains about 20 different Comfrey species. The family takes its name from the beautiful kitchen herb. I always admire this plant's optimism to crown its deformed, prickly, and stubborn self with such lovely deep blue flowers! This personality trait seems to run in the family because the pale violet flowers of Canadian Comfrey are also a contrast to its shapeless leaves.

Contrasts abound among members of the Borage family. Of its 1,600 species, few are familiar to us as medicinal plants although they include Comfrey (*Symphytum officinale*), Lungwort (*Pulmonaria officinalis*), Borage (*Borago officinalis*), Forget-Me-Not (*Myosotis* spp.), Bugloss (*Anchusa officinalis*), and Houndstongue (*Cynoglossum officinale*). They cover the color palette, often blossoming in red and withering in blue. With Comfrey, too, one cannot always tell if the flower is blue or red. Lungwort can even combine both colors, bearing red and blue flowers at the same time. Yin and Yang unite in these plants—the blue heavenly energy and the red earthly energy. The same polar energies are found in Comfrey's healing properties that can join and dissolve at the same time.

This balance play is revealed further by a closer look at another peculiarity of this plant family: All members have a high silicic acid content, a substance that assumes forms from the watery to the solid; in its hardest form, a rock crystal. It lends to plants the ability to absorb water. Comfrey has fleshy, watery leaves with its stem and root full of viscous mucilage. His preferred habitat is wetlands, along the course of a river, or in water-filled ditches. At the same time, the silicic acid—full of life—desires form. For Comfrey plants, this manifests as the innumerable sharp bristles on leaves and stem. In the human body, silicic acid can affect both soft and firm structures. It can have a form-giving, firming effect on soft connective tissue and support growth at the periphery on hair, skin, and nails. Likewise, Comfrey can dissolve swelling and bruises as well as strengthen and stabalize ligaments and tendons.

Allantoin is another substance found in Comfrey. It distinguishes this plant from others containing silicic acid and gives it medicinal properties all its own. Historically, we know that Napoleon's surgeon Larrey treated nasty, purulent wounds with fly maggots, a treatment probably learned from old folk medicine. Over a century later, in World War II, an American named Robinson watched Native American healers treat wounds with fly maggots. He discovered that the maggots contain allantoin, a crystalline oxidation product of uric acid that makes wounds heal faster. Although manufactured synthetically with success, allantoin from Nature was found to produce better results. Two plants that contain this ingredient in large amounts are Comfrey and Sanicle (*Sanicula europea*)—two plants that for centuries have been known to produce a similar effect. Hildegard von Bingen, the twelfth century medieval herbalist, called Comfrey "Consolida" (from the Latin *consolidare*, to join together). The little Sanicle herb, a plant that is all but forgotten, bears a white umbel and grows in wet woodlands and along creeks. And she received the name "Consolida minor."

As we know today, allantoin is also found in the bark of the horse chestnut tree (*Aesculus hippocastanum*), in wheat germ (*Triticum aestivum*), and in the urine of dogs. The allantoin content of Comfrey is especially high, and the combination of diverse medicinal properties gives Comfrey a more far-reaching effect than the isolated active ingredient. Allantoin cleanses wounds by removing destroyed tissue and by stimulating and speeding tissue repair. Combined with the silicic acid and its other elements, this makes Comfrey an especially helpful remedy for wounds with tissue loss. Furthermore, allantoin speeds the healing of fractures by stimulating the formation of callus. Callus is the name for the repair tissue that forms around a broken bone, joining it back together by bridging the gap. In this we find an explanation for the old Comfrey name Wallwort (*wallen*; to join, to grow together). But this does not exhaust the list of Comfrey's important ingredients. The plant also contains large amounts of mucilage and tannins, making him a remedy for stomach and intestinal disorders; especially for treating hyperacidity of the stomach, gastrointestinal inflammations, and ulcers in this area. The allantoin heals; the mucilage protects, calms, and absorbs the acid; and the tannins consolidate the mucous membrane.

Anyone who has processed fresh Comfrey roots—or chewed a piece of it—will recall the viscous mucilage of the plant. In the old days, tanners would extract this mucilage by boiling and using it to make leather soft and pliable. Likewise, weavers and spinners used it to moisten rough fibers like camel hair. Finally, painters brewed an intense red color from it by boiling the mucilage and mixing it with oils, pigments, or shellac.

HEALING PROPERTIES

Our earliest account of Comfrey's miraculous healing power is from the first century A.D. Dioscurides, a famous military physician, praised the plant in his *De Materia Medica Libri*. He and Comfrey were no doubt well acquainted for he probably dealt primarily with wounds, injuries, and fractures. And according to our modern understanding, these are Comfrey's most common applications. Forgotten for a while, Comfrey has experienced a revival. With a jar of Comfrey salve and a box of Comfrey powder in one's home pharmacy, a person is prepared for emergencies too numerous to list here. Once you know Comfrey's main ingredients, you can deduce the medicinal properties for yourself.

The American researcher, Edgar Allen (1892–1943), was well-known especially in the field of pharmacology. He called Comfrey "the Arnica" of bones and periosteum, of tendons, scars, and fibers. Consequently, we can use Comfrey for all conditions of the skeletal system: for injuries to the periosteum and bones, for inflammations of the knee joint, and for fractures. Tendons and ligaments are also healed and fortified by Comfrey. It is helpful for tenovaginitis, sprains, and overstretching. Wound healing is hastened by removing dead tissue and fluid and by stimulating tissue repair. From this, further areas of application can be deduced: wounds, leg ulcers, nail bed infections, ulcers, phlebitis, scar pain, hardened and poorly healing scars, pain after amputation, frostbite, and bruises.

How do we use Comfrey for all these conditions? Experience shows that concurrent internal and external application has the most favorable effect on the healing process. In addition to the external applications described, we can take Comfrey internally in the form of tincture, powder, or tea. For instance, I might prescribe 25 to 30 drops of Comfrey tincture taken three times daily. For Comfrey tea, a patient can brew one cup from leaves or root and drink it three times daily. However, in my experience the strongest effect is obtained from Comfrey powder. To speed the healing of large wounds, leg ulcers, and fractures, and following amputations and surgery, I give one teaspoon of the powder three times daily. People who have a hard time swallowing this sticky powder can moisten it with honey or tea and shape it into small pellets or wafers.

Apply Comfrey salve to wounds, scar pain, phantom pain, nail bed infections, athlete's foot, painful heel, and tenovaginitis. For disorders of the knee joint, bruises, leg ulcers, gout, arthrosis, and phlebitis, make a poultice of Comfrey powder dissolved in hot water. Better still, use fresh

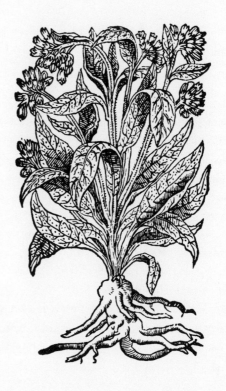

pulp from a crushed root: Dig out the root, clean and crush it, spread it on a cloth, and apply it, letting it take effect overnight when possible. Comfrey powder, ground from the dried root, can be mixed with hot water to form a stiff, viscous mush which can then be spread on a piece of cloth, applied to the affected body area, and again allowed to act overnight.

Comfrey soothes and strengthens the mucous membranes and eases inflammations. It is a good remedy for gastrointestinal conditions such as gastric or duodenal ulcers, enteritis, gastritis, heartburn, and excess gastric acid. For gum disease and periodontitis, rinse or brush with tea brewed from the root or with a tincture mixture of equal parts Comfrey and Tormentil tinctures. (*Important Note: When using Comfrey for internal consumption, as when preparing a powder or tea, only use Canadian Comfrey.*)

The following list compares various herbs used for healing wounds:

- Comfrey (*Symphytum officinale*): Regenerates tissue; heals bruises, especially where bone lies directly under the skin; for bone diseases, slows down the growth of malignant cells; heals dull injuries with tissue loss and old wounds. Use where Arnica is too harsh or causes allergies.

    Comfrey roots are available in herb stores as "Radix Symphyti." The homeopathic mother tincture "Symphytum" is processed from the fresh root.

- Arnica (*Arnica montana*): For injuries from blows, punctures, and cuts; bruises on soft tissue; strengthens arterial and venous vessels; for local application to inflammations from fresh wounds.

- St. John's Wort (*Hypericum perforatum*): For wounds and burns, especially where nerve endings are injured; neuralgias; for fresh frostbite and burns.

- Tormentil (*Potentilla erecta*): A hemostatic and astringent for heavily bleeding wounds.

- Calendula (*Calendula officinalis*): For poorly healing wounds, swellings, and inflammation of the lymph nodes and lymphatic vessels.

- Ground Ivy (*Glecoma hederacea*): For purulent, poorly healing wounds and burns.

- Hemp Agrimony (*Eupatorium cannabinum*): Use externally for poorly healing, infectious wounds; use internally to strengthen resistance.

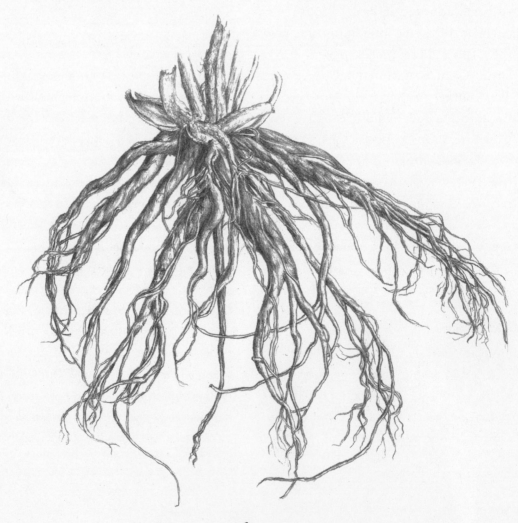

Important Note: Comfrey contains pyrrolizidine alkaloids which as an isolated pure substance can cause cancer. While this has not been proved for complete extracts, Comfrey preparations currently are forbidden in Germany and the United States. My comment is that cancer can be caused by almost any active ingredient isolated from a plant and given as a single substance in megadoses. In other words, it is the dosage that makes it poisonous.

Processing

To prepare salves and other external preparations, we can use the roots of either Common Comfrey or Canadian Comfrey. However, as I noted earlier, only Canadian Comfrey should be used in remedies to be taken internally. Canadian Comfrey contains more allantoin. Allantoin content is highest in early spring and in late fall when the plant's energies withdraw into the root. This is the best time to dig it up. A strong spade is called for because the root is big and bores its way deep into the ground while the upper part branches out. The root bark is dark brown to black, the inside whitish yellow and very slimy. After carefully digging out the root (saving a shoot to re-bury), wash it thoroughly and cut it into small pieces. Spread them on a piece of cloth to dry in the sun. Normally, we do not process medicinal plants this way because they lose valuable ingredients. However, Comfrey root is so rich in mucilage and water that it molds easily if not dried properly. In cloudy weather, spread the pieces on a baking sheet and place it in an unlit gas oven or very low-heat electric oven until dried. Slices of the root can also be hung on a string to dry. Store the dried root in a moisture-proof container with a tight lid.

For Comfrey powder, process the pieces of root with a mortar and pestle or in a coffee or spice grinder (cleaned of any residue). For Comfrey tincture, fill a dark mason jar with finely chopped pieces of fresh root. Top it off with grain spirits or vodka and let the jar sit, tightly lidded, for three weeks before straining. For emergencies one year I even kept a few Comfrey plants growing in a cellar sandbox—and, interestingly, they did well!

℘ Comfrey Tea

  1 teaspoon Canadian comfrey leaves
    (*S. Peregrinum* or *S. asperum*)
  1 cup boiling water

Pour boiling water over 1 heaping teaspoon of Comfrey leaves. Let steep, strain off the liquid, and drink. Three cups is a daily dose.

The leaves of Canadian comfrey contain vitamin B_{12}, allantoin, silicic acid, and protein. They can be used fresh in salads and to make fresh-pressed juice. When drying them, do it carefully because they mold easily. You can mix the dried leaves with other teas to make your own "house blend." Comfrey tea has a supporting effect for all of the previously discussed illnesses.

℘ Comfrey Salve

  1 pound fresh comfrey roots (500 grams)
  2.5 fluid ounces lanolin (70 grams)
  2 cups olive oil, cold-pressed
  0.6 ounce beeswax, grated (20 grams)

Wash and clean the comfrey roots and cut them into small pieces; set aside. Melt the lanolin slowly in a heavy pot over low heat; add the olive oil. Stir in the comfrey roots and heat for about 20 minutes, stirring constantly.

Do not let it boil! Strain the mixture through a cloth, pressing the liquid from the roots; reserve. Melt the beeswax in a double-boiler and stir in the olive oil mixture. Heat slowly until the ingredients are well blended. While it is still warm, fill small salve pots. Stored in a cool place, it will keep for about a year. (Note: For this salve, either Comfrey species can be used.)

✑ "MIRACLE" SALVE

    1 pound fresh comfrey roots (500 grams)
    2.5 fluid ounces lanolin (70 grams)
    1 cup calendula oil
    1 cup arnica or St. John's wort oil
    0.7 ounces beeswax (22 grams)
    2 teaspoons propolis tincture

Prepare the herbal oils from fresh plants. Propolis tincture is available in health food stores. Following the previous procedure for "Comfrey Salve," add the tincture to the mixture before filling the salve pots. This extraordinary salve is especially effective for treating wounds and open leg sores.

✑ SOME TIPS FOR MAKING SALVES

It is said that "cooking salves is a holy task" demanding concentration and devotion. Just as when baking bread, if you are distracted or in a hurry, the end-product will not turn out well. Therefore, take the necessary time. Harvest the plants with gratitude and process them carefully.

To avoid mold, rinse pots, bowls, salve pots, and cooking utensils with boiling water before you begin. Also, avoid metal containers because some ingredients react chemically with metal. It is better to use heat-proof porce-

lain or glass pots and wooden spoons. To fill my salve pots, I use a horn spatula. To weigh small quantities, use a letter scale; for larger amounts, a regular household scale. Strain the warm liquid salve through clean kitchen cloth (like cheesecloth) placed in a strainer. To test the finished salve's consistency, put a drop on a plate to cool and then rub the cooled drop onto your skin. If the salve is too firm, add a little more oil. If it is too soft, add some melted beeswax. Save small containers such as empty cosmetic or spice jars. Finally, store herbal salves in a dry, cool place.

COSMETICS

Comfrey soothes and heals sensitive and inflamed skin. For a mask, smooth fresh-pressed juice from Comfrey leaves over the skin and allow it to penetrate for 15 minutes.

As a massage oil, Comfrey makes a skin-care product that stimulates blood circulation and firms the skin. For stretch marks and scars, massage twice a day with Comfrey salve.

A Comfrey bath is a boon for the whole body. Its earthy smell can be refined by adding sweeter-scented essential oils.

✑ COMFREY MASSAGE OIL

    100 millileters calendula oil
        (3.3 fluid ounces)
    1 tablespoon fresh-pressed juice of
        Canadian comfrey leaves
    5 drops essential oil of rosemary

Mix all ingredients together in a jar with a tight lid; shake it vigorously until mixture is well blended. The oil keeps for about 2 weeks without preservatives and is an excellent massage oil for cellulite and for sagging skin that suffers from poor circulation.

ᚋ A Comfrey Bath

> 2 tablespoons mild herbal shampoo
> 6 tablespoons fresh-pressed juice of
>   Canadian Comfrey leaves
> 20 drops essential oil of your choice

Shake the ingredients vigorously in a jar with a tight lid and add to running bath water.

For an invigorating and refreshing morning bath, add rosemary oil (*Rosmarinus officinalis*) or lemongrass oil (*Cymbopogon citratus*). For a relaxing evening bath, balm (*Melissa officinalis*), Swiss mountain pine (*Pinus mugo*), or lavender (*Lavandula* spp.) make good additions.

For something more luxurious, add a few drops of jasmine oil (*Jasminum* spp.), geranium oil (*Geranium* spp.), or sandalwood oil (*Santalum album*). Men might prefer bergamot oil (*Citrus aurantium* spp. bergamia) or cypress oil (*Cupressus sempervirens*). For an "all natural" bath, eliminate the essential oil.

CULTIVATION

The cultivation of both Comfrey species demands deep soil because of the deep roots. Moist conditions are ideal but not necessary. Space the plants about three feet apart. All species can be planted throughout the year if the ground is open. Comfrey is a perennial plant propagated by root cuttings. Bury the cuttings about two inches deep and soon you will see the

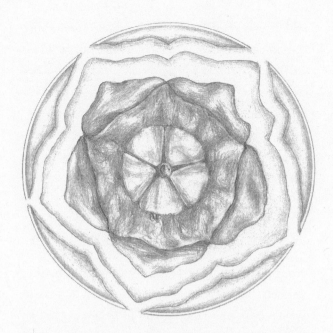

first leaves peer out from the earth. Water the young plants daily if conditions are dry. I fertilize my plants in the fall with compost and rock meal.

Canadian Comfrey leaves can be harvested several times a year. Removing the flower petioles increases leaf growth. After every cutting, Canadian Comfrey will produce new root leaves and Common Comfrey a new stem. Both plants soon form large rhizomes that can be divided for new root cuttings.

Comfrey is rich in minerals making it a valuable green fertilizer and compost plant. It promotes overall plant growth in the garden and enriches the soil. Its high potash content makes it especially suited as a fertilizer for potatoes. To do so, mulch the potato plot in the fall with Comfrey leaves and, when planting potatoes, add some dried leaves to the hole.

Use Comfrey as a liquid fertilizer for vegetables, especially tomatoes. For this purpose, fill a large non-metal container with rainwater and add a few handfuls of the leaves (preferably Canadian Comfrey). Let it ferment for a while and then dilute it for watering your plants. Because it speeds the process of decay, this mixture is also useful for watering your compost pile.

Common and Canadian Comfrey plants are commercially available in gardening centers and nurseries.

Veterinary Medicine

Not unexpectedly, Comfrey is useful for treating animals. In fact, Comfrey salve should appear in any stable's pharmacy to aid in healing wounds, inflammation, sprains, and infected udders. All animals thrive when fresh or dried crushed leaves of Canadian Comfrey are mixed into their fodder. And occasionally mixed into its food, a teaspoon of powder from the dried root or leaves of Canadian Comfrey will give a cat or dog a beautifully shiny coat.

Culinary Use

Young leaves, especially of Canadian Comfrey, make a good vegetable. Steam them like spinach. Or brown the chopped leaves in butter, add some vegetable broth, and sauté them until softened. At the end, stir in a little sour cream, lemon juice, and seasoning.

Or try this: Press several whole leaves together, dip them in pancake batter, and brown them on both sides until cooked through. They taste delicious!

BOTANICAL CHARACTERISTICS

Name: Symphytum officinale — Comfrey

Distribution: Europe to Siberia, Asia, and North America

Habitat: Wet meadows, along riverbanks, forest clearings

Description: Plant grows to 3 feet; large, broad-lanceolate, full leaves with a protruding mid vein, leaf bases extend down along the stem; stems and leaves hairy; whitish yellow or purple flowers, bell-shaped; thick, fleshy root, dark on the outside, whitish yellow inside.

Confusion with similar plants: Possibly with Bugloss (*Anchusa officinalis*) due to similar rough hairy leaves and red or blue-violet flowers; however, flowers are smaller than Comfrey's and are not bell-shaped. Bugloss is not poisonous.

Collecting season:
    Leaves – June to September
    Root – Early spring or late fall

Active ingredients: Allantoin, mucilage, tannins, silicic acid, choline, inulin, symphyto-cynoglossin

Astrological association: Saturn / Neptune

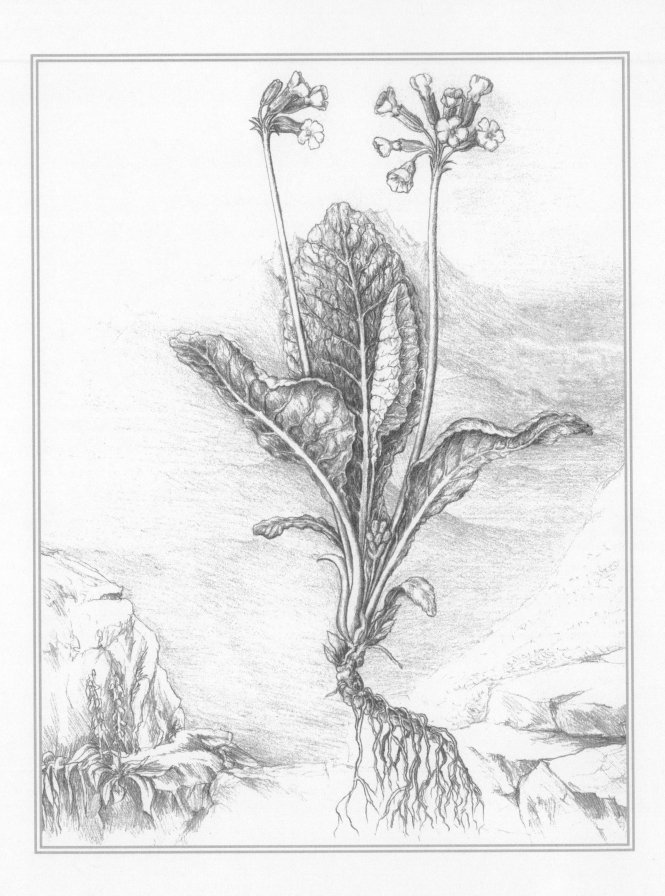

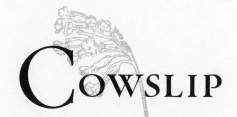

COWSLIP

Primula veris – Cowslip Primrose
Primula elatior – Oxlip Primrose
Oxlip, Peagle, "Heaven's Flower," "Key Flower"
Primrose family — Primulaceae

MORNINGS ARE STILL COLD at my alpine home. Hoarfrost covers the meadows and thick snow blankets the mountains' northern slopes. As winter silently withdraws, we wait expectantly for mottled colors to relieve the stark white. And in my mind's eye, I can see the warm yellow Cowslips that I discovered yesterday in a sunny glade.

A special magic seems to surround all spring flowers. Perhaps it is because, with their tender colors, they fill our hearts with joy and inspiration and let us forget winter's heaviness. Sky blue Hepaticas (or Noble Liverworts), sunny Coltsfoots, and dainty yellow Cowslips open up the colorful flower palette for the coming year. Some early plants, like Ramsons and Stinging Nettle, cleanse the body of waste products accumulated over the winter. But spring's fairy godmother also sends harbingers to cleanse our mind and spirit and to free us from gloom—and Cowslip is one.

The ancient Druids recognized Cowslip's soul energy. They combined her juice with that of five other plants to brew a honeyed "potion of enthusiasm" which was blessed by nine priestesses exhaling into it. This potion was said to capture all the inspiring and invigorating power of Cowslip. Long after these times, her potency was still known. Hildegard von Bingen, the twelfth century abbess whose writings preserve much pre-Christian wisdom, writes in her *Physica*:

> The "Heaven's Key" (a German name for Cowslip) is warm and gets all its power from the sun. In instances of melancholia and delusions, one should tie the plant over the heart.

For as long as can be remembered, Cowslip has been connected to female powers. Claimed by Venus and the Sun, she is tender with a sweet fragrance bathed in soft yellow hues. Freya was Cowslip's early patron. In her crown the Germanic Earth Goddess tucked a small key with which she could unlock the human heart. Eventually Cowslip was dedicated to Mary and given the name "Mary's Key to Heaven" with which followers believed she could open the celestial gates.

The powers attributed to the Cowslip that grew in Freya's magic garden were the stuff of legends. Originally, the goddess with her golden key—a symbol of the plant—could open and

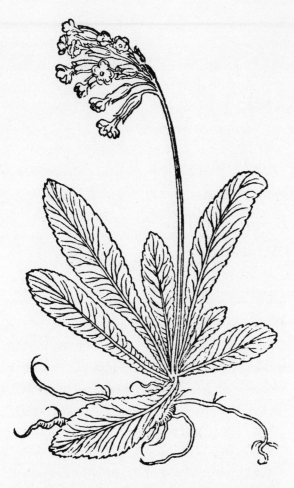

ize the life hidden within the earth that now would burst forth again. Round loaves of bread, symbols of the sun, were likewise blessed and eaten. Burning wheels were rolled down mountain slopes to symbolize the radiant solar path through the dark night of dying winter. Finally, Ostara's altars were decorated with her favored flowers, the Cowslip.

The joy I feel at the sight of my first Cowslip is part of the now forgotten sun festivals living on. Perhaps the magic laying over these spring flowers is a remnant of the veil of the old Sun Goddess—Ostara, who today we might call "Easter."

THE LAND OF COWSLIPS

Oh, the meadows! See the meadows!
See the meadows become green
and the yellow Cowslips flower again!

The pond glows black, still, clear and
the pasture stands with fluttering hair.
In the sky, blissful and quiet, sails on
its fast journey—a white flock of clouds.

Between buds in the Elder branches
sings a warbler. Wandering
on wet rises young lads, hats in hand.
And through girlish pigtails are
woven many a red and blue band.

Clouds pass, and the girls' dresses
are blowing, casting shadows
across the land of Cowslips.

Georg Britting

ready the human heart for the new year. Freya could also unlock Mother Earth and awaken the sleeping forces of Nature. Later tales had fairies and wood nymphs possessing a key that opened secret doors to vast treasures. Although warned by a fairy godmother not to leave it behind, many a shepherd did just that in his rush for the gold. And fret all he wanted, the door remained closed to him forever—the magic Cowslip key resting inside the treasure chamber.

As a sun-flower of spring, Cowslip is an integral part of one particular pre-Christian festival. Each year the eastern-rising sun was celebrated in the form of the Goddess Ostara (or Eostre) who symbolized the reawakening life-giving energy of the sun. Eggs were blessed to symbol-

HEALING PROPERTIES

The essential oils that give Cowslip its pleasant scent can soothe the mind and nerves. In fact, a tea from Cowslip flowers often alleviates a tension headache and defeats insomnia. In the recipe section is a sleep tea blend that I find particularly helpful.

A high content of saponins, mostly present in the root and calyx (not in the corolla), gives Cowslip demulcent and expectorant qualities. This makes it a good cough remedy especially when phlegm is present. Cowslip flowers with the calyx removed are used to treat migraines and kidney and bladder conditions. With the calyx, they are used as a demulcent and expectorant tea for cough and bronchitis.

Cowslip addresses other winter ailments as well. For example, when uric acid accumulates in the body, many people develop painful rheumatism and gout. In such cases Cowslip taken as a tea can influence the metabolism and flush out these waste products. (See the recipe for Uric Acid Tea.)

For rheumatic pains, nerve pain, and weak muscles, I recommend rubbing the affected areas with Cowslip oil. To make your own: fill a mason jar with fresh Cowslip flowers, pour cold-pressed Sunflower oil over them, and place the jar in the sun for two or three weeks. Strain the oil into a dark bottle.

In the past, Cowslip's soothing properties were used to cleanse and invigorate the mucous membranes of nose and sinuses. Ancient physicians had their patients sniff the finely ground powder or freshly pressed juice from the root. The juice in particular promotes vigorous sneezing, thereby stimulating the mucous membranes.

It is beneficial for chronic rhinitis and nasal stuffiness. For this purpose I put the finely chopped root through a garlic press and strain the juice through a cloth. Just sniffing a few drops is sufficient.

Cowslip roots have long been used in remedies and, due to their decimation, enjoy protected status in Germany. As always, check with your local library, park authorities, or nature societies before digging up roots or picking herbs in the wild. I recommend that you use only cultivated roots.

Our little spring-flowering plant is available from herb or health food stores in several forms: "Radix Primulae" (Cowslip root), "Flores Primulae cum Calycibus" (Cowslip flowers with calyx), and "Flores Primulae sine Calycibus" (Cowslip flowers without calyx). The homeopathic mother tincture "Primula veris" is prepared from the fresh flowering plant.

Note: Cowslip causes allergic reactions in some people so be sure to ascertain this before using it on yourself or others.

✂ COWSLIP TEA

2 teaspoons dried cowslip flowers
1 cup boiling water

Steep the cowslip flowers and boiling water for 5 minutes. Drink a few cups as needed, sweetened with honey. This tea is calming and promotes sleep, making it a remedial nightcap for those who toss and turn in bed.

A Sleep Tea

2 parts cowslip flowers (*Primula veris*)

2 parts hops fruits (*Humulus lupulus*)

1 part St. John's wort herb

(*Hypericum perforatum*)

1 part balm herb (*Melissa officinalis*)

This is a favorite sleep tea blend of mine. Keep the mixture on hand to prepare as you do the simple cowslip tea in the previous recipe.

A Sleep Pillow for Headaches and Insomnia

1 part cowslip flowers (*Primula veris*)

1 part lavender flowers (*Lavandula* spp.)

5 parts hops fruits (*Humulus lupulus*)

The effect of a sleep tea is enhanced by using a scented herbal pillow because the plants work all night. As we inhale, their fragrance acts directly on our brains and simultaneously through our lungs on the circulatory system to make a deep and gentle remedy. I make my pillows from beautiful mid-weight fabrics colored with natural dyes. They should measure at least 12 inches square and be stuffed with well-dried flowers.

Cough Tea

cowslip (*Primula veris*)

coltsfoot flowers (*Tussilago farfara*)

lungwort (*Pulmonaria officinalis*)

Nature presents us with spring flowers that make an especially potent cough mixture that also strengthens the lungs. Prepare this tea using equal amounts of the herbs.

Uric Acid Tea

1 part cowslip flowers (*Primula veris*)

1 part stinging nettle

(*Urtica dioica* / *U. urens*)

2 parts birch leaves (*Betula pendula*)

2 parts meadowsweet

(*Filipendula ulmaria*)

Pour 1 cup of boiling water over 2 teaspoons of the tea mixture. Let it steep for 5 minutes. Drink 3 cups daily.

Massage Oil

50 milliliters cowslip oil

(about 2 fluid ounces *Primula veris*)

50 milliliters St. John's wort oil

(*Hypericum perforatum*)

8 drops essential oil of mastic thyme

(*Thymus masticiana*)

3 drops essential oil of angelica

(*Angelica archangelica*)

10 drops essential oil of lavender

(*Lavandula* spp.)

In a jar with a tight lid, combine the ingredients and shake them vigorously until well mixed. Pour them into a dark bottle and store it in a cool place. (Use only pure natural oils.)

This oil blend is an excellent liniment rub for neuralgias and muscle weakness.

Winter Tea

30 grams aspen buds

("Gemmae Populi," *Populus tremula*)

20 grams cowslip flowers

("Flores Primulae," *Primula veris*)
20 grams blue mallow flowers
("Flores Malvae," *Malva sylvestris*)
10 grams linden flowers
("Flores Tiliae," *Tilia cordata*)
10 grams sweet woodruff
("Herba Asperulae," *Asperula odorata*)

This winter tea can lighten spirits during the coldest part of the year!

Make an herbal mixture of the ingredients listed. Add 1 teaspoon of the tea blend to cold water and bring it to a boil. Let it bubble briefly and then allow it to steep for 5 minutes. Strain it into a cup and drink the tea sweetened with honey.

Culinary Use

Cowslip has quite a few culinary uses. The young leaves can be added to salads, soups, and raw vegetable plates. The root was once used to improve beer. I even make my own liqueur from the sweet-flavored flowers using pear brandy, honey, peppermint, and vanilla. I also prepare a thick and delicious semolina gruel flavored with saffron and garnished with fresh Cowslip flowers.

With its good flavor and healthful properties, Cowslip wine has been popular for centuries. In his 1731 herbal, Tabernaemontanus recommends it for "gout, a stupid head, and clogged nerves." We also find that in 1698 and 1699 the ducal court chamber of Mecklenburg ordered the Neustadt office "to have a quantity of the so-called Cowslips delivered on behalf of the cupbearer of our court wine."

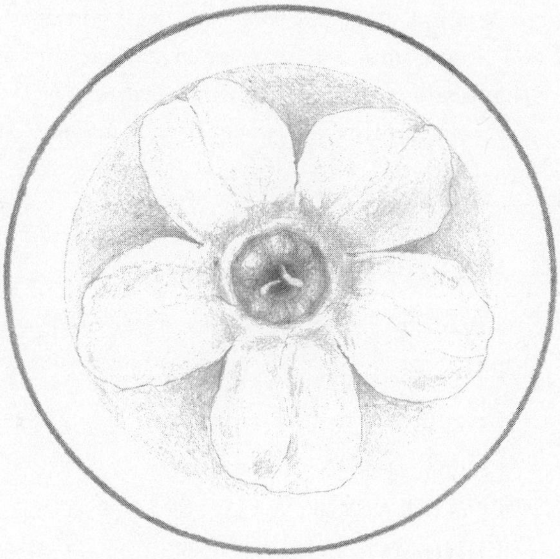

Cowslip Wine

1½ pounds unsulfured raisins
2 vanilla beans
1 gallon cold water
2 pounds sugar (or honey)
5 cups fresh cowslip flowers
1 small bottle of liquid yeast used to make wine (for white wine, use sweet)
1/10 ounce tartaric acid
1 package of baker's yeast

Add raisins and vanilla to cold water, bring it to a boil, and let it bubble for 15 minutes. Carefully strain the hot juice into a clean pot, add the sugar, and stir until it dissolves. Mix in the cowslip flowers, cover the pot, and let it steep for several hours. Strain the juice again. Mix the liquid yeast, tartaric acid, and baker's yeast into a small amount of the juice until it dissolves; stir this back into the pot. Pour this mixture into a glass carboy and attach a cork with a fermenting tube or airlock. Let it ferment for 4 to 6 weeks in a place with an even temperature. Pour the wine into dark bottles and let it continue to ferment in a cellar for 3 months or longer. (For further instructions on making wine, call your local wine-making store.)

℘ Sweet Cowslip Cream

> 1 vanilla bean
> 2 cups dried cowslip flowers
> 1 pint milk
> 1 ounce cornstarch
> a pinch of saffron
> 3 teaspoons honey (or to taste)

Slice the vanilla bean open and add it to the cowslip flowers and milk. Slowly bring this to a boil, stirring constantly. Transfer it to a bowl, cover it, and let it cool before straining the mixture through a cloth. (Remember to squeeze the flowers to remove their full essence.) Dissolve the cornstarch into a small amount of cooled milk; reserve. Dissolve the saffron in a teaspoon of boiling water; reserve. Slowly reheat the remaining milk, adding the saffron and cornstarch. Simmer the mixture, stirring constantly, until it thickens; add the honey. Pour the cream into individual dessert dishes or a large glass bowl; chill. Serve garnished with whipped cream, slivered almonds, and cowslip flowers.

CULTIVATION

Both *Primula elatior* and *P. veris* species are available as seeds as well as starter plants. The modest Cowslip thrives well in the dense soil of rock gardens or wild gardens to delight us as early as April with her beautiful yellow blooms. Decorative varieties in other colors are available.

Because the numerous primrose species are especially susceptible to mildew, water them occasionally with a liquid manure or tea made from Horsetail (*Equisetum arvense*). Fresh manure or dung, however, increases Cowslip's susceptibility to bacterial diseases.

BOTANICAL CHARACTERISTICS

Name: *Primula veris, P. elatior* — Cowslip

Distribution: Temperate zones in Europe, Asia, the Americas

Habitat: Meadows, deciduous forests, wet locations especially on calcareous and basaltic soils

Description: Both species share certain characteristics: leaves are strongly wrinkled, hairy, and arranged in a rosette; hairy flower stalks and flowers condensed in a nodding terminal umbel. Distinguishing traits: *Primula veris* has strongly scented flowers ranging in hue from deep yolk yellow to orange; they have a bulging, green calyx; flower stalks grow 4 to 8 inches tall; earlier blooming (March to April). *P. elatior* has pale yellow, subtle scented flowers with a slender, green calyx; flower stalks can reach 12 inches; later blooming (April to May).

Confusion with similar plants: None

Collecting season for flowers: March to May

Active ingredients: Saponins, essential oils, vitamin C, bitter compounds

Astrological association: Sun / Venus

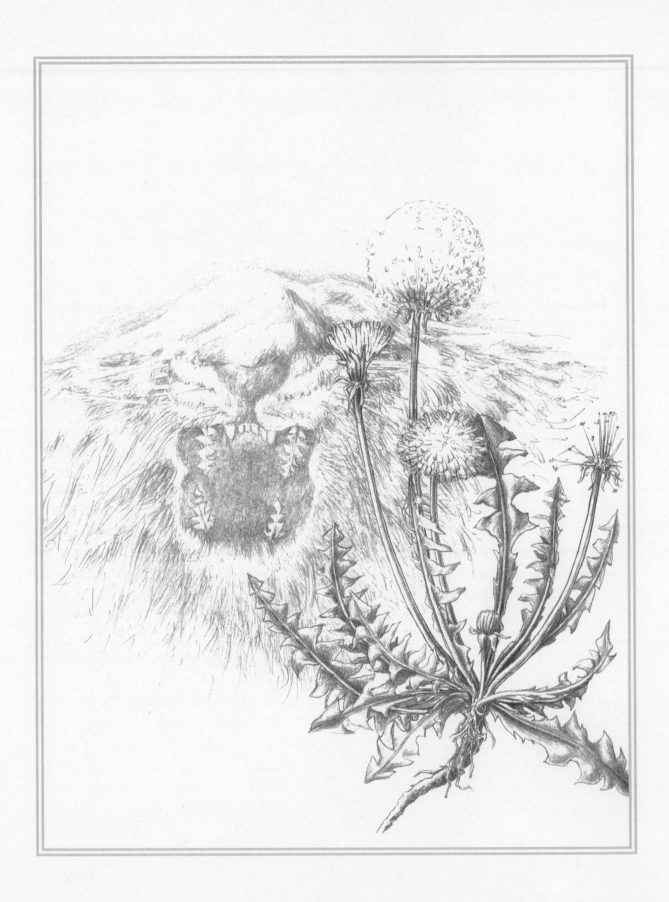

DANDELION

Taraxacum officinale

Piss-a-beds, Blowball, Cankerwort, Lion's Teeth, Priest's Crown, Puffball,
Swine Snout, White Endive, Wild Endive

Daisy family — Compositae / Asteraceae

WHEN MAY TRANSFORMS THE MEADOWS into golden Dandelion carpets, it is as if the Sun herself had fallen to Earth. Thousands upon thousands of flowers open to the light, alerting everyone to the promise of approaching summer.

But would anybody decorate a May birthday table with a Dandelion bouquet? As pretty as the yellow flowers may look from afar, we still consider them to be "weeds"—ones that occur en masse. Somehow this plant strikes us as primitive and common. Yet, despite this, from early childhood we take it to our hearts. Already deep into the contradictory character of Dandelion, maybe we cannot fully recognize the character of this plant. All Dandelion plants look alike to us—a "bulk weed." However, we are quickly convinced otherwise once we inspect a Dandelion meadow more closely. Indeed, no two leaves of this plant are alike! Each has its own teeth, indentations, and size, his shape revealing a very sensible reaction to the surrounding condition of soil, locale, climate, light, shade, and probably other factors as well. This sensitive

changeability contrasts with his common but showy vitality.

I have discovered Dandelion plants in wet, shady locations with leaves I could not initially identify because they were so lacking in indentations. And further up the mountains in rocky soils, I have stumbled upon Dandelions with pointy leaves incised so deeply that they truly lived up to their vernacular name of "Lion's Teeth."

And there are more contradictions: Above the simple, hollow, crude tube-like stem sits a most bright sun-flower. Would we be more inclined to place Dandelions into a vase were their stems more graceful? Although the flower is a pretty yellow, its smell is not as pleasant as we might expect in a spring bouquet. But observe the sensitivity of these flowers: They vibrate with the rhythm of the day, opening in the morning sun and closing in the afternoon or during a rainstorm. In bad weather, they prefer staying closed rather than opening up and not finding the sun. Finally, even the so-called crude stem pays attention to the neighboring plants, adjusting his height to theirs.

In maturity, the calyx closes around the flower and the stem becomes longer, bends, and lets the entire flower head hang sadly to the ground. This is when it appears as if all the Dandelions have disappeared from the meadow, their yellow beacons extinguished—and it becomes Beak Chervil's turn to paint the meadow white. When the Dandelion fruits ripen, the little head lifts itself again and opens like a grab bag to the most incredible plant creation we know. This common weed magically creates incredibly fragile spheres composed of delicate, pale silvery stars. They sit with their dark fruits atop a convex, white flower receptable waiting to release their delicate shapes to the Wind to carry over the meadows in a snow-like mist.

Dandelion contains much that is beneficial to our bodies: bitter compounds, choline, inulin, large quantities of minerals such as calcium, sodium, silicic acid, sulfur—and, in the fresh leaves, a high content of potassium. The bitter compounds stimulate the appetite and promote digestion. Choline affects the gallbladder and the intestines, often stimulating the mucous membranes of the large intestine in a laxative effect. It also has a relationship to the liver's lipid metabolism. Our daily requirement of choline is 2 to 3 grams (0.07 to 0.1 ounce) and a lack of it increases fatty degeneration of the liver. Dandelion can promote bile production in the liver and its secretion from the liver. Bile flowing from the gallbladder into the intestines aids the breakdown of lipids in food and prepare it for assimilation into the organism. Insufficient bile causes abnormal digestion. Medicinally, Dandelion is an effective remedy for all liver and gallbladder diseases.

In this herb we encounter another of Nature's rhythms. Dandelion roots are the main storage site of inulin, the tasteless white polysaccharide that can have a beneficial influence on carbohydrate metabolism—especially that of sugar. With only a 2% presence in spring, by fall the chemical composition of the roots will be 40% inulin! This makes Dandelion a potent dietary and medicinal plant for diabetics.

Dandelion also can stimulate our kidneys to excrete urinary waste products from the body. This diuretic effect can help in cases of chronic rheumatism and arthritis.

It would be unjust not to mention children in this chapter on Dandelion—he is, after all, one of their favorite flowers. Without a doubt, he is the first flower that we perceive consciously. As adults we have nearly forgotten the many uses we found for Dandelions: water pipes, whistles, trumpets, braided necklaces, even coils of little snakes that curl and twist when their stems are cut lengthwise and put in water. And blowing the many little parachute seeds from their stems in a single breath—who can forget? Lastly, do you remember the white milk that would drip on your hands? Well, this Dandelion "milk" contains a white latex that is particularly evident in the root and wall of the hollow stem. Children who suck on the stems can show mild symptoms of poisoning such as nausea, vomiting, diarrhea, and heart disorders.

HEALING PROPERTIES

Due to its large and well-balanced quantity of medicinal ingredients, Dandelion has a comprehensive effect on our bodies. Its blood-cleansing

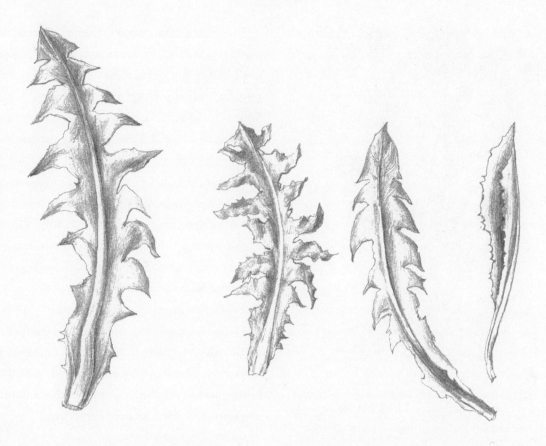

property is especially valuable in spring when it invigorates the body, improves digestive function, and stimulates the liver, gallbladder, kidneys, and bladder.

Eat salads of Dandelion in the spring when its leaves contain a large quantity of vitamin C. A four-week course of treatment with freshly pressed juice from leaves, flowers, and roots is most effective. Two or three tablespoons a day diluted with water are sufficient. Dandelion juice is also a good supplemental tonic and diuretic to use during a cleansing fast or weight-loss program.

The main target organs of Dandelion are the liver and gallbladder. It has long been used as a remedy for liver and gallbladder dysfunction, such as liver stasis, hepatitis, stagnation,

swellings, and inflammatory processes in the gallbladder, including relief from gallstones. For these illnesses, a spring treatment with the fresh juice is highly recommended. *Caution: Do not use Dandelion in cases of blocked bile ducts, intestinal obstruction, or the accumulation of pus in the gallbladder.*

Dandelion tea can be used throughout the year and you can easily make your own mixture. To benefit from the plant's entire palette of active ingredients, use leaves, flowers, and roots. Gather the leaves and flowers in the spring, carefully drying them and cutting them into small pieces. Dig up the root, clean it, cut it lengthwise, string it, and hang it to dry in a protected but airy place. Later, cut the dried root into small pieces and add them to the dried leaves and

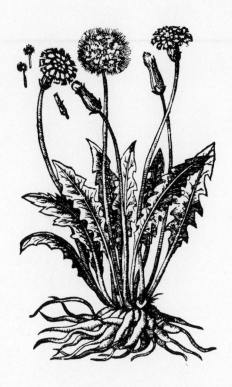

flowers. Pour boiling water over two teaspoons of this mixture, steep it, then strain it. For a course of treatment, drink three unsweetened cups daily for four to six weeks. Then stop for four weeks.

Tea made from the pure root has an even stronger effect. Spring is when the root contains the most bitter compounds; fall is when it has the most inulin. For Dandelion root tea, steep one heaping teaspoon in one cup of boiling water. As always, to gain full benefit from the bitter compounds, bitter teas like this one should not be sweetened. They have a special stomachic function and stimulate the appetite. Dandelion has such all-encompassing effects that I prefer using it as a single-herb tea. However, I also prescribe herbal blends for particular conditions. For example, I might recommend the use of a certain herbal blend for liver disease along with a pure Dandelion tea.

Some archaic names for Dandelion refer without ambiguity to his next area of application—the old English name "Piss-a-beds," the French *pisenlit*, and the German "Bed-wetter." Dandelion stimulates the kidneys and bladder and acts as a diuretic for dropsy and bladder problems. Earlier I mentioned its suitability for flushing out waste products and cleansing in rheumatic and arthritic conditions. It is especially indicated in liver diseases combined with water retention.

With its inulin content, Dandelion is good dietary fare for diabetics. Eaten as a salad, tea, or root vegetable (especially using roots dug up in the fall), it stimulates the pancreas.

Dandelion tea prepared from roots, leaves, and flowers is available in herb or natural food stores as "Radix Taraxaci cum Herba." The homeopathic mother tincture "Taraxacum" is prepared from the whole fresh plant.

CULTIVATION

We all know that Dandelions grow everywhere. However, they thrive best in deep, humus-rich soil. Available commercially, seeds can be sown in the spring or fall. Later, thin the seedlings to a distance of four inches apart and, before they mature, cut off the seed heads—otherwise your garden plot will be covered with bright yellow flowers next year!

Note: If you cover the plants with cardboard or straw, the leaves will blanch out and taste like Chicory. To have healthy and delicious Dandelion salads throughout the winter, dig up the roots in the fall and transplant them to a small box of sand. Cover the box with paper, keep it in a cool place, and the roots will sprout.

VETERINARY MEDICINE

Dandelion has long been known as a good fodder for rabbits. However, other animals will also benefit from Dandelion administered as a general tonic. Like Stinging Nettle, it is suitable for poultry. And if you occasionally mix finely chopped Dandelion leaves and roots into their food, your dogs and cats will stay healthy and have a beautiful coat.

CULINARY USE

Dandelion's culinary uses are legendary. And I bet you will be tempted to try some of the recipes included here. As a vegetable, they are commonly served in the spring using the entire plant—leaves, flowers, buds, and roots. The tender young leaves taste wonderful in a salad. But once they flower, they turn bitter. The bitterness can be removed, however, by soaking them in water for two hours before their preparation.

℘ DANDELION SALAD

Cut the tender young leaves in crosswise strips like endive. Rub a stoneware bowl with a peeled garlic clove and place the salad greens in it to marinate covered for 30 minutes. Meanwhile prepare a dressing of oil, vinegar, mustard, sour cream, and herbs of Provence; dress the salad. Cut smoked meat into small cubes and sauté them lightly before tossing with the salad.

You can have Dandelion salad in the winter by digging up the roots in the fall, planting them in boxes of sandy soil, covering them with paper, and allowing them to sprout in a cool place.

℘ BUTTERY DANDELION BUDS

Gather the small flower buds in spring. Drop them into boiling water and cook them quickly. When they are tender, drain them well before sautéing them in a little butter. Serve at once with salt, pepper, fresh parsley, and lemon juice to taste.

℘ STEWED DANDELION ROOTS

Dig up the roots, clean them carefully, and cut them into small pieces; sauté them in butter. Add a little vegetable broth, soy sauce, and a chopped clove of garlic and simmer until cooked through. Season with gomasio (a sea salt and roasted sesame seed condiment available at your health food store) and sour cream. This is delicious served with venison or grain dishes.

℘ DANDELION ROOT COFFEE

Dandelion roots make a healthy coffee substitute. Dig up the roots in early spring or in late fall. Wash them carefully, cut them into small pieces, and lay them out to dry. When well dried, slowly roast them on a baking sheet in the oven, stirring often so that they cook evenly. Store the roots in an airtight container and grind them as you do coffee beans before use. To prepare: quickly boil 1 teaspoon powdered root in 1 cup water. (Steeping it too long makes it bitter.)

℘ DANDELION FLOWER HONEY

6 handfuls fresh dandelion flowers
   (*Taraxacum officinale*)
1 handful dried meadowsweet flowers
   ("Flores Filipendulae,"
   Filipendula ulmaria)

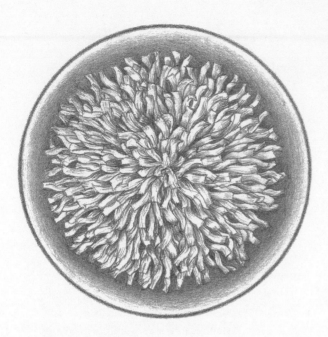

water to make 6½ gallons, bring it to a boil, and stir in the sugar until it dissolves. Add the lemon and orange juices, fermenting yeast, and nutrient salt tablets. Pour into a glass fermenting jar fitted with an air-lock. Let the mixture ferment for 4 to 6 weeks before siphoning it into clean bottles. Store the wine in a cellar for several months before drinking.

(Steinberg is a type of wine as well as the name of a supplier of wine-making ingredients. This recipe calls for a yeast used in making white Reisling-style wine—that is, sweet and fruity.)

2 quarts water

4 pounds granulated sugar

juice of 2 lemons

Soak the flowers together in cold water in a covered pot for 2 hours. Bring the mixture to a boil and let it bubble for 15 minutes while stirring. Strain the liquid, pressing the flowers well to capture their essence. Return the liquid to the pot, add the sugar and lemon juice, and cook until the sugar forms threads. Pour into jars.

❧ ENGLISH-STYLE DANDELION WINE

9 pounds dandelion flowers

16 pounds granulated sugar

juice of 2 lemons

juice of 2 oranges

fermenting yeast "Steinberg"

4 nutrient salt tablets

Cover the dandelion flowers with boiling water; let it steep for 1 day. Strain and add

Botanical Characteristics

Name: *Taraxacum officinale* — Dandelion

Distribution: All temperate zones

Habitat: Meadows and waysides

Description: Leaves in a basal rosette, and depending on the habitat, more or less deeply serrated; stem about 4 to 12 inches tall, round, hollow, and smooth; yellow ligulate flowers in a large solitary head; a "blowball" of many rays is formed when seeds mature.

Confusion with similar plants: None in the spring because similar-looking plants do not have white latex. Confused in the fall with the nonpoisonous Fall Hawkbit (*Leontodon autumnalis*), whose stem is not hollow.

Collecting season:

    Leaves and flowers – Spring
    Root – Spring or August to October

Active ingredients: Bitter compounds, choline, about 18% sugar in spring, inulin (in spring 2%, in fall 40%), flavonoids, vitamins, minerals

Astrological association: Jupiter / Mars

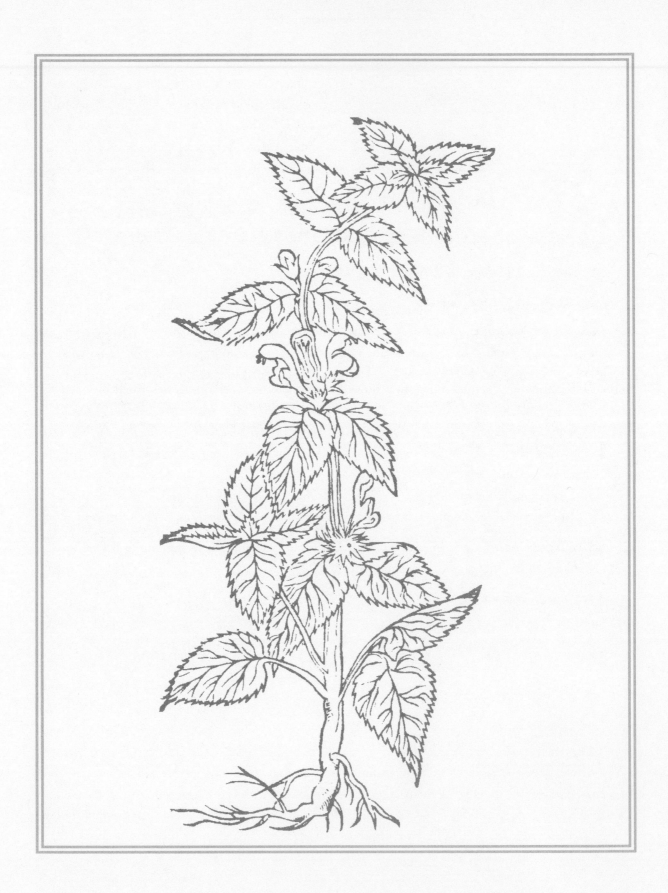

DEAD NETTLE

Lamium album

White Dead Nettle, Archangel, Blind Nettle, Stingless Nettle, White Nettle

Mint family — Labiatae / Lamiaceae

THOSE WHO DO NOT LOOK CLOSELY, especially in spring, could confuse White Dead Nettle with Stinging Nettle—but only those without an eye for the different personalities exhibited by these plants. Stinging Nettle, for instance, focuses on developing her leaves and filling them with Fire energy. Always ready for the attack, she craves places that are dry and warm.

In contrast, Dead Nettle's element is closer to Water—viscous, gentle, cooling. While her nettle-like leaves stand crosswise-opposite on a square stem, they are covered with a light fluff and not with Stinging Nettle's painfully aggressive hairs. The leaves, cool and soft to the touch, even have a scent. A member of the Mint or Labiatae family (*labium* is Latin for "lip"), Dead Nettle has lovely, white "lip-flowers" that perch atop her leaves, usually blooming in groups of three to seven from the leaf axils of the upper leaves. They appear to grow in a whorl around the stem. (The botanical term for this is "apparent whorl.")

The ancients considered Stinging Nettle to be the male counterpart to Dead Nettle's feminine nature. According to the Doctrine of Signatures, a system of superstitions described by Nicholas Culpeper in his seventeenth century herbal, a plant's medicinal use was determined by some element of its appearance. Dead Nettle's signature, in this case, was the pale white flowers said to resemble female sexual organs in shape. (Still administered primarily to women, she is an effective remedy for treating leukorrhea and strengthening the uterus.) The ancients saw in her that undefinable something imprinted on plants of Venus and the Moon.

I am overjoyed whenever I encounter a cluster of Dead Nettles! She grows mostly in groups and, compared to the more austere Stinging Nettle, presents herself with good cheer and devotion. The ancient Chinese called her the "Herb of the Smiling Mother." The medieval abbess and healer Hildegard von Bingen believed her power could be transferred to humans and wrote: "Whoever ingests her loves to smile, for her warmth, which affects the spleen, cheers the heart."

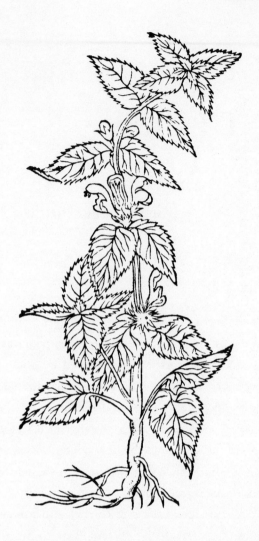

chest of the fat bumblebees who, as they suck, pollinate by pressing their backs against anther and stigma. Further inside, the flower tube narrows and bears a ring of fine hairs. This is a last safety measure to keep unwanted smaller insects away from the desired nectar. The bumblebee carries the only key to Dead Nettle's "honey lock" although some burglars obtain access with force. For instance, attracted by the sweet scent, a honeybee sometimes bites holes in the flower tube to reach the honey. Pure vandalism, this method does not pollinate the flower.

Let me introduce a few sisters of White Dead Nettle that I frequently meet on hikes. The most inconspicuous one is Henbit Dead Nettle (*Lamium amplexicaule*), frequently growing in fields, gardens, and vineyards. Her upper leaves surround the stem holding tiny flowers of pink to carmine red that grow in apparent whorls from the leaf axils. This nettle rarely grows higher than a foot.

An old field weed, Purple Dead Nettle (*Lamium purpureum*) is more commonly known. We find her in the nutrient-rich loamy soils of waysides, waste areas, and fields. Her leaves are similar to Stinging Nettle—but without the sting. Her flower-lips are purplish red, a hue that even tinges the stem tip and upper leaves. In true nettle fashion, the leaves stand in crosswise-opposite rows and the flowers in apparent whorls. A mature plant grows 4 to 10 inches tall. Medicinally, she is used for a dark vaginal discharge and as a remedy for burns.

A true beauty among nettles is Archangel Dead Nettle (*Lamium galeobdolon*). We meet her mostly in mixed woodlands and deciduous forests where she finds the moist, mulch-containing

In the animal world, Dead Nettle's special relationship is with the bumblebee. She loves these unperturbed insects and allows only them to pollinate her flowers. Their long proboscis lets them manage her deep flower tubes and reach the sweet nectar whereas the wings of the butterfly are a hindrance. Obligingly, Dead Nettle has adapted the shape of her flowers to provide a horizontal lower lip as a comfortable bench for her favored bumblebee guests. The green dots and lines on this landing field are honey marks that show the way. The flower's lateral lobes are just the right distance apart to fit the head and

soil she loves. Surprisingly, her flowers are golden yellow. And unlike White Dead Nettle, she is not fanatically attached to bumblebees, shaping her tubular corolla a bit shorter to allow other bees access to her nectar.

HEALING PROPERTIES

While scientists are not entirely clear about Dead Nettle's active ingredients, we know that this plant contains mucilage, tannins, saponins, and essential oil. Used almost exclusively in gynecological cases, it is a remedy for leukorrhea and fluor albus. In old herbal lore, White Dead Nettle is used for white fluor, the golden Archangel Dead Nettle for yellow fluor, and the Purple Dead Nettle for reddish brown fluor. One should always ascertain the cause of a malady before prescribing a particular remedy. For instance, in cases when the fluor albus results from fungal infection or a trichomonad, Dead Nettle would apply only as an adjunct treatment. However, it is helpful for constitutional fluor, which is a disposition toward leukorrhea and is usually recommended for pale, young female patients. (The tea blend described in the chapter on Lady's Mantle is more appropriate for older women.) As a course of treatment, a decoction prepared from Dead Nettle flowers can be taken internally as a tea and administered externally as a vaginal douche.

As a woman's plant, Dead Nettle is also a practical skin-care product. The cool tea is a good cleanser for oily skin. Similarly, used as a hair rinse, a tea made from equal amounts of Dead Nettle flowers and Coltsfoot flowers (*Tussilago farfara*) reduces oil and prevents the hair from getting oily again too soon.

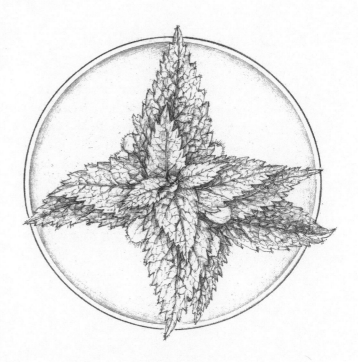

Gathering Dead Nettle flowers is labor intensive, making the purchased tea expensive. But allowing plenty of time, you can easily gather enough for your own needs. Do so on a sunny day, carefully plucking the flowers and spreading them out to dry.

Dead Nettle flowers are available in herb or natural food stores as "Flores Lamii albi." The homeopathic mother tincture "Lamium album" is prepared from fresh leaves and flowers.

✌ YOUNG WOMAN'S TEA AND DOUCHE

2 teaspoons dried dead nettle flowers

1 cup water

Pour boiling water over the dried flowers, cover, and let the mixture steep for 5 to 10 minutes. As a tea, a daily dose is 3 cups. As a douche, use the tea at body temperature once or twice a week.

৪৯ Dead Nettle Burn Gel

Another area of application is burns. (In folk medicine a plant so cool and mucilaginous would certainly make a good burn remedy!) To prepare a burn gel, gather dead nettle plants in full bloom. Place them in a pot on the stove, cover them with water, and boil the mixture for several minutes. Remove the pot from the heat, cover it, and let it cool for about 2 hours. Remove the gelatinous mass and store it in sterile jars. It is very helpful for sunburn and similar skin irritations.

BOTANICAL CHARACTERISTICS

Name: *Lamium album* — Dead Nettle

Distribution: Europe, Asia, America

Habitat: Garden fences, hedges, meadow banks

Description: 1 to 2 feet tall; Stinging Nettle-like, but without stinging hairs; square stem, leaves are stalked, ovate, serrated along the edges, and crosswise-opposite; white lip-shaped flowers in apparent whorls in the leaf axils. Flowering time is April to October.

Confusion with similar plants: With Stinging Nettle (*Urtica dioica*) in spring before Dead Nettle flowers. Dead Nettle does not sting.

Collecting season: Flowers – April to October

Active ingredients: Mucilage, saponins, essential oils, tannins

Astrological association: Venus / Moon

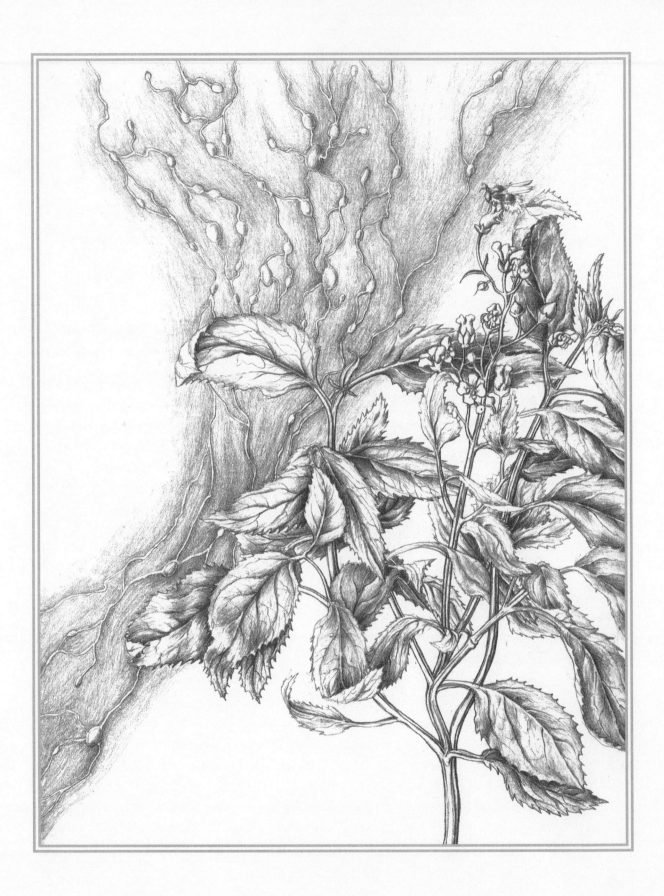

FIGWORT

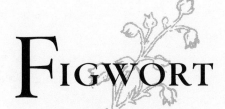

Scrophularia nodosa

Common Figwort, Wood Figwort

Throatwort, Scrofula Plant, Carpenter's Square, Heal-All

Figwort family — Scrophulariaceae

CAST ASIDE ANY EXPECTATIONS right away—Figwort is feast for neither eyes nor nose. Her leaves and stem when crushed between your fingers emit a putrid smell. And the root! Its pale white or yellowish flesh pours forth a foulness when processed into salves. To top it off, Figwort is considered to be poisonous. However, as with people, each plant has its purpose and, in this instance, a great remedy hides within the dark, offensive form. Having personally felt her power in my body when she healed me from an illness, my heart opens every time I meet her.

Figwort belongs to those forgotten medicinal plants that were once highly valued for their healing properties. The Greek physician Dioscurides, who practiced in Rome in the first century A.D., praised her in his *De Materia Medica*. And those who claim to have never seen her have probably passed her many times. She is still quite common, choosing to grow in thickets and ditches, in wet meadows and wastelands. Every year she sprouts a new stem from her root that can reach a height of four feet. This somewhat rigid stem is exactly square. You can easily feel it with your fingers and this is one way to distinguish Common Figwort (*Scrophularia nodosa*) from "Winged Figwort" (*S. umbrosa* or *S. alata*). The latter's stem, as her German name suggests, has tiny wing-like strips running along the edges. Another species, Water Figwort (*S. aquatica*), chooses to live in ponds, riverbanks, flooded meadows and the like. Long ago, she was the "Figwort woman" to Common Figwort's "Figwort man." However, Common Figwort is the only one used for healing purposes.

Except for their smooth surface, Figwort's long egg-shaped leaves are similar in shape and size to those of Stinging Nettle. Leaf pairs sit opposite each other on the stem at a right angle to pairs growing above and below. Their dark green color has the black hue that is characteristic of all Saturn plants. Figwort is one of the few plants in nature that bear brown flowers. Their brownish purple color and fascinating shape are easily appreciated with a magnifying glass. The inflated throat opens to a mouth with two lips, the upper lip dividing into two lobes and the lower one into three. This shape is adapted to the wasp, her insect of choice for pollination.

The flower's shape will remind you of her cousin, our garden-variety Snapdragon (*Antirrhinum majus*). Other Figwort family members are Mullein (*Verbascum thapsiforme*), Toadflax (*Linaria vulgaris*), Foxglove (*Digitalis grandiflora*), Speedwell (*Veronica officinalis*), Rattleweed (*Rhinanthus minor*), Eyebright (*Euphrasia officinalis*), and Hedgehyssop (*Gratiola officinalis*). Their strangely beautiful flowers seem friendlier than Figwort's. Consider the sparkling sun-eyes of Mullein, the innocent blue eyes of Speedwell, the merrily twinkling flower dots of Eyebright, and the tiger-striped purple blooms of Common Foxglove.

Interestingly, Foxglove contains large amounts of cardio-active glycosides—which Figwort has in very small quantities. If ingested in high concentrations, they stimulate the heart and produce unwanted side effects. This makes Foxglove both a dangerous poison and a powerful remedy. Most specific heart medications prescribed by today's orthodox medical professionals contain Foxglove glycosides in synthetic form. In turn, modern herbalists do not use Foxglove because of its reputed toxicity.

This is where we witness the close relationship between poison and remedy. Dosage decides the direction. Paracelsus (1493–1541) postulates this age-old wisdom when he writes that all things are poisonous—only the dose makes them otherwise. Therefore it is important for medicinal herbalists to know the proper application and dosage of a healing plant. Even harmless Chamomile can be damaging when consumed improperly and in excessive amounts. In overdoses, opposite effects can occur, causing a plant to produce exactly the disease that it is supposed to treat. Even non-toxic plants should not be used extensively for more than six weeks. If the disease shows no improvement, another plant should be tried.

But let us return to Figwort, who seems to have been used in the past for magical purposes. Old German names such as "Witches' Herb," "Nightshade," and "Smoke Herb" suggest her use as an amulet against sorcery. Hieronymus Bock hints of this in his 1577 herbal—although he gives no further details:

> Women tie Figwort to the cattle . . . chase away worms and maggots with it . . . [and] carry out strange superstition with [it].

Another name for Figwort—"Red Urine Herb"—arose from observing that her ingestion by grazing animals caused blood to appear in their urine. Today we know that this is due to the herb's high concentration of saponins. Lastly, she was called "Sow Herb" because she was said to cure mange in pigs.

The secret of her healing power is easily discovered when we dig up her brown root with its fig-like knobs. (Hence her English name of Figwort and her German one of *Braunwurz* or "Brown Root.") Ancient herbalists repeatedly assure us that Figwort's root is a potent ally. It is a stocky rhizome made up of swollen tubers strung together, dark brown outside with yellowish white flesh. In fact, the root looks so much like the connected lymph nodes of the human body that they took it as a sign from God of its purpose. And, indeed, Figwort has long proved to be a remedy for swollen glands, having a dissolving effect on stagnant lymph fluid which thereby allows the glandular swelling to subside. She is used mostly for swollen tonsils and for swollen lymph glands around the female breast and genitals. Her scientific name of *Scrophularia nodosa* comes from the Latin term *scrofula*, referring to swellings of the neck's lymph nodes.

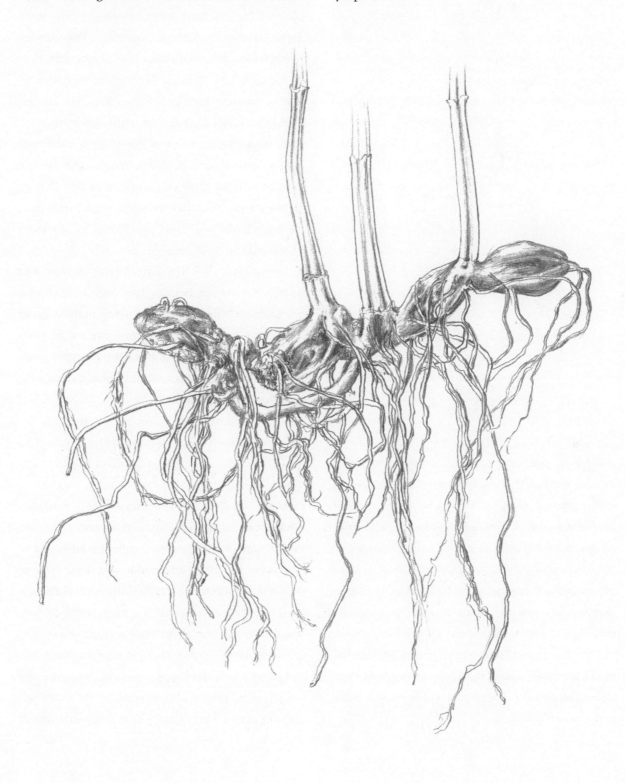

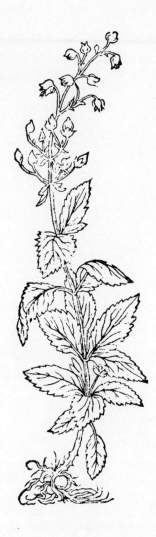

From their sturdy wicker hampers, the medieval root diggers offered Figwort alongside Angelica, Comfrey, Tormentil, and Saxifrage. Originally, only the roots of healing plants were gathered for medicinal purposes. Dioscurides wrote in the *Pharmaceutics* that most of the 600 or so remedies of plant origin recommended in that tome were prepared from roots. Hence, the first herbal books were actually "root books." *Rhizomika*, or those knowledgeable in medicinal plants, called their booths *rhizomotoi* from the Greek *rhiza* for root and *temnein* to cut. Part of a long tradition, they roamed woodlands and pastures gathering roots and herbs to sell from door to door or at local fairs.

Nowadays, "herb women" with baskets full of their wares can be found in front of the main entrance to Munich's big shopping mall. A quiet island in the surging crowd, they are a relic from the past as they sit in colorful dirndels with kerchiefs and red noses—but offering, alas, only the roots of horse radish.

The old ones saw in Figwort a twofold astrological relationship—to Saturn because of her stern, gloomy radiance and to Venus because of her spongy, white root flesh. Accordingly, Saturn represents the contracting, hardening energies of the body while Venus is assigned the glandular system, sexual organs, skin, bladder and kidneys, and venous system. From this we can deduce that Figwort treats hardened glands like tonsils, the thyroid, and glands in the breast and genital area. At the same time, it stimulates and strengthens the bladder and kidneys and heals certain skin diseases.

HEALING PROPERTIES

Figwort has long been a remedy for scrofula, a congenital disposition to react to stimuli (often minor ones) with tedious inflammations. The condition primarily affects the lymphatic system, mucous membranes, and skin. Its signs are lymph-node swellings on the neck, swollen tonsils, chronic head colds, facial eczema (especially around the nose, mouth, and ears), cradle cap, constantly inflamed eyes, rickets, and, in the past, goiter, which was thought to be a swollen thyroid gland. People so afflicted should consider drinking a cup of Figwort tea daily for three weeks, repeating the treatment every season.

Besides Figwort, other medicinal plants are used to treat scrofula. They are Walnut leaves (*Juglans* spp.), Oak bark tea (*Quercus* spp.), Acorn coffee (which is especially suited for children), and Speedwell Beccabunga (*Veronica beccabunga*). This last plant is best ingested daily in the form of freshly pressed juice—one or two tablespoons diluted in water—or as a fresh salad.

For scrofulous skin symptoms you can apply Figwort externally in a bath, a salve, and a plaster. To prepare a plunge bath, boil equal amounts (500 grams or about a pound) of Walnut leaves and the Figwort plant without the root in water. Strain off the liquid and add it to the bath water. For partial baths, dilute the decoction. For washing eczema, skin lichens, and ulcers, steep 100 grams of the Figwort root in one liter of cold water and let it stand overnight before using the strained liquid.

Figwort's antibiotic effect on germs that cause skin diseases explains its longstanding usage for rashes. You can apply Figwort salve to facial eczema, swollen glands (especially tonsils), hemorrhoids, ulcers, skin lichens, rashes, and ear eczema. Calendula (*Calendula officinalis*) and Sweet Clover (*Melilotus officinalis* or *M. albus*) are used for inflammations and swellings in the lymph area as well. Figwort is used for lingering and congenital illnesses of the lymphatic system and the skin.

In addition, Figwort has a stimulating and strengthening effect on the bladder and kidneys. The glycosides it contains make it suitable for treating mild heart conditions that call for stimu-

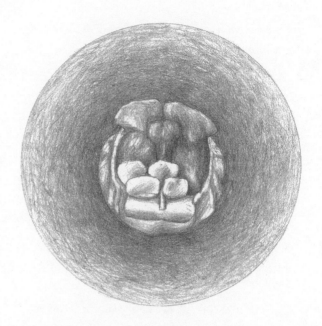

lating the metabolism and eliminating water retention in the body. For this purpose, use Figwort as a tea or tincture.

In traditional Chinese medicine, Figwort (*S. ningpoensis*) is a standard remedy. Because of its ability to stimulate the pancreas, it is used in the treatment of diabetes. Known as *huyên sâm* or *xuan shen*, it is also a remedy for fever and sadness, swellings and pain of the throat, furuncles, and to aid digestion.

October is when I go digging for Figwort roots. After cleaning them carefully and cutting them into small pieces, I allow them to dry thoroughly on a piece of wire mesh stretched over a frame. To prepare the tea, I pour a cup of cold water over a teaspoon of finely chopped dried root and let it stand overnight. The next morning I strain off the liquid and drink it in small sips throughout the day.

In addition to the herb's internal applications, her root has long been made into a salve for external use. One of the old herbalist-writers who praised it highly felt compelled to divulge the following recipe:

> From Figwort, [one can] make an exquisite and trusted salve for all kinds of scabs and mangyness thus. In May, take the herb with the roots already washed and cleansed, then crushed and the juice pressed out. This same juice keep over the year in a narrow jar well plugged. One can prepare a salve from it by taking the pressed juice, wax, and tree oils in equal amounts heated together on coals well tempered to a salve. I tell you in truth that great abscesses as one would deem for leprosy have been healed when salved with it.
>
> Out of Christian love not wishing to keep it to myself,
>
> *Hieronymus Bock 1577*

I make Figwort salve according to the directions for salve preparation given in the chapter on Comfrey (see "Some Tips for Making Salves"). Her root, like Comfrey's, is gathered in the early spring or late fall for this purpose and then is extracted in lanolin and oil. Likewise, Figwort tincture can be prepared as is Comfrey tincture. The dose is 10 to 15 drops three times daily.

In herb stores Figwort is available as "Radix Scrophulariae" and the homeopathic tincture "Scrophularia nodosa" is prepared from the fresh plant.

Cultivation

As Figwort is a favorite food of worms, caterpillars, and snails, I advise you to plant her at some distance from your garden. She prefers moist, humus- and nutrient-rich soil and sunny places but will thrive in partial shade. Well-worked soil will allow the roots to grow bigger. Lastly, observing that Figwort is not very neighborly—perhaps due to her Saturn nature, I recommend keeping other plants at arm's length. Seeds are commercially available.

Veterinary Medicine

Amulets of Figwort root were once used to protect animals from disease. Long associated with pigs (remember her old German name "Sow Herb"), mangy animals were washed with a strong tea prepared from the plant's leaves and roots. And her salve has proved helpful for eczema and skin rashes in animals in general.

BOTANICAL CHARACTERISTICS

Name: Scrophularia nodosa — Figwort

Distribution: Europe and Asia

Habitat: Thicket, ditches, riverbanks, wasteland

Description: A 2- to 4-foot tall plant; its square stem has few branches; opposite-facing pairs of lanceolate-ovate leaves with serrated edges; purplish brown flowers in terminal panicles: the seed capsule ovoid, pointed, with small seeds; the rootstock is greyish brown, knobby, and thick with an unpleasant smell. Flowering time is June to September.

Confusion with similar plants: Only with other Figwort species (see text)

Collecting season:
    Upper parts – June to July
    Root – October to November or early spring

Active ingredients: Saponins, glycosides

Astrological association: Saturn / Venus

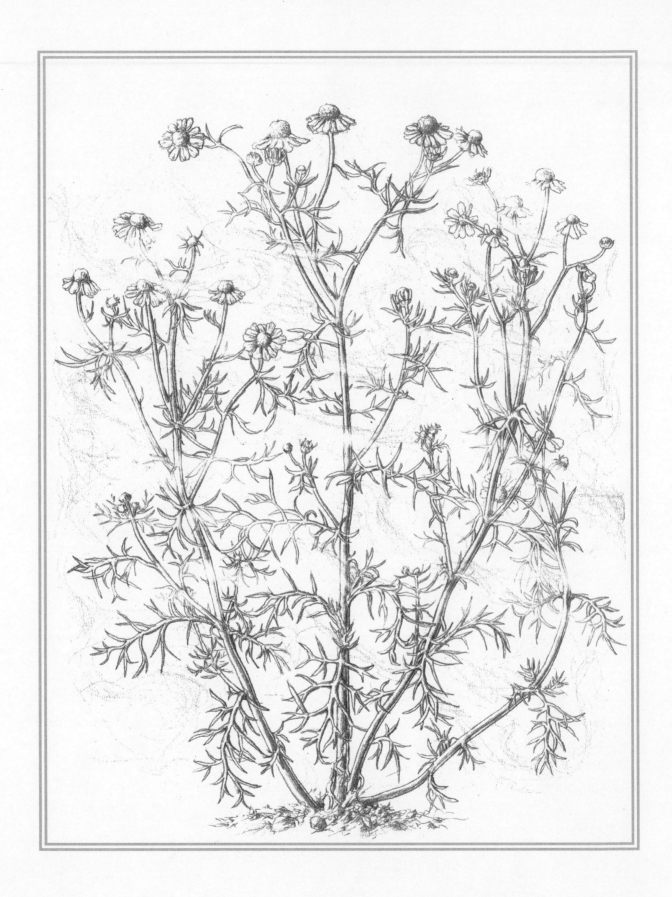

German Chamomile

Chamomilla recutita
(*Matricaria chamomilla, Chamomilla matricaria, Matricaria recutita*)*
Wild Chamomile, Scented Mayweed, Feverfew
Daisy family — Compositae / Asteraceae

God bestowed to Chamomile
the gift to still the body's aches.
But, she flowers, thrives, and waits in vain
for someone with a stomach pain.
For people in their pain do not believe
in what they can so easily obtain—
they want a pill.
If you will, leave me alone with Chamomile.

from Karl-Heinz Waggerl's
Humorous Herbarium

MANY PEOPLE ARE FAMILIAR with the scent of Chamomile flowers. From early childhood on, it is something connected with certain images and sentiments—a comforting, warm promise of well-being. Most of us first remember a steaming cup of Chamomile tea brought to our bedside to soothe a stomachache for, from infancy to old age, this herb soothes our pains, relieves cramps, and heals wounds. And so she has served humankind since the Neolithic period.

Modern skeptics scoff at claims that a simple botanical can heal so many ills. In his poem, Karl-Heinz Waggerl noted that people do not want to believe in something so readily available. We would rather have a processed "medically correct" pill with side effects that go unquestioned. Yet once we are attuned to our body's signals and have some herbal awareness, a simple cup of hot herbal tea will often cure the problem.

Fortunately, not everyone has forgotten Chamomile's beneficence. In many kitchen cabinets sits a package of Chamomile flowers still reached for at the first signs of stomachache or general discontent. In fact, Chamomile tea is one of the most popular products in natural food stores. In contrast to the fate of other medicinal plants, her healing power is undisputed scientifically. Chemical analysis confirms the empirical knowledge of thousands of years. Ancient Egyptian, Arabic, Babylonian, Greek, and Roman herbalists and physicians administered Chamomile the same way we do today.

Matricaria, German Chamomile's early Latin genus name, means "mother" (*mater*) and

---

*Other botanical names found in some herbals

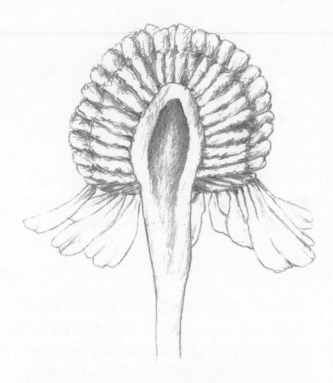

"uterus" (*matrix*), pointing to Chamomile's most important original use. The "Mother's Herb" helps dysfunctions of pregnancy, labor and birth, and postpartum because of its anti-inflammatory, analgesic, and disinfecting properties. In infants and toddlers, it heals chafed skin and alleviates stomachaches, cramps, and teething pains.

The main active ingredient is the deep blue chamazulene, an essential oil with azulene obtained through the steam distillation of the flowers. Only this process brings out the oil. With its disinfectant, anti-inflammatory, and sedative qualities, it soothes pains and alleviates cramping. Its warm scent is somewhat reminiscent of apples and gives it the name we know today. "Chamomile" comes from the Latin *camomilla*, a variation of the Latin-Greek *chamaelan* meaning "apple" (*melon*) and "on the earth" (*chamai*).

Chamomile contains other important medici-

nal ingredients such as flavons, bitter compounds, tannins, and coumarin. They indicate that she is a remedy for stomach and intestines and can heal inflamed mucous membranes.

In Germany, Chamomile's popularity is enormous and cultivation cannot meet demand. As with other medicinal herbs, it is cheaper to import her. Our Chamomile flowers, for instance, come mostly from the Balkan states, Italy, and South America. But many countries that sell herbal products use toxic pesticides that are illegal in Germany and North America. Business ethics, however, do not prevent us from exporting these pesticides to Third World countries whose products—coffee, fruit, herbs, and tea—return these dangerous substances (like DDT) to our tables. And we wonder why there is so much DDT in mothers' milk!

Interestingly, medicinal herbs in the Federal Republic of Germany are not governed by a law concerning these substances. Chemical analysis in 1972 through 1974 found high residues of chlorinated hydrocarbon in Chamomile flowers. Moreover, to make the mechanical harvesting of flowers more efficient, the Chamomile cultivated in large monocultures is being defoliated with the highly toxic Agent Orange.

I strongly advise only the purchase of products derived from certified organically grown Chamomile. Furthermore, anyone with a garden can grow her. It is not difficult—about 20 square feet can supply a family. You can also gather smaller quantities of Chamomile yourself.

In the old days, Chamomile gatherers headed for the closest cornfield where she grew as a weed, healing the soil by redressing disturbed mineral balances and killing off soil toxins. A traditional companion of grain crops, Chamomile boosts the growth and yield of wheat spikes and, in turn, gains her highest content of active ingredients. Nowadays, a search for Chamomile in our cornfields would be in vain. She is highly sensitive to chemical fertilizers and pesticides and has disappeared from these cultivated areas. Instead we find her along waysides, in meadows, and around dumps and wastelands.

In early spring before she blooms, we might pass her without recognition. Most people are familiar only with her flowers but, having a Chamomile bed in my garden, I have observed the plants more closely. By the fall, small plants spring up all over the garden from the seeds of her withered plants. With apologies, I pull up most of them or soon my herbal garden would only contain Chamomile! I recognize the small, tender leaf rosettes with their finely divided, filigree-like leaflets. They are soft and almost fleshy in comparison to similarly shaped but rough Yarrow leaves. When you rub them under your nose, these leaflets smell more like spinach than Chamomile. The young rosettes winter over —even the heaviest snow and coldest frost will not harm them. In springtime, when the sun regains her power, a light green, round, fleshy stem emerges from the rosette that can grow 20 inches tall. This stem branches out into more side shoots, many originating from the leaf axils.

The finely divided leaflets are two or three times pinnate, showing more spaces than actual leaf and a green color that is friendly and light with hints of yellow. Overall, Chamomile appears airy and lofty, seeming to shun a heavy contact with Earth. On the terminal ends of her graceful, thin stems float beautiful flowers reflecting the plant's undivided love for the sun. The dainty blooms look like tiny suns, their white florets radiating from a golden yellow center. From these flowers emanate the familiar Chamomile scent—the warming and soft sweetness of summer. We can almost "sniff" the soothing, softening effect this plant has on our bodies.

Initially flat, the flower heads soon arch upward as the white ray flowers bend down. Using our thumbnail to dissect a flower in the middle, we find that its head is hollow in the center as if the flower, like the leaflets, seek airiness inside. From May to August, these tiny flower-suns appear over and over until the last one forms its seeds. The fruits of the Chamomile plant are small, crooked, moist, and slimy formations that fall to the ground, soon sprouting into the dainty rosettes that were discussed earlier. The mother plants wither and die.

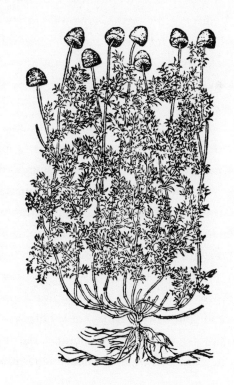

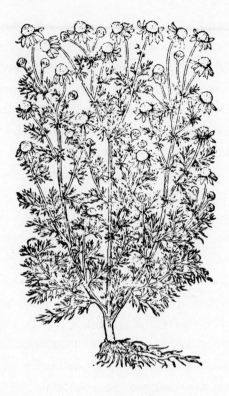

German Chamomile has a few doubles with whom she is frequently confused. Features of what I consider this true Chamomile safely distinguish it from her false "cousins": her hollow receptacle, strong aromatic scent, and the white ray flowers that bend backward at the end of their flowering time.

German Chamomile is easily confused with Field Chamomile (*Anthemis arvensis*), a plant that is not used medicinally. Field Chamomile is more common than the true Chamomile in Germany. Her German name "Dog Chamomile" derives from her odor, which is similar to dog's urine. She grows 8 to 20 inches high with yellow flower heads surrounded by white ray flowers. Her flower head barely arches upward and is solid and marrowy inside—not hollow. The white florets stand out horizontally; the leaves are soft, green, hairy, undivided, and feathered

one to three times. A final distinguishing mark: The receptacle bears small, chaffy scales between the single flowers, which true German Chamomile lacks.

The scentless Mayweed (*Matricaria inodora*) also closely resembles German Chamomile. Her name tells us that she smells only vaguely like our "Mother's Herb" and is taller—up to two feet high—and much coarser. She has yellow disk flowers, white ray flowers, and a solid receptacle. This plant is not used for healing purposes.

"The Chamomile Who Lost Her White Flowers" could be the title of a fairy tale about Pineappleweed, also called Rayless Mayweed (*Chamomilla suaveolens*, *Matricaria matricarioides*, or *M. discoidea*). Her story takes us to her original homelands of East Asia and North America and back to the nineteenth century when she was first carried to Germany from across the sea. Specifically, she was brought to Berlin's old Botanical Garden. The story goes that she spread from there across the entire city, out along roadsides, and subsequently across the entire country. Today we find her everywhere. She does not bear white ray flowers but is content with her inconspicuous greenish yellow and much-arched flower heads. She is coarser and stockier, growing close to the ground. The hollow receptacle is like that of German Chamomile but her essential oil contains no azulene, thereby denying her anti-inflammatory properties. However, she does have healing qualities as an anthelmintic for expelling parasitic worms, especially maw worms and pinworms. (In such cases, three to four cups of herbal tea is sipped daily.)

Roman Chamomile or Common Chamomile (*Chaemaemelum nobile*, *Anthemis nobilis*) is rarely encountered in the open country. Originally a native of Mediterranean regions, she has been cultivated in Germany since the sixteenth century. With her beautiful shape and double white flowers, she is a popular and traditional planting of rural gardens where she grows easily in a sunny, warm spot. She is 8 to 12 inches tall, has a hairy stem and leaves that are twice pinnate, and her receptacle is conical and solid inside. She bears broad, white ray flowers. Like German Chamomile, she emanates a pleasant aromatic scent that conveys its healing power especially through the essential oil. Roman Chamomile has the same medicinal properties as German Chamomile although weaker. Less expensive than German Chamomile, she is preferred for baths and washes.

HEALING PROPERTIES

German Chamomile's anti-inflammatory, calming, carminative, and vulnerary properties are used mostly in gynecological and pediatric medicine.

Its anti-inflammatory quality helps for inflammations of the skin and mucous membranes, especially of the stomach and intestines. We can use it for acute or chronic conditions of the stomach and intestines, for gastritis, and gastric and duodenal ulcers. It heals inflamed mucous membranes and simultaneously soothes pain and cramping. Dr. R.F. Weiss writes in his *Textbook of Phytotherapy* (1974): "Chamomile is one of our best and most suitable remedies for influencing acute and chronic inflammatory conditions of the stomach's mucous membranes." For treating these conditions, we use Chamomile tea prepared by pouring boiling water over two teaspoons of the flowers and steeping it covered. A daily dose is two to three cups taken in small sips throughout the day.

We also can treat the inflamed oral mucosa with Chamomile tea. For stomatitis, an uncomfortable inflammation of the mouth's mucous membranes, and canker sores, the mouth is rinsed with the tea or a liquid Chamomile extract ("Extractum Chamomillae fluidum") that is available from a herbal pharmacy. To make an oral rinse, stir half a teaspoon of Chamomile extract into one glass of water.

Inflamed and itching eczema and all inflammatory skin diseases, lichens, and skin injuries can be treated with Chamomile. Apply it externally for disinfecting and anti-inflammatory treatments in the form of packs, baths, and compresses using a strong tea, diluted Chamomile tincture ("Tinctura Chamomillae"), or a liquid Chamomile extract. Chamomile is administered internally with other specific herbs for skin diseases such as Wild Pansy (*Viola tricolor*), Burdock (*Arctium lappa*), and Stinging Nettle (*Urtica dioica*).

Due to its antispasmodic properties Chamomile is a good remedy for all cramping pains, especially for abdominal cramping in children. At the same time it has a carminative effect of relieving flatulence. In pediatric medicine we use Chamomile as a tea or syrup. The syrup "Sirupus Chamomillae" is available in naturopathic pharmacies in Germany and is ingested by the tablespoon. We can increase its effect by placing a hot Chamomile sachet on the painful area. For this purpose, fill a small cloth bag with Chamomile and heat it in the oven. To treat abdominal cramps, mix equal parts of Chamomile flowers and Silverweed (*Potentilla anserina*) to make a tea. Chamomile is a classic remedy for teething pains in children. For this, we use Chamomile in its homeopathic form or as teething tablets. For dosages, check with your homeopathic practitioner or homeopathic pharmacy.

For irritability, restlessness, colic, and restless sleep, as well as for discomfort during pregnancy, concurrent external application of the essential oil is helpful. The essential oil of Roman Chamomile has proved especially effective psychologically. Essential oil of Chamomile ("Oleum Chamomillae aeth.") is available in herbal pharmacies. I vaporize it by putting about 10 drops in a pot of hot water placed near the bed. You can also pour the oil into an aroma lamp especially designed for this purpose.

Gather flowers for Chamomile tea in sunny, warm weather when they are in full bloom. Spread them thinly over a wire screen and dry them carefully in a shady, airy place away from direct sun. The flowers absorb moisture easily and should be stored in a dark container with a good lid.

Because the boiling process destroys the medicinal essential oils (including the azulenes) in Chamomile tea, it is advisable to brew the dried flowers in hot water and let it steep covered for several minutes. And be sure to drink it hot. On a cautionary note, too much Chamomile can bring the opposite effect. Rather than healing pain, cramps, and restlessness, too much of it can cause such problems. Only drink three cups a day and do not make Chamomile tea your herbal beverage of choice for daily consumption. In particular, do not give it regularly to children.

For packs, baths, and compresses we can use the more reasonably priced Roman Chamomile available in natural food stores as "Flores Chamomillae romanae." Put three tablespoons in one quart of water for compresses and when treating wounds. For a relaxing bath that soothes the nerves, place a cloth sachet filled with Chamomile flowers into the hot bath water or add an infusion with hot water.

Note: Do not administer the steam of Chamomile in cases of conjunctivitis, blepharitis, or any other inflammations of the eyes because it can worsen these conditions. Instead, use Eyebright (*Euphrasia officinalis*), Fennel (*Foeniculum vulgare*), Rose leaves (*Rosa* spp.), and rosewater.

❧ Antispasmodic Chamomile Body Oil

- 10 drops essential oil of chamomile
- 10 drops essential fennel oil
- 2 fluid ounces cold-pressed olive oil or sunflower oil

Put the ingredients into a jar with a tight lid and shake vigorously. Use as a liniment for cramping pains of the digestive organs or lower abdomen. For small children, add only half the amount of essential oils.

❧ Chamomile Oil

Place freshly crushed chamomile flowers in a clear mason jar and cover them with cold-pressed sunflower oil or olive oil. Place the jar, tightly lidded, in a sunny place for 2 or 3 weeks. Strain the oil and discard the flowers, pressing them out well. Add a few drops of essential oil of chamomile.

Use as a liniment for back pain, sore muscles, neuralgias, kidney pain, facial neuralgias, abdominal pain, and diaper rash.

✌ CHAMOMILE TINCTURE

Fill a dark mason jar with freshly crushed chamomile flowers and enough vodka or a fruit liqueur to cover. Replace the lid tightly and let the mixture steep for 2 or 3 weeks. Occasionally shake the jar. Strain the tincture and pour it into dark dropper bottles. For internal use, take 20 drops 3 times a day. For external use, add ½ teaspoon to a glass of water.

✌ CHAMOMILE SYRUP

100 grams fresh chamomile flowers

50 milliliters vodka or other grain spirit

200 milliliters distilled water

300 grams sugar

Crush the chamomile flowers in a mortar, moisten with the alcohol, pour the mixture into a jar, and top off with distilled water. Place the jar, tightly lidded, in the sun for 2 days and shake it occasionally. Strain off the flowers and dissolve the sugar in the liquid by bringing it to a simmer, stirring constantly. Pour the syrup into bottles and store in a cool place. Administer by the tablespoon especially to children.

COSMETICS

Chamomile flowers are a wonderful beauty aid. They cleanse and soothe the skin and heal inflammations. Tolerated by every skin type, they are particularly suited for the care and cleansing

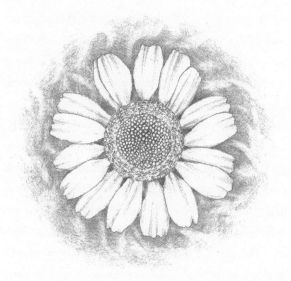

of sensitive, dry, chapped skin. Use them in steam baths, cremes, compresses, and packs. Rinsing the hair with Chamomile tea lightens blond hair.

CULTIVATION

Chamomile should not be missing from any garden. It heals not only people but also the soil and neighboring plants. It was once believed that this herb possessed such strong healing powers that, to strengthen a sickly plant, one only had to grow Chamomile next to it. Such superstitions are not laughable because we now know that Chamomile has an inhibitory effect on nematodes within a radius of three feet and really can strengthen soil and other plants. Chamomile also absorbs lime and passes it on to other plants. Finally, its antiseptic qualities have a beneficial effect on the growth of nearby plants. Chamomile is an especially good companion plant for cabbage and onions, strengthening them and keeping away pests.

Chamomile is easy to grow and self-seeds profusely. For medicinal purposes only the flowers are needed and a patch of 20 to 30 square feet is sufficient to keep a family in supply. Roman Chamomile is an evergreen perennial. However, German Chamomile is an annual, dying off the second season. It loves deep, nutrient-rich soils and lots of sun. Starters planted in the fall will winter over without harm and develop into full-grown Chamomile plants the next year. Seeds can be sown year round by lightly pressing them into the soil—Chamomile needs light for germination. (I mix the fine seeds with some sand to prevent the small plants from growing too closely together.) Water them carefully so that nothing washes away. Later, thin the plants to eight inches apart. Harvest the flowers only during sunny weather, about three to five days after the flowers open, when they have their highest content of essential oils. Grown in containers, Chamomile flowers make a beautiful addition to balcony or patio.

VETERINARY MEDICINE

The benevolent Chamomile is helpful in treating animals. Here, too, we can rely on its powers to soothe cramps, relieve flatulence, and heal wounds. We administer the tea internally and apply it externally to cleanse and heal wounds. Colic in horses is aided by a steam bath with a hot Chamomile infusion. For this purpose, we can place a pot of hot water and Chamomille flowers under the horse and allow the steam to rise up over the area of complaint. Chamomile tea also helps dogs with intestinal trouble and diarrhea. My own formula for diarrhea in chickens is to administer Chamomile tea in the form of the homeopathic remedies Chamomilla 4x and Ipecacuanha 4x (five drops each).

BOTANICAL CHARACTERISTICS

Name: Chamomilla recutita, *Matricaria chamomilla*, or M. *recutita* — German Chamomile

Distribution: Europe, North Africa, the Americas, and Australia

Habitat: Fields, waysides, meadows, and wastelands

Description: Grows 4 to 20 inches tall; round, glabrous, erect stem, much-branched; leaves are greenish yellow, two to three times pinnate with small, linear leaflets. Flowers terminal with golden yellow disk flowers and ligulate bright white ray flowers, receptacle is hollow and cone-shaped. Flowers from May to August or September.

Confusion with similar plants: With Field Chamomile (*Anthemis arvensis*), Roman Chamomile (*Chaemaemelum nobile/Anthemis nobilis*), Scentless Mayweed (*Matricaria inodora*), Rayless Mayweed (*Chamomilla suaveolens*). German Chamomile has a hollow receptacle and aromatic scent.

Collecting season: May to July; gather flowers only in bright sunshine because constituents decrease in rainy weather.

Active ingredients: Essential oil with azulene (0.3 to 1.5%), flavonoids, sesquiterpenlactone, coumarin, bitter compounds, mucilage, umbelliferon, and herniarin

Astrological association: Sun / Venus

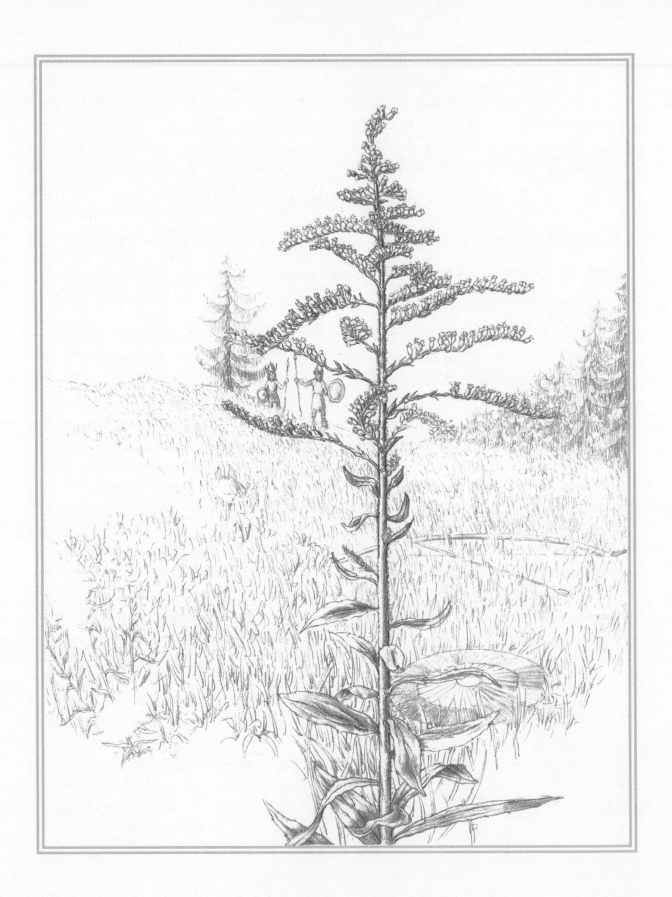

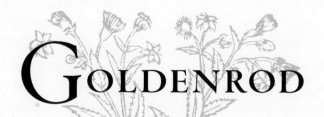

GOLDENROD

Solidago virgaurea

European Goldenrod, Common Goldenrod, Woundwort

Daisy family — Compositae / Asteraceae

GOLDENROD HAS A PAGAN PAST. The ancient Germans considered her to be the best wound herb and, before engaging in battle, gathered Goldenrod as a precaution. In tribute, herbals of subsequent centuries called her "Pagan Woundherb," a name later christianized to "St. Peter's Staff Herb." Now as then, herbalists in rural areas prepare packs, compresses, and potions from the fresh and dried plants. Today in Germany she is commonly called "Fastening Herb" because she can fasten wounds together or "Golden Woundwort" because of her golden flowers. Consider what Tabernaemontanus wrote in 1731 in his *Perfect Herbal*:

> This herb receives its name not without cause. It is called Golden Woundwort inasmuch as it is completely healing and useful for both external and internal wounds due to the dry and astringent powers it bears. One can simmer the herb alone in wine or water depending on availability or combine it with other wound herbs such as Sanicle, Snowline Pyrola, Silverweed, Self-Heal, Beadruby, and Plantain. And thereby drink of it.

The name "Solidago" did not appear until the sixteenth century. Derived from the Latin word *solidare* ("to join"), it was a collective name for different wound herbs like Sanicle (*Sanicula europaea*), Plantain (*Plantago* spp.), and Twoleaf Beadruby (*Maianthemum bifolium*). Yet another Latin name was *Virga aurea* ("golden rod") because of the plant's long, golden yellow panicle of flowers. Hieronymus Bock complained of this diversity of names in his 1577 herbal. "Christen it as you may, it is still a noble wound herb!" he said. Finally, for us at least, two hundred years later Swedish botanist Carl von Linné (Carolus Linnaeus) established a system of nomenclature that we still use for plants. To Goldenrod he assigned *Solidago* as the genus name and *virga-aurea* as the species name.

Over the course of time, Goldenrod's principal area of application has shifted. The old herbals mention the plant's effect on kidneys and bladder as an aside. However, the German physician Johann Rademacher brought new attention to her great effectiveness as a kidney remedy. In his book *Empirical Medicine* (1937) he describes numerous cases of severe kidney diseases healed with Goldenrod. "This herb is quite an old and beneficial kidney remedy . . . It can restore normal function to diseased kidneys . . . For a long time I have used Goldenrod and have only positive things to say about it."

Today's naturopathic medicine still favors Goldenrod as one of the best kidney remedies. Dr. Rademacher pointed out that the Goldenrod tea available in Germany's herbal pharmacies was often altered with what he called "false" Goldenrod and urged the use of only "true" Goldenrod in the treatment of patients. Indeed, of the several species of Goldenrod native to Germany, he recommended that only *Solidago virgaurea* be used medicinally.

This has become a controversial issue because some healer-authors attribute the same or even higher medicinal qualities to certain "false" Goldenrods. I personally stick to the proved true Goldenrod for my teas and other kidney preparations, meanwhile growing other varieties in my garden for aesthetic purposes. To avoid contributing to the general confusion, I will describe the Goldenrod species because they are easily distinguished, none are poisonous, and I do not wish to deny the medicinal value of any Goldenrods. (In fact, my American readers will find it interesting to note that of the more than 80 species of Goldenrod, all but one can be found in North America.)

Seasonally, Goldenrod flowers from midsummer to late summer. At that time of year she adorns with radiant yellow her favorite habitats —open and dry woodlands, forest fringes, sandy dunes, and clearings. It seems as if the sun's full energy concentrates in their saturated yellow before Nature's vivid hues fade with the approach of fall and winter.

I remember picking bouquets of yellow Goldenrods on many a hot alpine summer's day. Conditions sufficient for her needs are nearly everywhere. I often find her in wastelands, along railway embankments, and on slopes where her fine root fibers protect the soil from eroding.

From her knotty root supplied with many side roots, the stem of European Goldenrod (*Solidago vigaurea*) rises 8 to 12 inches, and sometimes even three feet. Examine the stem closely, carefully feeling how it is firm, fine, and furrowed to the touch. It may be either slightly hairy or completely smooth. Narrower at the top, the elliptic or lanceolate leaves sit opposite each other and are serrated with a winged stalk. Further up, the stem branches out to hold the many golden yellow flowers that form a long, clustered raceme. The flowers develop from the bottom, then up along the stem. Looking inside the yellow flower heads, we find different shapes. In arrangement, they resemble the Arnica flower we met in an earlier chapter. The long ligulate ray flowers along the edge are all female. They surround a number of five-pointed bisexual disk flowers whose anthers, merged into a tube, stretch far up. (If you carry a magnifying glass with you, now is a good time to dig it out.) With very fine hairs, the pistil brushes out the pollen. Later, the side styles spread themselves wide to allow the pollen to fall inside.

Although Goldenrod's flowers have a pleasantly sweet and aromatic scent, the tea made from them is bitter and tart. Nevertheless, the numerous guests of the flowers—bees, butterflies, and flies—find sweet nectar at the base of her petals. When summer and fall are over, the golden flowers are transformed into fine, grayish white tufts of hairs. From the wilted flower springs a bushy crown of hairs called a pappur. Like tiny parachutes, these devices for flight carry the small fruits of the plant away with the wind. Withered, the plants remain visible long into winter when our alpine snows finally bend their stems.

For my ancestors, a Goldenrod was the species I have just described. Only in the last century were additional species introduced into Germany from the Western Hemisphere. In these instances, a few plant lovers who grew fond of the handsome Goldenrod species of North America brought them home to cultivate in their own gardens as decorative plants. The wind carried the seeds of the garden plants far across the land that was open and accessible to the new Goldenrod varieties. These so-called "false" Goldenrods have run wild and conquered all of Europe.

Reaching five feet in height, Giant Goldenrod bears the impressive name *Solidago gigantea*. Her stem is completely smooth and her leaves are conspicuously pointed. Higher up, the stem divides into many flower panicles, making this species bushier than her German cousin. Also called "Late Goldenrod," her flowers do not open until August, a month later than the original native European plant.

Canadian Goldenrod (*S. canadensis*) can grow even taller. Specimens of six and a half feet have been found! Her firm, erect stem is hairy from top to bottom and, like Giant Goldenrod, branches out into many protruding panicles of flowers at its terminal end. Although more numerous, her flowers are much smaller than those of the European Goldenrod. A closer look

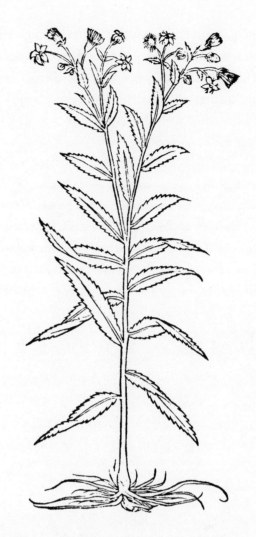

reveals yet another difference in the flowers—the ligulate ray flowers of true Goldenrod are clearly longer than the bracts of Canadian Goldenrod.

Native Americans used this plant to heal various illnesses. They applied the crushed flowers and leaves to bites and stings of various insects. Goldenrod, in fact, is one of the ingredients of old remedial preparations for treating rattlesnake bites. The Zuni Indians also chewed the flowers when they had sore throats.

A strongly scented species, Fragrant Goldenrod (*S. odorata*) has long been used in North America as a stimulating, perspiration-increasing remedy. This is the species so well known to hayfever suffers! This Goldenrod truly enriches our native flora, and while I am not allergic to it, many readers who suffer from this malady will not be thrilled to hear that its pollen is a main trigger for hayfever.

The greatest healing properties belong to the true Goldenrod (*Solidago virgaurea*). She is rarely cultivated commercially anymore and other species are usually offered as substitutes. However, if you have your own garden and are interested in the kidney-specific healing attributes of this plant, I urge you to cultivate it yourself.

HEALING PROPERTIES

I mentioned earlier that modern naturopathic medicine considers Goldenrod to be one of the best organ-specific kidney remedies. Like other herbal diuretics, it promotes the elimination of urine from the body, a process that can be useful in conditions like the following:

- when the body accumulates waste (as in diseases of the heart, liver, and kidneys)
- in inflammatory and chronic conditions of the kidneys, bladder, and urethra, and for kidney and bladder stones (in order to better flush out these organs)
- in metabolic diseases like rheumatism, gout, and skin diseases (in order to eliminate urea and toxic waste from the body)
- during a cleansing or weight-loss diet (in order to flush out broken-down toxic waste products)

Dr. R. F. Weiss (1974) subdivides diuretics according to their effect. Group One comprises plants with essential oils recognizable by their intense scent. Examples of this group are Juniper (*Juniperus* spp.) and garden herbs like Parsley (*Petroselinum sativa*) and Lovage (*Levisticum officinale*). Group Two contains diuretics whose effect derives from a high saponin content—for instance, Spiny Restharrow (*Ononis spinosa*), Field Horsetail (*Equisetum arvense*), Couch Grass (*Agropyron repens*), and European White Birch (*Betula pendula*). In Group Three we find Goldenrod along with Javatea (*Orthosiphon grandiflorus, O. stamineus*). The latter two plants not only have diuretic and anti-inflammatory qualities but specifically strengthen, heal, and regenerate the kidney tissue.

Goldenrod is used successfully for acute and chronic conditions of the kidneys; acute and inflammatory conditions of the bladder and kidneys; anuria (no urinary secretion) or reduced urinary secretion in the course of a kidney infection; the presence of protein in the urine; stones or gravel in the kidneys or bladder; as an additional means to flush out water in dropsy, rheumatism, gout, and metabolic disorders; and in Bright's disease (glomerulonephritis).

To make medicinal preparations with Goldenrod, it is best to gather them at the beginning of their flowering season in July and August. Cut off the top part of the plants a little below the bottom-most flowers. Tie them in bunches and hang them up to dry in a shady but airy place. (Note: Improperly dried plants will mold.) Plants for making tea should be picked fresh every year because they lose their diuretic quality after a year of storage. The herb, fresh or dried, can be used for a tea. A cold extract is more effective than an infusion made with boiling water. To do so, pour one cup of cold water over two teaspoons of the herb and let it stand overnight. In the morning, strain and drink the liquid. A daily dose is two to three cups.

The alcohol extract from the herb contains many constituents that some authors consider more effective than the tea. In former times it was popular to prescribe Goldenrod wine in cases of kidney stones and gravel. I have included recipes here for tincture and wine that you can prepare at home.

Javatea (*Orthosiphon grandiflorus, O. stamineus*) has an effect similar to Goldenrod's. However, it is a single-herb remedy for chronic diseases of the kidney; do not mix it with other herbs. Using two teaspoons of the herb per cup of water, prepare a cold extract as you do for Goldenrod. A daily dose is two to three cups.

The following list describes other medicinal herbs with diuretic properties. As with Javatea, you should only administer them as single herbs.

- Field Horsetail (*Equisetum arvense*) tea is administered for weakness of the bladder, skin diseases, and weakness of the connective tissue.
- Barberry (*Berberis vulgaris*) tea, juice, or marmalade affects the liver and gallbladder.
- White Birch / Silver Birch (*Betula pendula*) tea or juice is taken for rheumatism and skin diseases.
- Boldutree leaves (*Peumus boldus Molina*) tea is used for severe water retention.
- Borage (*Borago officinalis*) is a spice taken for the kidneys and bladder and while dieting.

- A tea of Common Burstwort (*Herniaria glabra*) and Bearberry leaves (*Arctostaphylos uva-ursi*) is administered for cases of acute cystitis.
- Stinging Nettle (*Urtica dioica/urens*) tea or juice promotes metabolism and affects the bladder, liver, and gallbladder.
- Stemless Carline Thistle (*Carlina acaulis*) tea affects the stomach and stimulates the kidneys and bladder.
- Dyer's Greenweed (*Genistra tintoria*) tea is taken for kidney gravel and water retention in diseases of the liver.
- Spiny Restharrow (*Ononis spinosa*) tea from the root is taken for water retention and skin impurities.
- Salad Chervil (*Anthriscus cerefolium*) is a spice used for the bladder and kidneys and while dieting.
- Garden Lovage (*Levisticum officinale*) is a spice that strengthens the stomach and stimulates the sexual organs, bladder, and kidneys.
- Horseradish (*Armoracia lapathifolia*) is a spice that strengthens the stomach (with lack of appetite) and affects the bladder and kidneys.
- Corn stigmata (*Zea Mays*) tea is administered in weight loss programs and for flushing out the system.
- Common Garden Parsley (*Petroselinum hortense*) is a spice that stimulates the uterus and affects weak menstrual flow, the bladder, and the kidneys.
- Garden Celery (*Apium graveolens*) is a vegetable for special diets and for the bladder and kidneys.

- Asparagus (*Asparagus officinalis*) is a vegetable for special diets and for the bladder and kidneys.
- Common Juniper (*Juniperus communis*) is taken for blood cleansing and the kidneys.
- Garden Onion (*Allium cepa*) strengthens the stomach and has a slight diuretic effect.

For the first-aid treatment of wounds, you can apply freshly crushed Goldenrod leaves. You can also make a strong tea from the herb to use in compresses or to cleanse wounds. From time immemorial Goldenrod has been used as a gargle for sore throats. For this purpose: combine equal parts of Goldenrod and Selfheal (*Prunella vulgaris*). Pour one cup of boiling water over two heaping teaspoons of the mixture and let it steep for 10 minutes. Strain the liquid to use as a gargle. On a final note, for a sore throat while travelling, you can chew the fresh flowers and swallow the fresh juice as Native Americans do.

Goldenrod is available in herb stores as "Herba Solidaginis." The homeopathic mother tincture "Solidago Virga aurea" is prepared from the fresh flowers.

Goldenrod Kidney Tea

2 parts goldenrod herb
(*Solidago virgaurea*)
2 parts birch leaves
(*Betula pendula*)
1 part spiny restharrow root
(*Ononis spinosa*)
1 part meadowsweet herb
(*Filipendula ulmaria*)

Use 1 heaping teaspoon of the mixture to make an infusion. Drink 2 to 3 cups daily.

Goldenrod Tincture

Fill a dark mason jar with freshly cut goldenrod herb. Pour in a 70% alcohol (like a grain spirit or fruit liqueur) to cover, close the jar tightly, and let the mixture steep in a dark, warm place for 2 or 3 weeks. Shake it occasionally. Strain the tincture into dropper bottles. A daily dose is 20 drops taken 3 times daily.

Goldenrod Wine

Fill a mason jar halfway with freshly cut goldenrod herb. Top it off with a liter of good white wine, close the jar, and let the mixture steep for 2 or 3 weeks in a dark, warm place. Strain the wine into another bottle. Drink 2 to 3 snifters daily.

Tea Blend for Bladder Infection

15 grams European goldenrod herb
(*Solidago virgaurea*)
15 grams rosemary leaves
(*Rosmarinus officinalis*)
15 grams rosehips (*Fructus Cynosbatum*, pharm.; *Rosa canina*, botan.)
10 grams white willow bark
(*Salix alba*)
10 grams common nasturtium flowers
(*Tropaeolum majus*)
10 grams common burstwort herb
(*Herniaria glabra*)

5 grams boldutree leaves
(*Peumus boldus Molina*)
5 grams short buchu leaves
(*Barosma betulina*)
5 grams purple echinacea root
(*Echinacea purpurea*)

Combine the herbs and store them in a tightly lidded container. To prepare a tea, pour 2 cups boiling water over 1 tablespoon herb mixture. Let it steep for 5 minutes before straining it. Drink several cups daily.

ᴤᴀ A Rheumatism Tea for Flushing Out Waste Products

goldenrod herb (*Solidago virgaurea*)
stinging nettle herb (*Urtica dioica/urens*)
white birch leaves (*Betula pendula*)
white willow bark (*Salix alba*)

Mix the herbs in equal parts and store the mixture in a tightly lidded container. To prepare a tea, pour 1 cup boiling water over 2 teaspoons herbal mixture. Steep, strain, and drink.

Veterinary Medicine

Goldenrod is also used to treat kidney diseases in animals. In such cases, we administer the tea or add the herb to the affected animal's fodder. Historically, the herb was used to treat wounds. For example, Hieronymus Bock reported using Goldenrod in 1577 to treat a horse that had been severely bitten by a wolf. For first-aid treatments, apply freshly crushed leaves and flowers to the wound.

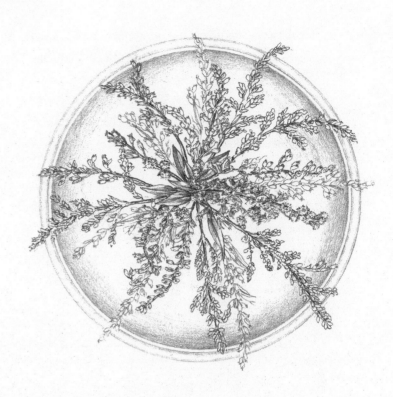

Cultivation

Goldenrod—European as well as Canadian—can be bought as seeds or as plants. It proliferates quickly and soon runs rampant, so be careful when cultivating it in a garden. It is a hardy shrub that is one of our most beautiful midsummer flowers. It goes well with tall, blue-flowering plants such as Larkspur (*Delphinium* spp.) or Aconite Monkshood (*Aconitum napellus*) and adds a sunny yellow to summer bouquets. It thrives everywhere but prefers dry, even sandy soils. Sometimes Goldenrod flowers into November. The seeds only germinate for a year. Sow them in March or April, later thinning them in June to a distance of 16 inches apart. Older plants are easily divided.

North American Goldenrod can grow everywhere although it flourishes more widely in the

Rocky Mountains and eastward. In Germany, several garden hybrids are available: "Goldfichte" ("Golden Spruce") has golden yellow flowers and grows to six feet; "Leraft" has butter yellow flowers and grows to 20 inches tall; and "Golden Gate" (called "Golden Mosa" in the United States) blooms a light yellow mimosa color and grows to three feet. Lastly, the shorter *Solidago virgaurea nana* is suitable for a rock garden. For more varieties, consult your local nursery or regional plant catalogs.

BOTANICAL CHARACTERISTICS

Name: *Solidago virgaurea* — Goldenrod

Distribution: Europe, the Americas, and Central Asia

Habitat: Dry woodlands, forest clearings, dunes, and waysides

Description: Grows 8 inches to 3 feet tall; erect, furrowed stem that branches only at the terminal end; leaves ovate to broad lanceolate, glabrous or sparsely hairy, roughly serrated (less so in the upper leaves); yellow flower heads in a dense, terminal panicle. Flowering time is July to October.

Confusion with similar plants: Other Goldenrod species (see text)

Collecting season: July to October

Active ingredients: Saponins, tannins, essential oil, flavonoid

Astrological association: Sun / Venus

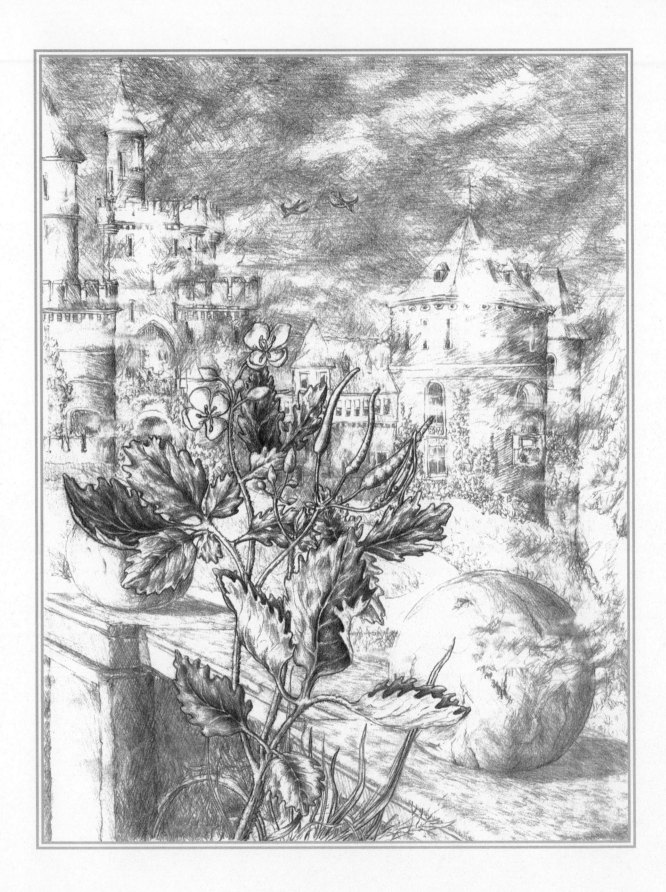

GREATER CELANDINE*

Chelidonium majus
Celandine
Chelidonium, Garden Celandine, Tetterwort
Poppy family — Papaveraceae

AN ACQUAINTANCE ONCE TOLD ME that he had given fresh juice of Greater Celandine to his wife—for her liver. My heart stood still. "Greater Celandine," it flashed through my head at lightning speed, "is a poisonous medicinal plant with immediate effect!" Like its cousin, the Opium Poppy, it contains toxic alkaloids, an overdose of which produces pain, a burning sensation throughout the entire gastro-intestinal tract, and severe bloody diarrhea with painful colic. Death is usually due to respiratory failure.

However, this person did not appear to be a grieving widower and so I inquired about the health of his spouse. She reportedly experienced a strong heat sensation in her stomach but now, having overcome the initial shock, she felt fine. Heaving a sigh of relief, I expressed amazement at this woman's tough constitution. It remains a puzzle to me how she could manage to swallow a whole glass of this caustic plant juice.

It seems that some people tolerate a medicinal overdose of Celandine without suffering harm.

Maurice Mességué reports a similar case in his *Dictionary of Medicinal Herbs*. While these two instances had happy endings, I still caution you against repeating the experiment on yourself or others. Greater Celandine is one of our strongest medicinal plants and must absolutely be administered in the proper dosage. Paracelsus' wisdom rings especially true here: Only the dose makes a poison. Used wisely, this "poisonous weed" becomes a valuable medicinal plant.

Physicians from many traditions have prescribed Greater Celandine as a dependable remedy. Paracelsus, the sixteenth century Swiss-born alchemist and physician, frequently administered it. Samuel Hahnemann, the founder of homeopathy, included it in his medicine chest. The great naturopathic physician C. W. Hufeland and his student Johann Rademacher relied on Greater Celandine for treating conditions of the liver, gallbladder, and spleen. Dr. Karl Daniel and pharmacist Dieter Schmaltz even wrote a book about the herb in 1939.

---

*Greater Celandine, or simply Celandine in some herbals, is not related to Lesser Celandine (*Ranunculus ficaria*), a healing plant in the Buttercup family.

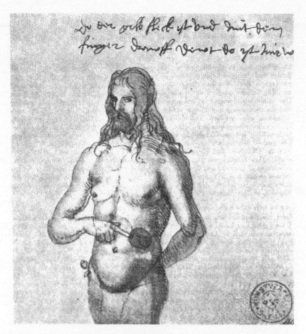

Perhaps the most famous patient to personally experience Celandine's effectiveness is Albrecht Dürer. Coming down with malaria on a journey, the Renaissance painter-engraver thereafter suffered from it chronically along with a spleen tumor and an enlarged liver. When he sent a self-portrait to his physician indicating the area of his pain, he was prescribed Celandine. Perhaps it was out of gratitude that Dürer later painted his beautiful image of this plant.

If you break a stem or leaf of Celandine, a bright yellow sap (latex) exudes from the ruptured area and changes to a dark orange when exposed to air. Caustic enough to dissolve warts and corns, we know today that its effect slows cell division and kills bacteria. The juice leaves colorfast orange stains on clothing and, in the past, was used to dye wool, fabrics, and even leather. When impregnated with alum and cream of tartar, wool takes on a bright orange hue. And Celandine juice tints wall paint beautifully. The most curious dye recipe—for hair, in this instance—is related by

Tabernaemontanus in his 1731 herbal. (Note: I have not tried this myself . . .)

> To make pretty yellow hair, take the root of Celandine and the root of Dyer's Madder, carefully cleansed and in equal proportions to your liking. Crush them into a fine powder and keep it. Then take a small cup full of Walnut oil, into which you put 1 *loth* [about 10 grams] each of fresh Celandine root and shavings of Boxwood, ½ loth of Roman cumin seed, 1 *guintlein* [equivalent unknown] of Saffron, and two spoons full of good white wine. Let these pieces boil together until the wine boils down, thereupon strain it through a cloth. With this oil, temper the aforementioned powder to make a pomade and smear or rub it well into the hair. Let it remain for a day and a night, and in the morning wash the head with suds made from Kölkraut stems, Ash, and Barley chaff.

The fresh juice of Celandine reminded the old herbalists of the bile in the human gallbladder. Similar in color, they were both caustic with a pungent and bitter taste. The golden yellow flowers likewise seemed to indicate that this was a plant with influence over the liver, gallbladder, and spleen. Paracelsus prescribed Celandine for diseases of the liver and gallbladder. He pointed to the plant's signs—or "signature," interpreting outer characteristics (shape, color, and taste) as well as internal properties (radiance and gesture). Only a person recognizing both levels could properly apply his Doctrine of Signatures, a theory developed by Paracelsus that incorporated his strong belief that God had placed all plants on Earth to benefit humankind. With the passage of time, however, fewer and fewer people were able to read a plant's inner signs and the system became confused and meaningless.

Secrets still surround Celandine. Some of the old names, stories, and legends take up the thread that broke long ago and spin it further. There are tales of the legendary "Goldherb" or "Goldwort" with whose aid one could make gold. Many sought this miracle plant and a lucky few found it. It was even told that a golden-haired fairy named Celandine led seekers to where the Goldherb grew.

We know that alchemists used plants who radiated the energy of certain planets in a particularly pure form. In Celandine they recognized the Sun's energy, and since gold was dedicated to this orb as well, it is said that they manufactured gold from it.

With roots dating back to ancient Egypt, alchemy is considered the forerunner of modern chemistry. Among other inventions and processes, it has given us porcelain and the production of phosphorus. Little is known about the alchemic medicine called spagyric that survives today except that it proves to be good medicine in the hands of natural healers. To treat disease, alchemists sought the pure essence of plants to use in the form of a "plant stone" or spagyric remedy. There are still companies that manufacture these remedies according to the old recipes in which plants grown in the wild are submitted to a process of fermentation and distillation. Their residues are dried, burnt into ash, and dissolved in the distillate. [Interested readers can peruse *Paracelsus: Essential Readings* by Nicholas Goodrick-Clarke, a Thoth Publications reprint.–Ed.]

The alchemists' regard for Celandine is expressed in the name they gave it—*Coelidonum* or "Heaven's Gift." They gathered the plants to prepare at their respective planetary hours. Accordingly, Celandine was picked when the solar energy in this sun-herb was especially effective: "At the noon hour, when the Sun is in Leo and the Moon is in Aries, we gather the Heaven's Gift."

We find Celandine in many old folk customs as a symbol of a peaceful, well-balanced life. Aggressive people, it was said, became calmer, their hatred and quarreling lessened, when they wore amulets of Celandine root. It is interesting that choleric, "gall-type" individuals tend toward emotional imbalances, venting consternation at an instant's notice, angered by anything and by anybody. (In German we say "their gall overflows.") Such people were urged to wear the amulets and allow the plant to bring the Sun into their hearts, freeing their spirits of melancholy and sadness. It was thought that Celandine directly brought the Sun into the liver and gall-bladder, both affecting the organs and calming the nervous system. With its fleshy, lobed, placidly scalloped leaves of strong growth power, it was considered a plant of vegetative energy, of the liver and gallbladder, bringing light and harmony into the metabolic process with its yellow juice and sunny flowers.

As do other plants, Celandine has a special connection to a particular creature of Nature. It is long remembered that the swallows showed humankind its effectiveness as a remedy for the eyes. From the writings of the Salerno school:

Celandine is healthy for the eyes,
as the swallows tell us.

The earliest account of Celandine and the swallows is credited to Aristotle in 350 B.C. The

Greek philosopher claimed that some blinded baby swallows were healed by their mothers with fresh Celandine. This story is still related in a passage from the herbal of Hieronymus Bock:

> To bitter Celandine have the swallows brought a good name because with mashed Celandine juice they wet the eyes of their young open again.

In the old herbals, introductions to the plant are usually followed with a thorough description of how to administer Celandine for curing problems like cataracts, glaucoma, night blindness, or conjunctivitis. For a long time it was considered

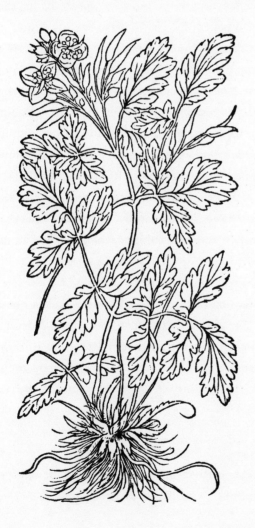

a panacea for eye diseases although I have never met anyone who observed these results. Regardless, I have planted Greater Celandine along a wall in my garden and will keep an eye on our barn swallows!

The story of Celandine and the swallows is often found in religious imagery as a healing symbol for "spiritual blindness." Since antiquity, Celandine and the swallows have shared historical significance. The swallow was called the "bird of light" and much later considered a symbol of Christ and the Resurrection. Swallows love the company of people and like to nest in stables and barns. Celandine, too, prefers our proximity and regularly follows human settlements. Along with Elder, Plantain, and Stinging Nettle it appears wherever humans dwell, even holding its post long after we abandon a place. Heinrich Marzell cites such an incident in his book *Unsere Heilpflanzen* ("Our Medicinal Plants"):

> This plant's occurrence in the middle of a forest is an odd phenomenon. But its appearance in the forest between Oppertshofen and Mauren (near Donauwörth in Swabia) was soon explained when, at the same spot at a depth of three to six feet, the walls of a Roman building were discovered. This attracted the interest of archeologists for several years.

In Europe, Celandine seems to prefer castles and old fortresses around whose walls you surely will find a few plants. When Peter Ebenhoch, this book's illustrator, was preparing to draw Celandine, he could not locate a single one in his area. I suggested that he visit an old fortress— and, indeed, there he found the desired herb in abundance. Likewise I recommend to readers who would get acquainted with Celandine in the wild to visit a castle—or the ruins of one—and look for a plant with bright yellow flowers growing near the walls.

Once the first snow melts, as early as January or February, Celandine puts forth from its root a light green leaf rosette. From that develops a plant that may later grow 18 inches high. The tender foliage resembles the lobed leaves of the Oak tree. The little known Gold Saxifrage (*Chrysosplenium alternifolium*) reminds us of Greater Celandine in its leaf shape and color. All three belong to the few plants that directly affect the spleen. However, in contrast to the leathery feel of Oak leaves, those of Celandine and Gold Saxifrage are soft, cool, and slightly fleshy to the touch.

Celandine's leaves are a gold-green hue on top with a glint of pale blue underneath. As the main stem rises, it branches out several times. Atop the juicy leaves sit the golden yellow, four-pointed, star-like flowers in loose umbels in pairs or in groups of up to six flowers. They appear so tender and fragile that the plant, as if to protect this treasure, bends the flowering stems at night and during a rainfall. As one flower wilts, a new one appears. From April to September we watch Celandine bloom continually until finally the last flowers are transformed into long, thin seedpods pointing straight up. Their small, black seeds are very oily and have fleshy white appendages inside that are a delicacy for the ants who carry them off, eating the white flesh and discarding the seeds. This is why Celandine flourishes in the most unusual places—in the hollows or forked branches of trees or in the cracks of a stone wall or high on a ruined tower.

HEALING PROPERTIES

Greater Celandine contains a number of alkaloids, bitter compounds, and flavons. Its effects are mostly attributed to the ten different alkaloids that have been identified in its latex. Similar to but much weaker than those of its cousin, the Opium Poppy (*Papaver somniferum*), Celandine's alkaloids act as mild sedatives and antispasmodics throughout the central nervous system. At the same time, Celandine promotes the emptying of the gallbladder by increasing the secretion of gall, kills bacterias, dissolves uric acid, slows cell division, and irritates the skin.

Celandine is poisonous in large quantities. Remedies prepared—particularly from the root —must be dosed carefully because the root holds a higher content of alkaloids than does the herb. The fresh juice can cause inflammation and allergic reactions in skin-sensitive people. To avoid a rash, wear rubber gloves when gathering it.

Modern natural medicine utilizes Celandine mostly as a liver and gallbladder remedy, a practice with a long tradition. It was already known that Dioscurides in the first century A.D. suggested drinking juice from the root mixed with Anise and wine for jaundice. The use of Celandine remains in today's folk medicine where, for example, people suffering from liver disease sometime are given omelets containing fresh Celandine leaves. Our respected, conventional physicians, however, have long forgotten Celandine. Only the physician Johann Gottfried Rademacher, a student of Hufeland and the poet Goethe's doctor, returned its well-deserved esteem.

Rademacher observed that with this herb he could heal jaundice in one-third the time usually required for remedies then commonly administered. But the challenge—and hence the cure—was in knowing the correct dosage. For a beneficial effect, he said, one must not be overly generous with it. As evidence, he cites the following case in the first volume of *Empirical Medicine* (1848):

> Once a man of common status from the Rhine came to see me, suffering from an advanced case of jaundice. Upon my inquiring if he had used any medicine, he answered, "Only a household remedy, namely the juice of Celandine, a thimble full four times a day." But his affliction grew worse rather than better. In two weeks his previous light yellow skin tone changed to dark yellow. In addition, the tension in his upper abdomen had increased so much that he did not trust the affair any longer and therefore desired my help. I gave an ounce* of tincture of Celandine to this man and had him take 15 drops five times a day. When he finished the ounce, he came to me once again. I heard from him that the free flow of gall into the intestinal tract had been restored because, according to his testimony, his excrement was brown again. I now gave him another ounce of the tincture with the instruction to use it only four times a day until the yellow color of his skin completely disappeared. This occurred without further difficulty.

This particular case shows that the wrong dose of a plant can produce exactly the disease that it can cure when administered properly. Rademacher's dosage for chronic liver disease is two to three drops of the tincture four to five times daily. He even describes the preparation of Celandine tincture, or what he calls "Tinctura Chelidonii:"

> Take fresh, flowering Celandine herb in any desired quantity. Crush it with a stone mortar, press it thoroughly, and mix the resulting juice in equal parts with highly distilled wine spirits [90% alcohol]. To extract the soluble parts of the drug, let it steep for several days, shaking it occasionally. Finally, strain the liquid through a fine cloth [or coffee filter].

This tincture relieves conditions such as inflammation of the gallbladder (cholecystitis), gallstones (cholelithiasis), discomfort after gallbladder surgery, and inflammation of the bile duct. Its antispasmodic properties are especially helpful for cramping gallbladder conditions that tend toward colic. It is also used for liver conditions such as an enlarged liver and jaundice, especially with severe yellow pigmentation (icterus) of the skin and the whites of the eye (sclera).

Important Note: Celandine's application for serious diseases of the liver and gallbladder should always be under the supervision of a naturopathic or allopathic physician.

The following is a list of other liver and gallbladder herbs that the reader may wish to investigate:

- Globe Artichoke (*Cynara scolymus*) for the liver.
- Running Pine (*Lycopodium clavatum*) for the liver.
- Barberry (*Berberis vulgaris*) for the liver and kidneys.

---

*A German ounce is about 31 grams; an American ounce is 28 grams.

- Surinam Quassia (*Quassia amara*) for the liver and dropsy.
- Boldutree leaves (*Peumus boldus Molina*) to stimulate the liver, gallbladder, bladder, and kidneys.
- Glossy Buckthorn bark (*Rhamnus frangula*) for the gallbladder and constipation.
- Turmeric (*Curcuma longa*) for the liver, and as a culinary spice for rice, eggs, and sauces.
- Hemp Agrimony (*Eupatorium cannabinum*) for the liver, spleen, and gallbladder.
- Yellow Bedstraw (*Galium verum*) for the liver, stomach, and gastroenteritis.
- Dandelion (*Taraxacum officinale*) for the liver, gallbladder, kidney, and pancreas.
- Milkthistle (*Silybum marianum*) for the liver, and to stimulate the endocrine system especially in women.
- Agrimony (*Agrimonia eupatoria*) for the liver and to stimulate the stomach.
- Peppermint (*Mentha piperita*) for the gallbladder and stomach.
- Black Radish (*Raphanus sativus var. niger*) for the liver, gallbladder, and as vegetable, salad, or fresh juice.
- Saffron (*Crocus sativus*) to alleviate cramping of the liver and gallbladder, and as a culinary spice for rice, egg dishes, white sauces, and desserts.
- Chicory (*Cichorium intybus*) for the liver, gallbladder, and spleen.

While it lacks the potency of the tincture or fresh juice, one can use the dried Celandine herb for tea. However, Celandine must be dried very carefully—if necessary, in an oven. It is best to gather the flowering plants on a sunny day around noon—and definitely not in the early morning when the plants are still wet with dew and more difficult to dry.

Greater Celandine is available in natural food stores or herbal pharmacies as "Herba Chelidonii" (the whole herb), "Radix Chelidonii" (the root), and "Tinctura Chelidonii Rademacheri" (Rademacher's tincture). The homeopathic mother tincture "Chelidonium" is prepared from the fresh root.

CELANDINE TEA

Pour 1 cup of boiling water over 1 rounded teaspoon of the crushed, dried herb. Let it steep for 5 minutes before straining it. A daily dose is 1 to 2 cups.

LIVER TEA

10 grams greater celandine:
Herba Chelidonii
(*Chelidonium majus*)
10 grams chicory root:
Radix Cichorii (*Cichorium intybus*)
15 grams milkthistle seed:
Fructus Cardui Marianae
(*Carduus marianus*)
15 grams dandelion herb and root:
Radix Taraxaci cum Herba
(*Taraxacum officinale*)
10 grams fumitory herb:
Herba Fumariae
(*Fumaria officinalis*)
10 grams boldutree leaves:
Folia Boldo (*Peumus boldus Molina*)

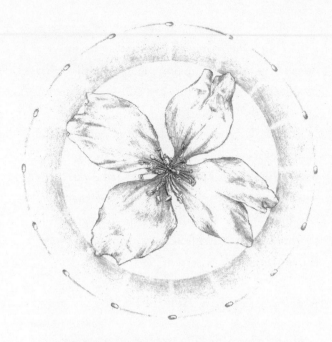

Celandine mixes well with these other liver and gallbladder herbs (for which I list both the pharmacological and botanical names).

Prepare the mixture and store it in a dry place. Pour 1 cup of boiling water over 1 teaspoon of the tea blend, let it steep, and then strain. Drink 2 to 3 cups daily.

❧ CELANDINE FOR WARTS AND CORNS

Celandine is an old folk remedy for getting rid of warts. For this purpose, apply the fresh juice flowing from the sliced stem to warts or corns. Repeat this application daily, being careful that the caustic juice not touch the surrounding skin.

❧ CELANDINE AS AN ANTISPASMODIC

Celandine's alkaloids have an antispamodic effect on the smooth muscles of the biliary duct and the gastrointestinal tract. Therefore, it is prescribed for conditions of these areas that involve cramping. Only recently has the antispasmodic and calming effect of this herb on asthma been brought to our attention, and it is now being used for asthma attacks, spasmodic coughing, and chronic irritating cough. Its cramp-soothing effects are by way of the central nervous system.

❧ COUGH DROPS

20 grams tincture of greater celandine (*Chelidonium majus*)

20 grams tincture of round-leaved sundew (*Drosera rotundifolia*)

10 drops essential oil of thyme (*Thymus vulgaris*)

Combine these ingredients in a jar and shake it thoroughly.

For irritating and spasmodic cough, a course of treatment is 10 drops ingested several times daily accompanied by drinking a tea of burnet saxifrage (*Pimpinella saxifraga*).

CULTIVATION

Greater Celandine is available as seeds or starters. It makes few demands on the soil, growing even in gravelly soil. It prefers to live in a place adjacent to the house or next to a wall in a shady spot. Sow the seeds in spring, later thinning the seedlings to about eight inches apart. Ants will happily spread the seeds. As a hardy shrub, it will come back the following year.

BOTANICAL CHARACTERISTICS

Name: Chelidonium majus — Greater Celandine

Distribution: Northern and central Europe, Mediterranean countries, Asia, and North America

Habitat: Especially near inhabited places, hedges, dumps, deserted ruins, castles, and fortresses

Description: Growing 12 to 20 inches tall, the plant has round, multi-branched stems; stem and leaves are slightly hairy; lower leaves are pinnate, upper ones are divided and sinuately (wavy) crenate, gold-green on top and bluish underneath; golden yellow flowers with 4 petals are arranged on umbels of 2 to 6 flowers; seeds appear in long upright pods. Flowering time is from April to October.

Confusion with similar plants: None due to the characteristic orange sap found in all plant parts

Collecting season: Fresh flowering herb in July according to the astrological notation cited in the text (namely at noon on sunny days . . .)

Active ingredients: Alkaloids 0.1–1%, flavonoids, saponin, carotinoids, and bitter compounds

Astrological association: Sun / Jupiter

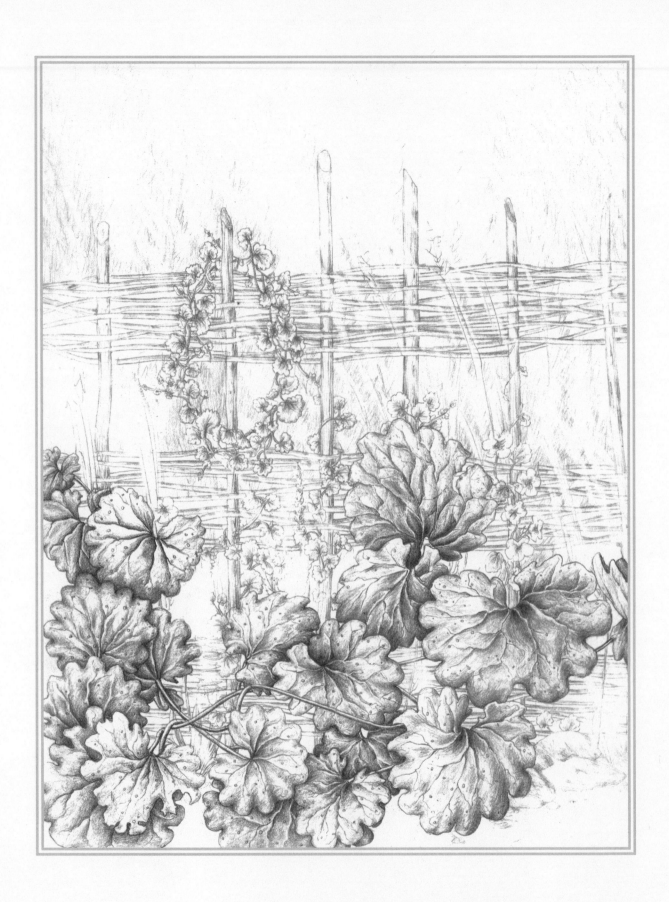

Ground Ivy

Glechoma hederacea (*Nepeta hederacea*)
Cat's Paw, Cat's Foot, Alehoof, Turnhoof, Gill-Go-by-Grounds,
Gill-Creep-by-Ground, Gill-Over-the-Ground, Gillrun, Hay-Maids, Hedge Maids
Mint family—Labiatae / Lamiaceae

THERE IS AN OLD GERMAN SAYING that a warm soup keeps body and soul together—especially one prepared from nine different kitchen herbs on Maundy Thursday.

It is not so long ago that people kept this custom of serving something green on the "Green Thursday" before Easter. Why that particular day? And why nine different herbs? The meaning has almost been lost over the course of time. To understand, we must return to when "Green Thursday Soup" still simmered in German stockpots. This ritual food was part of a communal meal as significant to my ancestors as the Holy Eucharist is to today's Christians. They believed that by partaking of Nature's life-giving, healing powers they entered into harmony with the gods. Eating this soup comprised of specific powerful herbs linked them to the good and sacred powers.

A primary ingredient in this powerful soup was Ground Ivy, another of the plants choosing to grow near human dwellings. In the olden days, people considered such plants to embody the favorable spirits of house and home who,

like good-natured elves, offered aid to people in times of need. On certain days connected to the cosmic powers these plants were thought to be especially strong and beneficial. Such a day, according to ancient wisdom, was Maundy Thursday. Others were feast days like the summer solstice (June 21st), the assumption of the Blessed Virgin (August 15th), and the birth of the Virgin Mary (September 8th).

Ground Ivy's name in German is *Gundermann*, which means "Pus Man." He is still addressed as a benevolent plant-elf and is thought to protect us from both harmful influences and consumptive diseases. He can heal serious wounds and give us strength in recovery. Ground Ivy was found in every Maundy Thursday soup. Our ancestors celebrated "Green Thursday" outside where Nature bestowed vigor and health after the long hard winter. People danced through the night in the forest wearing head wreaths of Ground Ivy to symbolize their connection with the gods and the power of nature. Once the priest uttered the blessing, everyone partook of this soup made with the strongest medicinal herbs of the season. When they arrived, the early Christians found this custom still very much alive in Germanic culture. They transformed the old tradition into *dies viridium*—the day of mercy when penitents were allowed to partake in the sacrament of Holy Communion again. This day also commemorated the Last Supper before the crucifixion of Jesus.

The mystery of the Green, the human experience of this divine energy—be it in the old or new religion—was summarized in the writings of the twelfth century German abbess, Hildegard von Bingen. Pagan and newer Christian outlooks as well as her personal experience and mystical vision come together in her words. Through them, we feel that people of all epochs have known the same divine forces. The abbess-healer wrote much about the power of the Green, calling it "a power from eternity, and this power is green." She spoke of the trust, hope, and ever-self-renewing forces that help all humankind.

> No tree will turn green without the force to be green. No rock lacks the green moisture. No living being is without this special innate force. Even living Eternity itself is not without the force to flourish and turn green.

People still desire to connect with this vital force. This is because those who unite with it no longer fear death knowing that Life eternally renews itself.

Today's herbal lore surrounding Ground Ivy and "Green Thursday soup" contains only a fraction of the original meaning. Tracking elements of this old rite of spring and renewal, we might wonder what became of the garlands woven from the plant's long, pliable stems

(knowing that in some regions Ground Ivy is still called "Wreath Herb" or "Earth Wreath"). In the Middle Ages people still connected Ground Ivy to the pagan nocturnal feast and dance of May Night (also called May Day Eve, the Germanic *Walpurgisnacht*, the Celtic Beltane)—in Germanic folklore, the night when all witches meet to dance and feast on a mountain called the *Brocken* as described in Goethe's "Faust." For centuries it was believed that a Ground Ivy wreath made at this time of year gave a person clairvoyance and the ability to recognize witches, as we learn in the following Saxon legend:

> Once upon a time, a maiden heard that a certain woman was a witch. To find out the truth, she made a wreath from Ground Ivy the Sunday after May Night, placed it on her head, and went to church. She was the first in and the first out and saw how the woman she suspected and many other village women rode out of the church on brooms and pokers. When the witches noticed the wreath of Ground Ivy she wore, they pounced upon it and beat it to shreds.

> from Heinrich Marzell's
> "Our Medicinal Plants"

The belief that Ground Ivy banished demons survived for a long time. One old spell even became a Christian blessing:

> Ground Ivy, I gather you
> In the name of Our Dear Lady
> and in the name of Our Lord Jesus Christ.

This particular blessing is in a manuscript dated 1617 from the abbey of Blasien. It was thought that Ground Ivy picked under such a benediction would protect one from evil and heal disease.

What a "milk spell" is we can hardly imagine. However, in the Middle Ages and well into modern times Ground Ivy was considered a magic charm for milk. If cows stopped giving milk, or if their milk was of poor quality and unsuitable for churning, then it was conceiveable that sorcery was the culprit. Ground Ivy protected against such. Countless milk spells have been preserved and recorded. This one is from a twelfth century Reichenau manuscript:

> When someone steals the milk, sprinkle holy water in the stable. Then take Ground Ivy, Duckweed, and salt and recite:
>
> > "Today I give you Ground Ivy, Duckweed, and salt,
> > Rise up through the clouds
> > And bring me lard and milk and whey."

To protect cows from enchantment when they were driven out to summer pasture, it was customary in many regions to do the first milking through a Ground Ivy wreath.

For ancient Germans, milk was a special and powerful panacea. It was the preferred medium to absorb a plant's healing properties and transmit them to those in need. Medicinal herbs were cooked in milk, and to this day a milk decoction remains the recommended method of preparation for certain plants like Silverweed (*Potentilla anserina*). My ancestors probably cooked Ground Ivy and other herbs in milk for their ritual meals—after all, the centuries-old milk magic is a primordial custom.

Ground Ivy was not only supposed to protect from evil but also to heal and strengthen the body. The kinds of diseases the "Pus Man" could cure has been preserved in his name. Purulent or pus-producing diseases linger and are notoriously difficult to heal. Ground Ivy was administered to wounds and diseases with purulent discharge or sputum, a custom still practiced in contemporary natural medicine.

Maundy Thursday is an especially auspicious day in the cycle of seasons still found in the weather rules of the German "Farmer's Almanac." Certain plants sown at this favorable time are said to grow strong and free from pests. Traditionally, Maundy Thursday soup contained nine different herbs. Nine, a number sacred to all cultures, was dedicated to the Mother Goddess, bestower and protector of new life. In "nine" the new is hidden; in "nine" one cycle ends and another begins. In many old religious rites this number connects people with the power of renewal. On Maundy Thursday, the first day of the annual seasonal cycle, people greeted the approaching spring. It was when they united with the awakening life-giving energies of Mother Earth through a celebratory ritual and the "soup of nine herbs." I am certain that the German expression "Ach du grüne Neune" ("Oh, you green Nine") reflects the nine herbs of the Maundy Thursday soup.

The nine herbs are long forgotten, although we can make some pretty good guesses. We know there was a good portion of Ground Ivy and, surely, the remaining eight herbs were among those plants who stretched early shoots toward the sun by Maundy Thursday. These might include Stinging Nettle, Ribwort Plantain, Daisy, Chickweed, Good-King-Henry, or Alpine Dock. Others might be those that, at the start of spring, we discover in the garden or around the house—small plants that would make a nourishing spring soup like Chervil, Yarrow, Beccabunga Speedwell, Dandelion, and Ramsons.

Many people had special recipes they touted for their Maundy Thursday soup. Naturalist Alexander von Humboldt swore so much by his spring soup that he prepared it daily every spring for several weeks. His particular pot herbs were Ground Ivy, Yarrow, Watercress, Plantain, and Daisy.

After this lengthy excursion into the magical history of a soup I urge my readers to acquire such a taste. This is because the herbs used in this savory green soup cleanse and strengthen the human organism when fatigue results from the changing seasons. Our bodies subsequently require some "green" stimulation, a need that

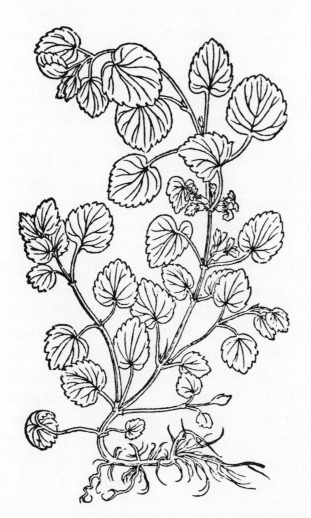

we should try to satisfy several times in early spring.

I have a personal story about Ground Ivy. Some years ago Franz Waldner related to me some plant lore from his Tyrolean homeland in the Siegerland. It included a so-called "Miracle Leaf" that I did not recognize as Ground Ivy until he showed it to me outdoors. "With the sun's help," he said, "you can make an oil from Miracle Leaf that heals severe wounds. I work at a blast furnace where burns are often deep, dangerous, and difficult to heal. However, the oil from this plant truly helps." Last year I remembered his words when I suffered a dog bite that became purulent. Snow still hid the Ground Ivy around my house because it winters over with only a few short stems and leaves. So Franz mailed me a vial of Miracle Leaf oil with which I dressed my wounds—and soon they healed well and fast.

Following a lot of construction work around our house, the ground was so disturbed that my usual Ground Ivy failed to reestablish itself. (This is why I sought in vain last winter for some.) Oddly enough, the following spring revealed an abundance of small Ground Ivy plants appearing all over my garden, and at summer's end many long, trailing vines covered the ground. I already have a few jars of fresh Ground Ivy leaves sitting atop the garden wall so that the sun can extract the healing oil. Sometimes one only has to wish for something!

HEALING PROPERTIES

Today we know that Ground Ivy's medicinal benefits are based primarily on its content of tannins, bitter compounds, and essential oil. It has anti-inflammatory, analgesic, and astringent properties; it expels phlegm, stimulates the bladder and kidneys, and stimulates and regulates the body's metabolism.

The old traditional indications have proved right again and again—Ground Ivy aids lingering diseases; conditions of chronic waste, rot, and purulent discharge; and chronic metabolic diseases. It is prescribed as an adjunct tonic for scrofula (especially in children), for purulent bronchial conditions with a disposition toward tuberculosis, for pus in the urine, for bladder and kidney diseases, for chronic rhinitis and cough, and for lung congestion. Ground Ivy can help where pus develops in the body or where a lingering metabolic disease exists.

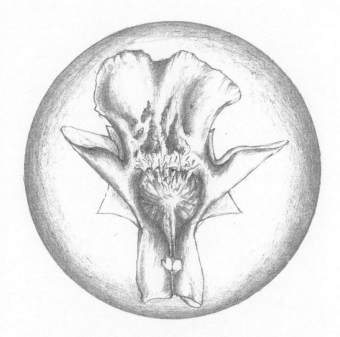

Best used fresh, Ground Ivy leaves fortunately are available year-round. For remedial preparations, juice the freshly gathered leaves and mix the juice with buttermilk in equal parts. A child's dose is one tablespoon taken three times a day. Adults can take three tablespoons three times a day. As an adjunct and follow-up treatment for tuberculosis, I recommend mixing Ground Ivy juice with goat's milk.

For a Ground Ivy tincture, mix freshly pressed juice in equal parts with 90 proof wine spirits. Let it steep for three weeks before straining it into dropper bottles. An adult dose is 30 drops taken 3 times a day; for children, it is 15 drops three times a day.

For treating purulent wounds, scars, eczemas, and injuries, the oil from the trees is best. (Rub the leaves between your fingers and you can feel that they contain oil.)

Traditionally, Ground Ivy is added to bath water to refresh the body's muscles and joints. It also strengthens the nerves and aids bladder and kidney conditions and pains related to rheumatism and gout. I boil five handfuls of Ground Ivy herb, fresh or dried, in five liters of water, straining it before adding to the bath water. For partial baths, use a smaller amount.

Ground Ivy tea is available in herb stores as "Herba Hederae terrestris" or "Herba Glechomae." The homeopathic mother tincture "Glechoma hederacea" is made from the fresh plant.

❧ Miracle Leaf Oil

Gather fresh ground ivy leaves in June and July. Wipe off any dirt without washing them. Fill a mason jar a third full with tightly packed leaves and place it in the sun where, after a few days, at the bottom a light-colored liquid will collect. This should be carefully strained into a dark glass vial and stored in a cool place. When needed, spread the oil on wounds several times a day.

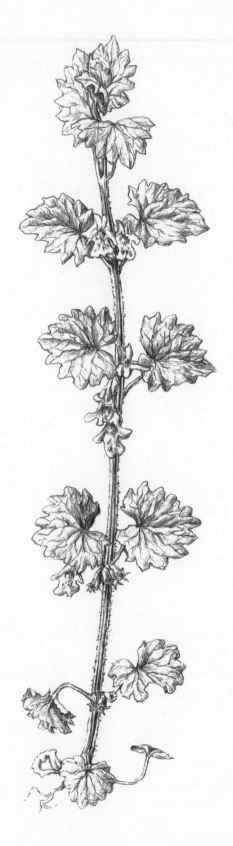

VETERINARY MEDICINE

Although Ground Ivy is not poisonous to people, it is toxic to many animals—especially horses. The bitter compound glechomin is supposedly responsible for most of this toxicity. According to Dr. Otto Gessner's "Poisonous and Medicinal Plants of Central Europe" (*Die Gift- und Arzneipflanzen von Mitteleuropa*, 1953), symptoms of such poisoning in horses include spreading limbs, rattled breathing, sweating, salivation, and circulatory problems. Miracle Leaf oil, however, can be administered externally to all animals to treat purulent wounds and eczemas.

CULINARY USE

As a culinary herb, Ground Ivy gives off an aromatic scent and flavor. In the past it was known as "Wild Parsley" because of its similar use. Ground Ivy can be gathered year-round. It is abundant in vitamin C and, fresh or dried, can be used to flavor salads, vegetables, soups, casseroles, and herb butter. Its acrid taste makes it ill-suited as a single vegetable although an herbal soup turns quite flavorful with its addition. It works especially well in bean or pea soups.

For a spring soup: mix Ground Ivy with other spring herbs like Daisy, Sorrel, Saltbush, Plantain, Chervil, Coltsfoot, and Lady's Mantle. Mince the herbs, sauté them with onion, and simmer them briefly in a vegetable broth (thickened with a roux if desired). Serve garnished with toasted croutons.

❧ GUACAMOLE WITH WILD HERBS

2 ripe avocados

1 garlic clove, crushed

dried red pepper or freshly minced chilies

sea salt and paprika

a handful of minced herbs
   (watercress, chervil, and ground ivy)

Peel and mash the avocado with a fork (or lightly in a blender). Add the garlic, fresh herbs, and spices to taste. This zesty dip can be served on fresh lettuce leaves and is a good accompaniment to salads and sandwiches or as a crepe filling.

CULTIVATION

Ground Ivy is commercially available as starter plants. It propagates quickly, forming runners up to three feet long above the ground from which new plants originate. In addition, its seeds are spread by ants. It winters over with a few leaves and puts forth new ones in spring. Its beautiful kidney-shaped leaves can cover a lot of ground although Ground Ivy prefers to grow along a fence or a wall. It tolerates sun and shade alike and makes a good ground cover around trees. In a moist, nutrient-rich habitat it thrives; in dry soil, it remains small. I hang Ground Ivy in a basket in front of my window inside the house where its fragile-looking branches cascade over the rim.

BOTANICAL CHARACTERISTICS

Name: *Glechoma hederacea* — Ground Ivy

Distribution: Europe, Asia, North America

Habitat: Walls, fences, wet meadows, open deciduous forests or clearings

Description: Ground Ivy creeps along the ground like Ivy. During its flowering time, individual erect stems hold noticeably smaller leaves. The square stem can reach to 3 feet in length, supporting buds that lay on the ground and fine roots where new leaf stalks originate. Leaves are crosswise opposite; the leaf stalk has a delicate furrow; the leaves are reniform (kidney-shaped) to cordate (heart-shaped) with a crenate margin covered with fine white hairs that give off an aromatic scent when rubbed. Blue-violet flowers grow in the leaf axils of apparent whorls.

Confusion with similar plants: With Speedwell (*Veronica officinalis*; not poisonous) whose flower stalks are much branched, leaves are obovate (upside-down and egg-shaped) and finely serrated; flowers are not labiate (lip-shaped) but funnel-shaped, pale blue to white in color. Speedwell lacks Ground Ivy's aromatic scent.

Collecting season: March to June (but in winter if needed)

Active ingredients: Tannins, bitter compounds, essential oil, and vitamin C

Astrological association: Venus / Mercury

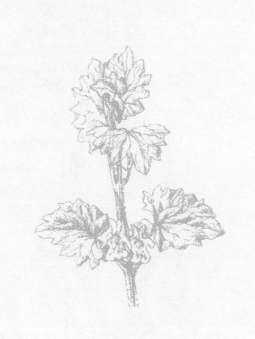

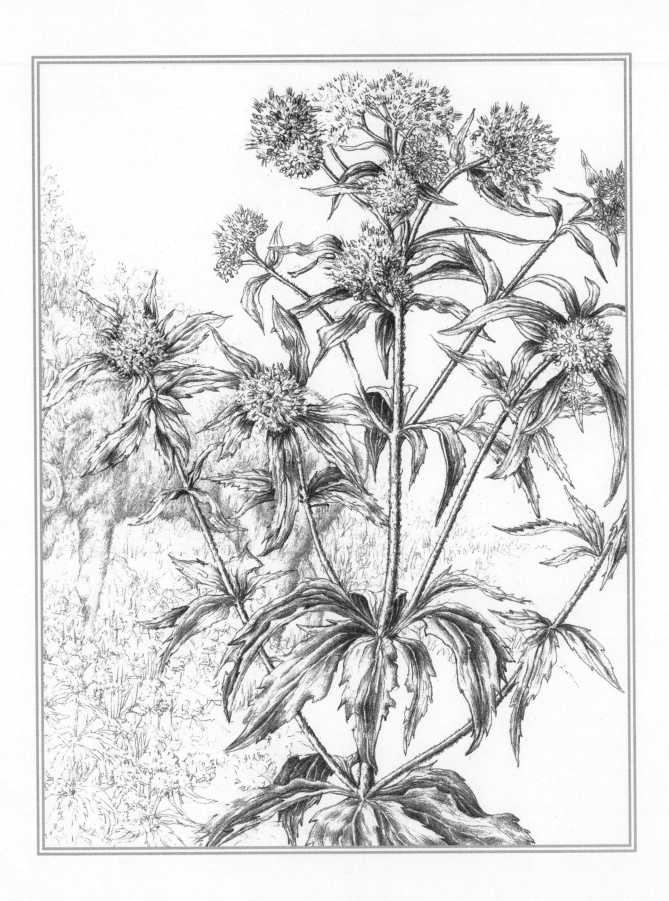

HEMP AGRIMONY

Eupatorium cannabinum

Water Hemp, Sweet-Smelling Trefoil, Water Maudlin

Daisy family—Compositae / Asteraceae

HEMP AGRIMONY IS ONE of the forgotten medicinal plants. Few people know it today even though it has a long and colorful history of healing—and a string of names.

A plant of the water element, its favorite habitat is damp or watery places. I really cannot overlook it, because down at the creek it grows in clusters. I have watched it now for a few weeks—watched it spread its big palm-shaped, filigreed leaves in a neat row along the tall stem. Their resemblance to the leaves of Hemp (*Cannabis sativa*) inspired the name "Water Hemp." Their similarity to the leaves of Wild Marjoram (*Origanum vulgare*) also gave the plant its German name "Water Marjoram." By July's end, it has grown high enough above the damp ground to unfold its flowers. Pale violet with a delicate trace of bordeaux red, their airiness lightens up the otherwise austere appearance of dark leaves.

These large umbrella-shaped flowers are actually composed of hundreds of tiny flower heads. Each of them, in turn, usually contains five narrow tubular florets surrounded by a green bract. The entourage of guests who visit the flowers of Hemp Agrimony are a varied lot— honeybees, bumblebees, flies, different insects, and beautiful butterflies. Later in the fall, the flower completely dissolves, shooting countless little seed-containing fruits through the air on tiny, hairy parachutes.

Historically, Hemp Agrimony is connected with a creature larger than its small nectar seekers. Tabernaemontanus, the eighteenth century herbalist, has this to say about our plant called by old German names like "Deer Clover," "Deerwound Herb," and "Deerheal":

> For it has been observed by huntsmen that the wounded deer eat the Hemp Agrimony, healing themselves with it. This is why it has also been called Deerwound Herb.

This was not the first time that people noticed animals instinctively seeking out a certain plant for their ills. Perhaps the hunter who observed the injured deer in Tabernaemontanus' report tried the same herb at home and noticed its healing capacity. Modern natural medicine has absorbed this old wisdom and confirmed it anew.

In fact, many natural remedies that strengthen a diseased body contain Hemp Agrimony. Deer have long held the reputation for being able to find hidden mineral springs and medicinal plants. My German ancestors venerated the deer as a sacred animal dedicated to the God Freyr. Its antlers were thought to be a sort of antenna with which it could contact higher powers. As we have learned in other chapters, such pagan beliefs were frequently assimilated into Christian mythology—in this instance, as the legend of St. Hubertus, who beheld a cross between the antlers of a deer. Today the deer bearing a white cross is the commercial logo of Jägermeister, a German stomach bitters. Quite an evolution, isn't it!

We can learn about medicinal plants by observing animals more closely. In our own era, the highly effective liver remedy Boldu (*Peumus boldus Molina*), a shrub native to South America, was discovered this way when some sheep suffering from a liver disease were separated from their flock and surprisingly regained their health. It was discovered that they had eaten from a hedge of Boldu that was in the enclosure. It is now proved that Boldu can heal the human liver and gallbladder as well. Modern wildlife biologists have observed how sick animals instinctively eat plants that they otherwise leave untouched: some birds use ant poison as a remedy for rheumatism, wolves with upset stomachs eat plants that induce vomiting, injured chamois roll in Alpine Plantain, and sheep with intestinal problems eat Yarrow. This list could go on and on, no doubt added to by the readers of this book.

Hemp Agrimony received its modern German name, "St. Kunigund's Herb," from the thirteenth century saint, who was the spouse of Heinrich I and a cofounder of the Bamberg cathedral. The third day of March is dedicated to her, St. Kunigund's Day, and is an important date in the traditional German rural almanac. Accordingly:

> When Kunigund is cold and chilly,
> She will feel it for 40 more nights.

> Thunder on Kunigund and Cyprian means
> You should leave your gloves on.

Like its saint's day, St. Kunigund's Herb seems to have had a relationship to the weather—yet other old German names are "Thunderherb," "Weathershrub," and "Cold Weatherwort." Hemp Agrimony was no doubt used in rituals performed on March 3 to influence the weather in a favorable manner. In fact, we know that many weather rituals took place in fields and gardens at the beginning of the seasonal cycle around the time of the first spring sowing. We note this again in the chapter on Mullein, another "weather" herb.

From the earliest known times and well into our modern era our forebearers believed that the weather and other natural phenomenon could be influenced by magic. Every culture had its priestesses, priests, shamans, or rainmakers who could contact the powers that influenced the events of Nature. People saw these powers personified in certain gods—the ancient Greeks honoring Zeus and Iris; the ancient Germans, Donar and Mother Holle. One old German legend—the "Rain Trude"—was recently reintroduced by the German writer Theodor Storm in his fairy tale of the same name.

Christianity has been unable to eliminate all of these old customs. In Germany today we still find instances of weather singing, weather riding, weather bells, and weather prayers. Some shamanistic tribes still have practicing rain-makers who either successfully perform their roles or receive the proverbial "boot"!

We know that the Celts, when praying for favorable weather, called upon Cernunnos, one of the oldest known divinities in the European geographical region. We find him crowned with deer antlers in Paleolithic cave paintings. Later the Celtic druid-priests of northern Europe were called Cernunnes ("deer"). The deer antlers they wore during rituals and festivals symbolized their connection with the cosmic powers. The Cernunnes brought various offerings and used certain plants to invoke good weather—and I would not be surprised to find Hemp Agrimony, then called "Deerherb" or "Blue Coolweather," among those ritual weather plants.

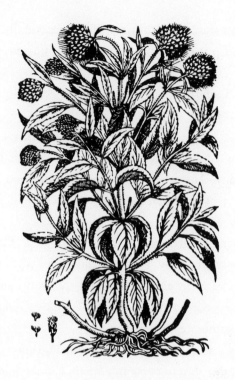

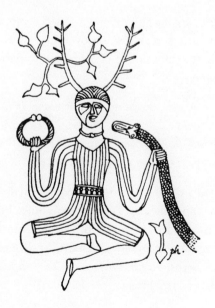

HEALING PROPERTIES

We know that the ancient Greek physicians often used Hemp Agrimony to treat dysentery, liver diseases, ulcers, and snake bites. Having fallen into oblivion, Hemp Agrimony is now experiencing a quiet renaissance in modern naturopathic medicine. How many of us know that it is Hemp Agrimony hiding behind the "Eupatorium" listed among the ingredients of many homeopathic flu remedies?

Nowadays, naturopathic medicine uses it primarily for acute cold, especially when there is fever, malaise, and aching bones. Hemp Agrimony can activate the body's natural immunity and is said to make fever more bearable. At the first signs of flu, drink a cup of tea made from Hemp Agrimony accompanied by the homeopathic preparation from this herb,

Eupatorium 4x, 10 drops, three times daily. We can also use combination cold and flu remedies that contain Eupatorium. (American readers may find the North American species Boneset *Eupatorium perfoliatum* used in their homeopathic preparations.) During the illness, we can sip two cups of Hemp Agrimony tea throughout the day. The tea has also proved effective as a tonic to strengthen the body following illness or surgery.

Hemp Agrimony is also used as a blood-cleansing remedy. I recommend it for all imbalances of liver, gallbladder, and spleen because it cleanses the liver, stimulates the secretion of bile, and stimulates the spleen.

As a water-loving plant, Hemp Agrimony has a relationship to the water balance in the body. It stimulates the kidneys and bladder and is used as a diuretic in cases of water retention. It is also helpful in the early stages of dropsy.

Let's remember what the hunters observed and imitate the deer because Hemp Agrimony is indeed a vulnerary remedy for healing wounds that has been around for a long time. We can wash wounds (especially purulent ones) with the tea, and at the same time, strengthen our immune systems by taking the tea internally. This hinders infection and allows the wounds to heal quicker. By stimulating the liver, gallbladder, and spleen, Hemp Agrimony also increases the production of white blood cells, which are primarily responsible for healing wounds. Other modes of action involved in the use of this plant remain unknown because the chemical constituents of Hemp Agrimony have not been fully researched.

We can gather the plants when they are in full bloom—from July to September, cutting the hard stems about a hand's width above the ground and then hanging the entire plant or laying them out to dry in loose bunches. When they are thoroughly dried, remove the flowers and leaves and break the stem into small pieces.

Hemp Agrimony is a Native American medicinal herb. The native species is Boneset (*Eupatorium perfoliatum*), which is commonly used for homeopathic preparations. Native Americans used this species for fevers, to ease pains, and for colds. The immigrants quickly learned of this medicinal use and Boneset became one of their most commonly used herbal plants. It was once the best known remedy for fever and colds. In 1699, it was brought to England where knowledge of its effectiveness quickly spread.

Hemp Agrimony is available in herb stores as "Herba Eupatorii cannabini." The homeopathic mother tincture "Eupatorium cannabinum" is prepared from the fresh flowering herb.

❧ Hemp Agrimony Tea

To prepare: Steep 1 teaspoon dried hemp agrimony in 1 cup cold water overnight, straining it in the morning and drinking it without warming it.

Note: Always prepare this particular herb tea as a cold extraction. Boiling the plant or pouring boiling water over the dried herb destroys its active ingredients.

A daily dose is 2 cups taken in small sips throughout the day. Do not overindulge thinking that more is better—overdosing can lead to nausea and vomiting. Finally, as with other bitter herbs, do not sweeten the tea—it is supposed to taste bitter.

❦ A TEA TO STRENGTHEN THE SPLEEN AND SUPPORT DETOXIFICATION

10 grams hemp agrimony herb
  (*Eupatorium cannabinum*)
10 grams shore gumweed herb
  (*Grindelia robusta*)
20 grams chicory root (*Cichorium intybus*)

Pour 1 cup of water over 1 teaspoon of the combined herb mixture. Let it steep for 10 minutes and strain the liquid. A daily dose is 3 cups.

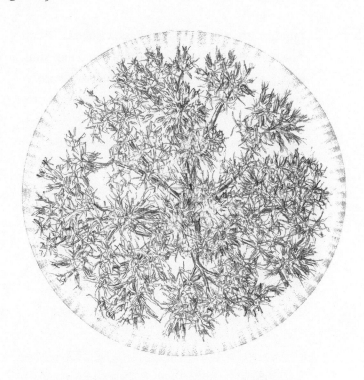

COSMETICS

Hemp Agrimony is helpful for dilated and broken capillaries. The enlarged red blood vessels in the skin, especially on the face, are caused by a congestion of blood in these capillaries. The three plants most recommended for treating this condition are Hemp Agrimony, Sweetclover (*Melilotus officinalis*), and Southernwood (*Artemisia abrotanum*). The fresh herb of Hemp Agrimony is applied to the respective body area for 15 to 20 minutes, Sweetclover is used as a compress, and Southernwood is used as a salve.

CULTIVATION

A hardy shrub, Hemp Agrimony prefers wet soil although it will thrive in sunny and partially shady areas. It quickly propagates itself, forming big clusters of plants. As mentioned previously, the flowers will attract a variety of insects—especially honeybees, bumblebees, and butterflies.

Dr. Madaus writes in his *Textbook of Biological Remedies* about fertilizing Hemp Agrimony: "I have tested the effect of nine different kinds of fertilizers on the development of this plant's essential oil. Unfertilized plants held the highest content (0.36%) of the oil; the percentage in fertilized plants sank as low as 0.16%."

Hemp Agrimony is available as seeds. Sow them in early spring and thin the seedlings to 16 inches apart. The plant flowers from July to September.

Earlier I mentioned Boneset (*Eupatorium perfoliatum*) as being one of the best known American varieties of this genus. Long used by the Native Americans, the herb was also called Thoroughwort, Feverwort, and Indian Sage. It was extremely prevalent as a medicinal plant a hundred years ago in the American Civil War, when it was used to break fevers, as a substitute for quinine in malaria cases, and popularly thought to aid the setting of broken bones. Today "regarded as a weed with an interesting past," this plant grows in swamps and marshy land throughout the eastern part of the continent—from Canada to Florida and west to Nebraska and Texas. Crowned with white tubular flowers, it grows three or four feet in height. (My source for this information is *The Rodale Herb Book* [1974], a fascinating guide to the cultivation, use, history, and lore of healing herbs in America.)

BOTANICAL CHARACTERISTICS

Name: *Eupatorium cannabinum* — Hemp Agrimony

Distribution: Europe, Asia; the native North American species is Boneset (*E. perfoliatum*).

Habitat: Riverbanks, open woodlands, wetlands

Description: Grows to 5 feet with erect, red-tinged, hairy stems, branched toward the top. Leaves are elongated, pointed, and serrate, similar to Hemp leaves; pink flowers in compound terminal cymes; fruits bear a white pappus and are spread by the wind. Flowers from July to September.

Confusion with similar plants: With Valerian (*Valeriana officinalis*), which has the typical Valerian smell and differently shaped leaves. Flowers are similar but pale pink; Hemp Agrimony's are dark pink.

Collecting season: Flowering herb from July to September

Active ingredients: Bitter compound glycosides, Eupatorin, resin, tannins, and essential oil

Astrological association: Neptune / Jupiter

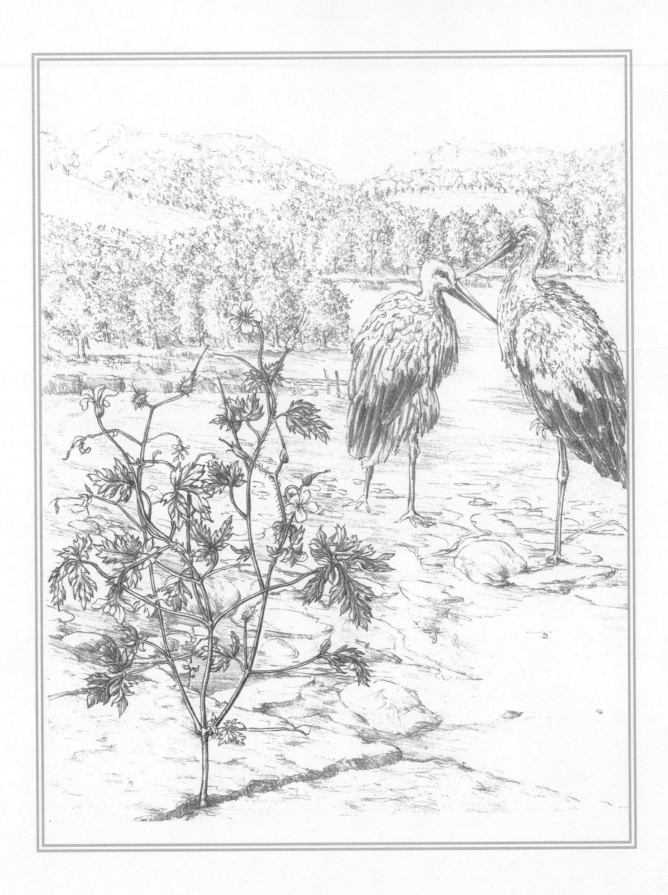

HERB ROBERT

Geranium robertianum

Storkbill, Dragon's Blood, Wild Crane's Bill

Geranium family — Geraniaceae

THE PROUD GERANIUMS on our balcony have a strong-smelling little brother who hangs out on walls, along fences, and in shady woods. While some accuse Herb Robert of smelling like moths and old billy goats, few know his name, let alone his healing powers. But the Geranium family resemblance cannot be denied. All members share the unmistakable characteristic of bearing fruit that resembles what my German forebearers thought of as a stork's long beak. However, reminding the ancient Greeks more of the bill of a different bird, its botanical family name comes from their word for "crane" (*geranos*).

Geraniums, or Pelargoniums as they were called, are not native to northern Europe. They cannot survive the cold winters there and must winter over somewhere safe from frost. They were introduced to England from what is now the Cape Province of South Africa in the early eighteenth century. In the mid-nineteenth century they reached Germany, quickly becoming so popular that every flower fancier wanted them. But it was not for their small, pale pink flowers

that Geraniums were so beloved. No! It was for the sweet fragrance of their leaves. For Scented Geraniums have a fresh, vigorous underlying scent that, depending on the variety, Nature combines with that of roses, citrus, pine, even cinnamon, ginger, or nutmeg and many more. In fact, two large, lemon-scented Geraniums sit near the window by my desk, filling the entire room with their cheerful fragrance.

This could move me to fill a few more pages with exuberant praise for Scented Geraniums. But I will be brief because this chapter is really Herb Robert's, their little brother. I will only add that Geranium oil derives from the leaves of Scented Geraniums grown primarily in Africa, Spain, and on the isle of Réunion in the West Indian Ocean. This oil, "Oleum geranium," has a strong, uplifting effect and is used in aromatherapy with great success to treat depression. It also has antiseptic and healing qualities when applied externally. Lastly, when vaporized in a room, it repels flies and moths. Although they faded from fashion to be replaced by the more colorful flowering Geraniums, these nostalgic scented varieties are enjoying a renaissance among plant lovers.

About Herb Robert's fragrance nothing very flattering can be said. One of his common German names—"Stinking Stork's Bill"—says it all. I personally find the adjective somewhat exaggerated although, admittedly, Herb Robert does smell, well, a bit sharp. However, its effect on the human soul is similar to that of Scented Geraniums—almost all of the old herbalists praised Herb Robert's effectiveness as a remedy for melancholy.

Hildegard von Bingen recommended a mixture of Herb Robert, Pennyroyal, and Rue for this purpose 800 years ago. Paracelsus later prescribed the same mixture to his melancholic patients to be eaten powdered and sprinkled on bread. According to the sixteenth century alchemist, this mixture strengthened the heart and made one happy.

And so, plants with opposite scents, Scented Geranium and Herb Robert, have the same effect on our moods—one through fragrance and the other via the stomach. In the course of this chapter, we will encounter greater similarities between these two plant siblings who appear so different. Maybe by the end, we will no longer turn up our noses at the stinky brother.

Herb Robert is native to my alpine region of Germany. In contrast to Pelargoniums, he is not a shrub but an annual plant. At the end of the year's cycle, he dies. We find Herb Robert on old walls and piles of rocks, near fences, in the forest. He loves the crevices between bricks, his long, thin, whitish brown root squeezing into the tight cracks in the wall. I wonder how such a delicate root can hold the often large, spreading tuft of a plant from inside the wall. Earlier, during years of starvation, people ate the root of Herb Robert as a vegetable. In some areas he is still called by names like "Heaven's Bread," "Adebar's Bread," or "Misery Bread." The Romans particularly liked this vegetable; their so-called *pulmenia* was a popular garnish. The fresh roots taste like parsnips and they are a delicacy when cooked or baked in a béchamel sauce.

At the upper end of the taproot just above the ground, the round stems originate, branching out like rays. Often deep red especially at their base, they are covered entirely by stiff, white hairs that give Herb Robert an appearance of fragility. On some plants, the leaves also are blood red, the depth of color seemingly related to soil conditions. The rockier and drier the soil, the darker are the plants.

His size also depends on the soil. In nutrient-rich, moist earth he can reach a height of 20 inches. In dry, stony dirt he is smaller. Herb Robert's leaves are more delicate than the Geranium's because he does not require protection from the scorching, dry heat that the Geraniums have adapted to in their places of origin. A leaf of Herb Robert is triangular in its general outline and consists of three to five separate leaflets. Botanists call this particular shape "pinnatisect-lobed." A reader who cannot picture this will find it better to simply examine a leaf. The delicately shaped, blood red leaves retain their color when pressed, and I use them to decorate homemade stationery and paper lampshades.

The flowers of Herb Robert are truly charming, sitting in pairs at the terminal ends of the flower stalks. Their five petals are pink or crimson, and a closer examination reveals three white veins in each. Some Scented Geraniums have similar pale pink flowers but Herb Robert's have a unique feature. At the time of maturation the style protrudes above the stamens to bear five curved stigmata. It extends to the structure that is shaped like a stork's bill. When mature, the carpels detach, the flexible bill-shaped fruits curve upward, and the seeds are scattered in the air.

Alfileria (*Erodium cicutarium*), which is also called "Heron's Bill" or "Stork's Bill," is a close relative in the Geranium family about which I can tell an odd tale of my own experience. Alfileria's seeds have a spiral-shaped awn (or "bill") that seemingly drills itself into the ground with the changing humidity—straightening when wet and curling up when dry. Several years ago I discovered a strange weather dial on a house in Austria. Fastened inside a glass box was a paper disk marked with indications like "Fair," "Bad," "Humid," and so on. In the center of this disk was a tiny corkscrew "bill" from an Alfileria fruit! The owner of this botanical weather dial assured me that it predicted the weather as accurately as a barometer. Because there are perhaps 20 different Geranium species in Central Europe, the reader who would seek out Alferia for such a weather dial should look for a plant that usually bears three or more purple flowers with white patches on a leafless flower stalk. Its leaves, rough and hairy, are smaller than Herb Robert's. We can find him along waysides or growing as a common weed among root crops.

Oddly enough, of all the Geranium species, our small, smelly Herb Robert is the one primarily used for medicinal purposes. Many mysterious names point to his history and healing properties: "Anthrax Herb," "Rupert's Herb," "Robert's Herb," "Scab Herb," "Red Flow Herb," "God's Grace Herb," "Warts Herb," and "Orvale."

We will start with Orvale—perhaps the oldest name passed down to us. Here we enter the fairy realm to meet those sprites of the water and air called Orvales with their power to heal certain diseases, especially in animals. Herb Robert was mysteriously connected to these spirits who worked their healing powers through this plant.

In the past Herb Robert was used mostly in veterinary medicine, especially for the treatment of blood in the urine (hematuria) and infectious diseases. This wisdom seems very old and probably dates back to Germanic and Celtic herbalism. As early as 1731, Tabernaemontanus comments in his herbal that these applications derive not from classical sources but from folk medicine.

> The name of this herb "God's Grace," by which it is known to the common man, gives sufficient notice that it is a name granted for the manifold powers and virtues with which it is endowed by Almighty God. It is rarely administered by physicians of our time who do not know its action and properties, inasmuch as in their writings they do not even consider the internal actions of this healing plant.

> First peasants had to show how it to use it beneficially and without danger to the body for, until then, it had solely been used for external ills. Daily experience testifies that this herb is of great benefit to cattle. Primarily when they have retention of urine, one gives the Rupert's Herb to them crushed into a pow-

der and mixed with warm wine . . . Therefore, have industrious husbandmen also considered this and planted the herb in meadows so that, from it, hay gains such strength that it does much good to the cattle in relieving kidney stones and also preventing them.

My German ancestors tried to heal anthrax, a dangerous infectious disease in animals, with the herb Orvale. His old German name "Biswurm Herb" reminds us of this because *biswurm* was the old name for anthrax. Likewise, "Red Flow" is an old name for this disease, and Herb Robert is still known in some regions of Germany as "Red Flow Herb."

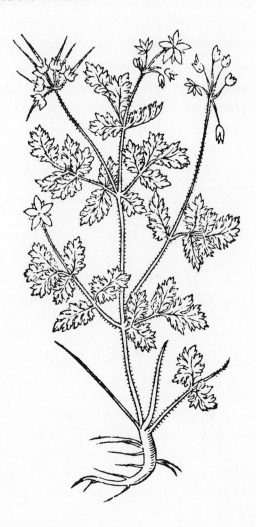

Eventually, the old beneficial pagan spirits who had worked their influence through plants were replaced with Christian saints. Today we still connect the power of a particular saint with certain plants; for example, St. John's Wort or Lady's Mantle. The Orvales, whose power once was envisioned in Herb Robert, have long been replaced with Saint Ruprecht (or Robert), an archbishop of Salzburg who, according to legend, healed his ulcers and canker sores with Herb Robert.

Some authorities, however, consider the species' epithet *robertianum* a reference to the red color of the plant and not to Saint Robert. And it really is striking how blood red some Herb Robert plants are. This was considered an unmistakable signature by the old alchemists-herbalists who felt that this plant could surely heal "red diseases." Therefore, the *Herba rubra* ("red herb") was used to alleviate bloody diarrhea and to treat open sores, especially open leg ulcers. The plant was said to be especially powerful in healing red rashes and eczema, hence its old name "Scab Herb."

Besides the shape of the fruits that resemble a stork's bill, there was supposedly another connection between our plant and this lucky bird, the bringer of children. In earlier times, women who were unable to conceive a child were advised to drink Herb Robert tea and to wear an amulet made from its root. And such healing powers make it easy for us to understand why Herb Robert was once called "God's Grace Herb."

HEALING PROPERTIES

Like the old medieval herbalists who followed Paracelsus' Doctrine of Signatures, we can trust the signature of Herb Robert and use the "Herba rubra" to heal bleeding, diarrhea, ulcers, skin rashes, and other so-called "red diseases."

Modern naturopathic medicine recognizes Herb Robert as an effective remedy for diarrhea, especially when there is blood in the stool. This is because the plant's bitter compounds and tannins have astringent and blood-staunching properties. It is likewise helpful for chronic inflammation of the stomach and small intestines and is frequently used to treat stomach flu.

Herb Robert can be taken as tea, wine, powder, tincture, or juice. I prefer the wine or tincture for internal ingestion and find that the fresh juice works best for external applications.

When gathering fresh flowering plants to administer internally, choose large green ones; for external applications, look for small blood red ones. Hang the whole plants in bunches to dry like laundry on a line in an airy place. When they are thoroughly dried, cut them into small pieces and store them in an airtight container.

To treat chronic inflammation in the gastro-intestinal tract, I recommend administering Herb Robert in the form of a medicinal wine (also the mode of preparation recommended in the old herbals). I make a simple wine at home by filling a large jar half and half with freshly plucked, chopped Herb Robert and a good red wine. Then I let the mixture stand for two weeks before straining it into a carafe or corked bottle. Because red wine has an astringent and calming effect on the gastric membranes, I suggest sip-ping this herbal wine by the snifter before meals.

For external applications, the freshly pressed juice of Herb Robert is best. (Although throughout the long winter months, a strong tea or the tincture will have to suffice.) You can either apply the juice directly to the area being treated or use it in compresses. I find that it helps to heal wounds, ulcers, canker sores, eczemas, stubborn skin diseases, erysipelas (known as "Red Flow" in German), and sore nipples.

And let's not forget Herb Robert's application for melancholy and sadness. A predisposition for this state of mind is often related to an accumulation of toxins in the body. Herb Robert's ability to stimulate the metabolism may explain this medicinal use. Paracelsus recommends a mixture of dried herbs to be ground into a powder and sprinkled on bread; namely, equal parts of Herb Robert, Pennyroyal (*Mentha pulegium*), and Rue (*Ruta graveolens*). Others swear by the same herbal blend prepared as a medicinal wine.

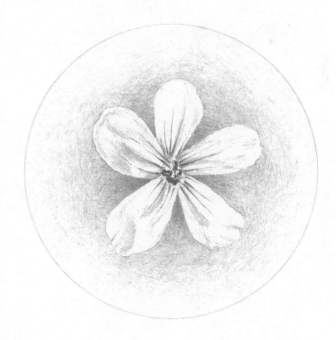

Herb Robert is available in herb stores as "Herba Geranii Robertiani." The homeopathic mother tincture "Geranium robertianum" is prepared from the fresh flowering plant.

❧ Herb Robert Tea

Use 2 teaspoons of the dried herb per cup of cold water, letting the mixture steep overnight. Never boil it! A daily dosage is 2 cups (or for acute cases, 3 or 4 cups).

❧ Herb Robert Tincture

Prepare the tincture by filling a dark mason jar with fresh, chopped herb Robert and enough grain spirit or fruit liqueur to cover. Let the mixture steep for 3 weeks, shaking the jar occasionally. Strain the tincture into dropper bottles. In acute cases, take 20 to 30 drops every hour.

This tincture is a great addition to a first-aid travel kit!

❧ Wine for a Happy Heart

herb robert (*Geranium robertianum*)
rue (*Ruta graveolens*)
pennyroyal (*Mentha pulegium*)
1 liter good red wine

From an old recipe: Take a handful each of the fresh flowering plants, chop them up, and put them in a jar. Pour the red wine over them, letting the mixture steep for 2 weeks. (*Note:* rue and pennyroyal are available as garden plants.)

Veterinary Medicine

Herb Robert is an old remedy for cattle. Considered a tonic, it has been used by farmers for a long time to treat blood in the urine, the retention of urine, and kidney infections. The freshly pressed juice is effective for treating wounds and ulcers in animals as well as people. Finally, skin rashes in pigs can be rubbed with the fresh juice.

Cultivation

Herb Robert is an annual that winters over in some areas. You will find that it self-seeds and propagates easily and quickly. It prefers well-watered soil and shady places but will grow in arid, sunny spots as well.

Lovely growing from the the cracks of a wall, pretty decorative varieties are available as seeds or starter plants. For a rock garden, try a low-growing variety such as the Dwarf Blood Red Geranium (*Geranium sanguineum var. prostratum*) with its pale pink flowers. The Lilac Geranium (*G. grandiflorum*), a brown variety (*G. phaeum*), and the beautiful blue-flowering Meadow Geranium (*G. pratense*) are striking in a wildflower meadow.

BOTANICAL CHARACTERISTICS

Name: *Geranium robertianum* — Herb Robert

Distribution: Europe, North Africa, Asia, and North America

Habitat: Walls and rock crevices, woods, hedges, wastelands

Description: Plants grow 4 to 20 inches high with reddish, thin, stiffly branched stems; leaves, stems, and sepals are covered with soft hair; leaves are triangular in shape, divided into 3 to 5 lobes, pinnatified-cleft; flowers are pink, crimson, or violet with 5 petals and 3 white veins; fruits are bill-shaped, pointed, about ¾ inch long.

Confusion with similar plants: Possibly with other Geranium species although the medicinally used Herb Robert has reddish stems and a particular sharp, acrid smell.

Collecting season: April to September

Active ingredients: Bitter compounds, geraniin, tannins, and essential oil

Astrological association: Mars / Venus

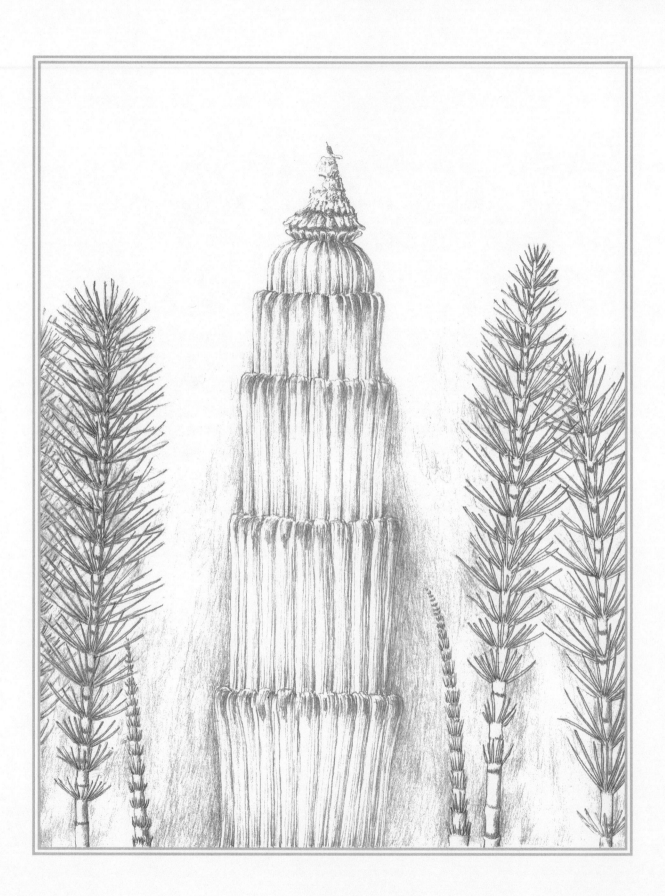

HORSETAIL

Equisetum arvense

Common Horsetail, Field Horsetail, Shave Grass, Horsetail Grass,
Horsetail Rush, Scouring Rush
Horsetail family — Equisetaceae

MILLIONS OF YEARS BEFORE the human race set foot on Earth, Horsetail flourished. In his odd archaic shape, we see 400 million years of history. Four hundred million years! Would such a staggeringly distant past ever reveal its secrets to us! And yet, today we can picture what Earth was like at the beginning of Horsetail's history. In our greed for natural resources we have dug down into the "Age of Horsetail"—to mine the pit coal that originated in the giant Horsetail and Fern forests of the Carboniferous period, at the birth of our world's history.

Now an odd little plant, then Horsetail was a stately tree towering a hundred feet in the air. Paleontologists have reconstructed his appearance from specimens of petrified plant fossils found especially in coal seams. The prehistoric coal forest that extended north to the Norwegian archipelago of Svalbard in the Arctic Ocean consisted primarily of giant Horsetails, Clubmosses, and Ferns. If we could time-travel into these huge swampy primordial forests, they certainly would appear very peculiar to us. This is because in all of this luxuriant vegetation we would not find a single flower. The fragrant and colorful beauty that so delights our hearts had not yet evolved. The Mosses, Ferns, and Horsetails of the Carboniferous forest reproduced asexually via spores. Today these plants (or rather smaller descendants of those gigantic trees) reproduce in the same way. It is an exciting story.

In March or April, pale stems about eight inches high appear in meadows and fields with their strange spikes on top. These are Horsetail's spring stems that bear no chlorophyll, a green plant's pigment. Without chlorophyll they cannot convert sunlight into chemical energy and process the substances they need for life. So where do they get their energy? When we go to the trouble of digging up a stem, we discover a multi-branched network of roots that can spread six feet deep. From their black, pencil-thick rhizomes hang small tubers that, like tiny potatoes, contain starchy reserves. Here is the stem's storehouse. This rootstock makes Horsetail nearly indestructible because neither plow nor hoe can destroy the deep-growing ramified roots. Today the king of the primitive forest is considered a weed.

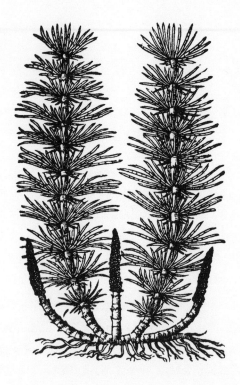

The brownish yellow, hollow, unbranched spring stems bear sheath-like brown leaves that look inflated. The pointed teeth on the sheaths often grow in pairs; the stem in between is grooved lengthwise. The individual sections of stalk are boxed in the sheaths that give Horsetail its German name *Schachtelhalm* ("Box Blade"). When you try to tear apart a young stem using both hands, it always breaks at the lower end of a section because it grows from there and is still soft. The stem's cone-shaped terminal spike is composed of numerous small scale-like leaves (sporophylles), each bearing a tiny hexagonal lamella on a stalk. On the inside of each lamella hang 12 white spore sacs (sporangia). Examining the spores under a magnifying glass, we see tiny pellets each with a band (elater) wound around itself. When mature, the spores dry and we recognize two bands crossing each other,

fixed at the center. As the spores unroll, the bands stretch with a movement that opens the spore sac. The wind now does its duty as, with the naked eye, we see a blue-green dust blow away.

The sporophyll branch/spring stem, its task fulfilled—dies. The spores carried to the ground grow into tiny plants (gametophytes). They do not in the least resemble the mature Horsetail. They instead look like small Lichens or Mosses. Fertilization occurs only when female and male gametophytes stand close together, and even before they jump from the seed capsules a few have attached themselves with their little band-arms and are carried off together. Female gametophytes are delicately fringed on their upper end and excrete a sour juice that attracts the zoospores, which are corkscrew-shaped, flagellated, sperm-like motile creatures. They swim to the female gametophyte where the egg-cell nestles in a swollen widening. Zoospore and egg fuse, creating a new Horsetail plant.

New shoots from the rootstock appear above ground. These summer stems are abundant with chlorophyll and replenish the plundered larder (the reserves in the root tubers). Horsetail's summer stems resemble small fir trees. Light and delicate, they grow 4 to 20 inches tall with rough grooves and bear stems rising in whorls that branch at every node. The single twigs are arranged in whorls as well. The Horsetail plant has neither flowers nor distinct leaves, consisting purely of an arrangement of stems whose construction is abstract and formal.

Those who study planetary signatures in plants recognize Horsetail as a plant of Saturn. Saturn symbolizes contraction and hardening, the power of giving form, abstraction, and minimalism. In contrast to Jupiter and Venus, he is reduction to the essential. Thus, in his shape, Horsetail limits himself to necessity. His concern is only with structure and not with the design of soft shapes, bright flowers, and fragrances noted in Venus and Jupiter plants. He is rough and hard to the touch. At the level of the human body, Saturn is related to things firm and structural—bones, teeth, joints, skeleton. In fact, the stems of Horsetail are connected by joints.

Horsetail's character is evident if we slowly bake one of its summer stems on a cookie sheet. What is left is a clear and glassy skeleton consisting mostly of silicic acid (up to 97%). In its purest form, silicic acid occurs as quartz crystal, a hard and cool rock. Less pure and precious is flint, which also consists mostly of silicon. Silicic acid is firming, dry, and cold in keeping with its Saturn quality. In both organic and inorganic states, it is hexagonal in shape. (Look at a quartz crystal's hexagonal cross section.) And in winter, which is the season of Saturn, water forms hexagonal structures in snow and ice.

We might now ask: What kind of diseases respond to the Saturnine contracting and synthesizing energy of silicic acid or Horsetail? Silicic acid has a relationship to the body's connective tissue. This type of tissue is the opposite of the Saturnine principle—soft, pliable, moist, and flexible as it surrounds the body's organs and firm parts. When it weakens, silicic acid can give new impulses for stabilization. It stimulates the metabolism of the connective tissue, promotes the excretion of waste products, and stabilizes its structure. Wherever waste products accumulate, especially in the joints, silicic acid can stimulate

their excretion. These qualities strengthen the bones, tendons, and ligaments.

Almost 50% of Earth's crust is silicon in an inactive form that does not bond with other elements. In plants, however, silicic acid is partially active, and in the case of Horsetail about 10% is extractable. Therefore, we prepare a tea from Horsetail not as an infusion but as a decoction. This means that we boil it for at least 20 minutes to allow as much of the silicic acid as possible to dissolve.

With a magnifying glass we can see small glassy pellets of silicic acid on the Horsetail shoots. In earlier times, people used this quality to practical advantage. It made a wonderfully fine "sandpaper" with which to polish pewter (hence, its German name *Zinnkraut* or "Pewter Herb"). We can also use it with care to polish aluminum, copper, and other metals. It is said that cabinetmakers and makers of musical instruments have long used Horsetail to polish delicate wooden surfaces.

There are many different species of Horsetail, some of which are considered toxic. However, if we learn to distinguish them, nothing adverse will happen. In some areas Horsetail used to be called "Cow's Death" because symptoms of poisoning were observed when the plant was used as fodder. Although Horsetail was considered dangerous to cows, it was thought to strengthen horses. There was even a saying about Horsetail—"Horses' bread, cows' death."

According to Dr. Otto Gessner's book on poisonous and medicinal plants of Central Europe (*Die Gift- und Arzneipflanzen von Mitteleuropa*, 1953), symptoms of poisoning did occur in horses and sheep. The so-called "staggering disease" has the following symptoms: increased excitability, cramps, disturbed coordination of movements, and death due to paralysis. Today this poisoning is attributed to a chemical constituent of Horsetail—the alkaloid equisetine that derives from a parasitic fungus (*Ustilago equiseti*) that grows on the plant. This fungus especially attacks Marsh Horsetail (*Equisetum palustre*), Sylvan Horsetail (*E. silvaticum*), and Scouring Rush (*E. hyemale*). Forming brown spots on branches and twigs, it attacks the plants only in late summer. To be totally safe, we should only gather Horsetail before late July after first examining the plants for brown spots. For remedial teas and baths, Field Horsetail (*E. arvense*) is preferred.

For identification purposes, I will summarize the different Horsetail species:

Field Horsetail (*Equisetum arvense*) grows in fields and meadows. In March or April, the pale spore-bearing stems appear like blades with spikes. The unbranched stem has sheaths with 6 to 12 teeth. Later, green stems with grooves grow with branches extending 4 to 20 inches high. At their lowest point, sections of the side branches are longer than their respective sheaths.

Sylvan Horsetail (*E. silvaticum*) you will find in humid forests growing 6 to 24 inches tall with stems that are more delicate than those of Field Horsetail. The sheaths of fertile stems are swollen, bulging, and reddish brown in the upper portion with three to six blunt teeth. Branches of infertile stems arch downward. The whorled branches divide in two, a distinguishing feature between this and all other Horsetail species with their undivided branches. Two different kinds of branched stems appear in spring:

infertile ones with a green tip and pale green fertile ones with a spiked tip. (*Note: Do not gather this Horsetail species.*)

Scouring Rush (*E. hiemale* or *E. hyemale*) grows in moist shade forests. Fertile and infertile shoots have the same shape, and evergreen, the stems winter over. (In Germany we call it "Winter Horsetail.") Growing four feet tall, the green unbranched stems are rough and hard with flat ribs. The teeth of the sheaths attach tightly and are usually black at the top and bottom and whitish or reddish in the middle. These teeth fall off early, leaving behind a black, grooved edge on the stem. The spore-bearing spike is short, blackish, and fertile in May or June. This species is similar in effect to Field Horsetail but weaker. Be sure to examine each plant carefully for brown spots. In China, a well-known powdered herbal formula containing *Equisetum hiemale* is sprinkled into wounds to stanch bleeding. Homeopathic medicine uses Scouring Rush instead of Field Horsetail. This species is the one most commonly found in North America.

Marsh Horsetail (*E. palustre*) prefers the wet swampy habitat of fens and bogs. It can grow 8 to 28 inches tall and fertile and infertile stems look alike. Undivided branches grow in whorls from the nodes and have 6 to 10 green white-edged teeth. (Field Horsetail has dark brown teeth.) The sheaths are longer than the lowest section of the branch and new shoots are ribbed. The spore-bearing spike is blackish. (*Note: Do not gather this type of Horsetail. In German it is called* Duwock *in reference to "Duwockian" or "staggering disease" in livestock.*)

Swamp Horsetail (*E. limosum*) is a rare plant that can grow five feet tall in standing water.

Its fertile and infertile stems are like those of Scouring Rush (*E. hiemale*) with smooth stems and sheaths that have 10 to 20 narrow black teeth. It sometimes grows short side branches. (*Note: Do not gather this type of Horsetail.*)

Giant Horsetail (*E. telmateia*) likes the shady wetlands along riverbanks. It is the largest species native to Germany, growing to four feet tall with thick stems. Fertile stems are unbranched; infertile stems are whitish with green whorled branches. A few days after releasing its spore dust, a thick, juicy sporangia spike collapses and rots. This species is preferred for use in herbal baths.

When out hiking, you may not remember all this information. So please be sure to at least follow these guidelines: (1) never gather Horsetail in wooded or swampy places and (2) never use plants that have brown spots.

silicic acid than older plants. Those who are able to distinguish the various Horsetail species and need fresh plants for treatments later in the year can still gather them then. However, be sure the plants have no brown spots (and I will continue to reiterate this point). I personally have seen cases where even the external application of Horsetail infected with this fungi has led to allergies. For baths use Giant Horsetail, whose large stems are more practical for a full body bath.

To harvest, cut the plants above the ground, tie them in bunches, and hang them up to dry. I like to place them decoratively against a white or pastel wall. Once dry, discard any stems that have turned brown and store the remaining ones for tea.

Horsetail is indicated whenever there is a weakness of the body's connective tissue. This type of tissue occurs everywhere in the body.

Healing Properties

Horsetail's medicinal properties are primarily attributed to its high content of silicic acid. This has a blood-stanching (hemostatic) quality and a firming effect on tissues. The plant also contains flavons that firm the blood vessels and minerals like calcium, phosphorus, magnesium, and aluminum.

We should gather Field Horsetail in spring and early summer. Scouring Rush has the same applications as Field Horsetail but its effects are somewhat weaker. I use Scouring Rush to treat disk problems and to strengthen the musculoskeletal system. According to Dr. Lohner, the young Horsetail shoots contain more soluble

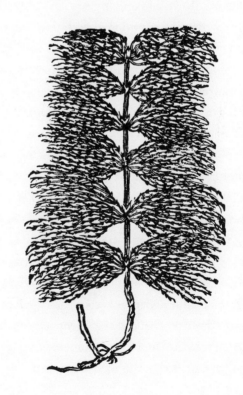

Although it is soft and pliable, it forms the firm parts of our bodies—bones, cartilage, tendons, teeth, hair, and nails. It is a part of the organs that it surrounds, connects, or separates and plays a major role in water balance, in storing fats, and in the body's own defense against toxicity and bacteria.

A course of treatment with Horsetail helps to strengthen, firm, and cleanse the connective tissue. We use it for flaccid tissue, impure skin suffering from poor circulation, brittle hair and nails, bad teeth and gums, disk lesions, weak connective tissue, and problems of the feet and calves (such as varicose veins, leg ulcers, and fallen arches). Besides ingesting the herbal decoction or juice, we can apply Horsetail externally in the form of full body baths, sitz baths, foot baths, wraps, or compresses. The effect of this ancient plant is strongest when administered internally and externally at the same time.

For sagging tissue and skin with poor circulation, I recommend taking frequent full body baths with Horsetail and dry-brushing the skin every morning.

Folk medicine has long used Horsetail to stanch bleeding and old herbal texts praise this particular quality. Two thousand years ago Dioscurides pointed it out. Pliny even claimed that, to stanch bleeding, one merely had to hold Horsetail in one's hand. Albertus Magnus in the twelfth century A.D. praised the hemostatic action of this herb but, as with many other medicinal plants, Horsetail's reputation fell out of memory. Again it was the German herbalist-cleric Pfarrer Kneipp who reintroduced this great remedy into natural medicine, reporting numerous cases in which he stanched bleeding in short order.

The fresh juice is used mostly to stanch bleeding. For this purpose, juice the fresh plants in a juicer. In acute cases, administer one tablespoon hourly; otherwise, the dosage is one tablespoon taken three times daily.

The freshly pressed juice promotes blood-stanching and stimulates the white blood cells that strengthen the body's defenses. Simultaneously, the flavons firm the blood vessels. The pressed juice can be administered internally or externally for all types of bleeding as an adjunct for internal bleeding, heavy menstrual bleeding, a tendency to nosebleeds, and bleeding hemorrhoids. For sties, blepharitis (inflammation of the eyelid), and especially for itching eczema and skin rashes, use a strong tea of Horsetail in a bath or compresses.

A tendency to blepharitis always indicates a scrofulous disposition. German physicians Kobert and Kühn have tested Horsetail's age-old application for pulmonary tuberculosis and have confirmed that extended treatment with Horsetail tea has a firming effect on weak lung tissue. The increased production of white blood cells strengthens the body's immunity against the tubercle bacillus. Horsetail is indicated as an adjunct and follow-up treatment for pulmonary tuberculosis, and Doctors Kobert and Kühn recommend a silica tea blend (adding two other native plants rich in silicic acid) for a long-term course of treatment. I include their recipe in the following section.

Proved effective for all chronic conditions of the bronchi, Horsetail is also a good adjunct therapy to other plants that have specific expectorant and anti-inflammatory properties.

Still another area of application for Horsetail is kidney and bladder disease. In fact, Parson Kneipp, who I mentioned earlier, called the plant "unparalleled, irreplaceable, and invaluable" for such conditions. He prescribed Horsetail for pain due to urinary and kidney stones and gravel, kidney and bladder weakness and related inflammations, and for retention of urine. He reported that a 70-year-old man who suffered from urinary retention, after the external application of steam from Horsetail tea, was able to urinate again within approximately 20 minutes!

Horsetail firms the bladder and kidney tissue and has anti-inflammatory, analgesic and diuretic properties. I prescribe it regularly to patients as a basic therapy for weak bladder, irritated bladder, bladder infection, kidney weakness or infection, and bladder and kidney stones. A course of treatment with teas ingested internally should always be supported by sitz baths or steam applications of Horsetail tea.

For administering steam to the pelvic area, there are several methods that work. You can use a chair with holes drilled in the seat, a wicker chair without a cushion, or an old chair with the seat removed. Alternately, you can sit on a slatted wooden crate turned upside down or even perch between two chairs (although there is the disadvantage of being unable to fully relax during the treatment). Put three handfuls of Horsetail, fresh or dried, in approximately one gallon of water; boil it for 20 minutes and place the pot under the chair or crate. Undressed from the waist down, the patient sits on the chair covered with large towels to prevent the steam from escaping. This steam bath is a boon to bladder infection, exposure to cold, burning pain with

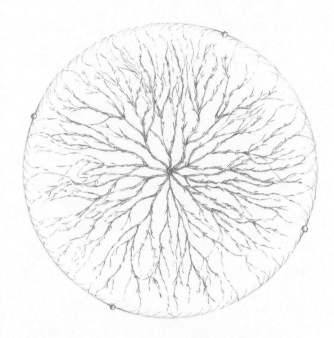

urination, and retention of urine. To treat cramping pains in the bladder, kidneys, or uterus, add a handful of Chamomille flowers (*Matricaria chamomilla*) to the hot decoction.

Horsetail is available in herb stores as "Herba Equiseti." The homeopathic mother tincture is prepared from fresh Field Horsetail (*Equisetum arvense*) and Scouring Rush (*E. hiemale*).

❧ HORSETAIL DECOCTION

Use 2 teaspoons of horsetail for each cup of water. First cover the herb with cold water and then bring it to a boil. Covered, let it simmer for at least 20 minutes to allow as much silicic acid as possible to be extracted. Strain the liquid and drink 3 cups daily.

❧ A BATH FOR SWEATY FEET

Bring to a boil 2 handfuls of horsetail in 5 liters of cold water, reduce the heat, and let it simmer, covered, for 20 minutes. Add 2 tablespoons pineapple weed (*Matricaria matricarioides*) and 1 tablespoon sage (*Salvia officinalis*). Cover and let the mixture steep before straining it to use as a foot bath. Repeat 2 or 3 times a week.

Wear only wool or cotton socks and go barefoot once in a while. Do not apply sweat-suppressing remedies—foot sweat is an outlet and indicates a disturbed metabolism, especially a weakness of the liver. One should instead support the excretion of toxic waste through the colon, kidneys, and skin.

✌ A Compress for Inflamed Eyelids

1 teaspoon horsetail (*Equisetum arvense*)
1 teaspoon fennel (*Foeniculum vulgare*)

Cover the herbs in 1 cup of cold water, bring the mixture to a boil, and simmer it covered for 20 minutes.

Soak some clean cotton or gauze in the strained liquid and apply it as a compress to the affected eyelid. Utilize the herbal mixture at as warm a temperature as safely possible and change the compress when it cools.

✌ Kobert-Kühn's Silica Tea

37.5 grams field horsetail
  (*Equisetum arvense*)
75.0 grams prostate knotweed
  (*Polygonum aviculare*)
25.0 grams ochre-yellow hempnettle
  (*Galeopsis ochroleuca*)

Three times a day, steep 1½ teaspoons of the herbs in 2 cups cold water. Bring the mixture to a boil and simmer it uncovered until the liquid is reduced by half.

Cosmetics

Horsetail baths and compresses aid sagging and impure skin by increasing the skin's resistance. Horsetail tea can be used as a hair rinse in cases of dandruff and oily scalp. A course of treatment with the tea likewise strengthens hair, skin, and nails. For swollen, red eyelids apply a compress soaked in Horsetail tea.

Cultivation

You would be ill-advised to plant Horsetail directly in a cultivated vegetable or flower garden because its highly invasive nature sends deep and widely branched rootstock to all corners. Instead, find a place for it in a wet spot where it can expand and make an interesting addition to the garden flora. Scouring Rush (*Equisetum hiemale*) with its long, undivided stems is suitable for planting around the edges of a pond. It can also be planted in water-tight containers.

As a point of interest, Horsetail is a valuable natural herbicide. You can spray a decoction on tomatoes for blight and on roses and berry bushes infected with powdery mildew. Horsetail plants are commercially available.

BOTANICAL CHARACTERISTICS

Name: *Equisetum arvense* — Horsetail

Distribution: Europe, northern Asia, northern Africa, and North America

Habitat: Sandy, loamy fields and waysides

Description: The spring stems are 4 to 12 inches tall, pale brown without leaves; hollow and ribbed, the stem is divided in many sections by nodes surrounded by serrated sheaths; at the terminal end there is a cone-shaped, spike-like sporangia. In May the summer stems appear 12 to 20 inches high like small fir trees with many nodes and whorled branches whose length decreases at the terminal end.

Confusion with similar plants: With other Horsetail species (see text)

Collecting season: Summer stems: May to July

Active ingredients: Silicic acid, flavons, and many trace elements

Astrological association: Saturn

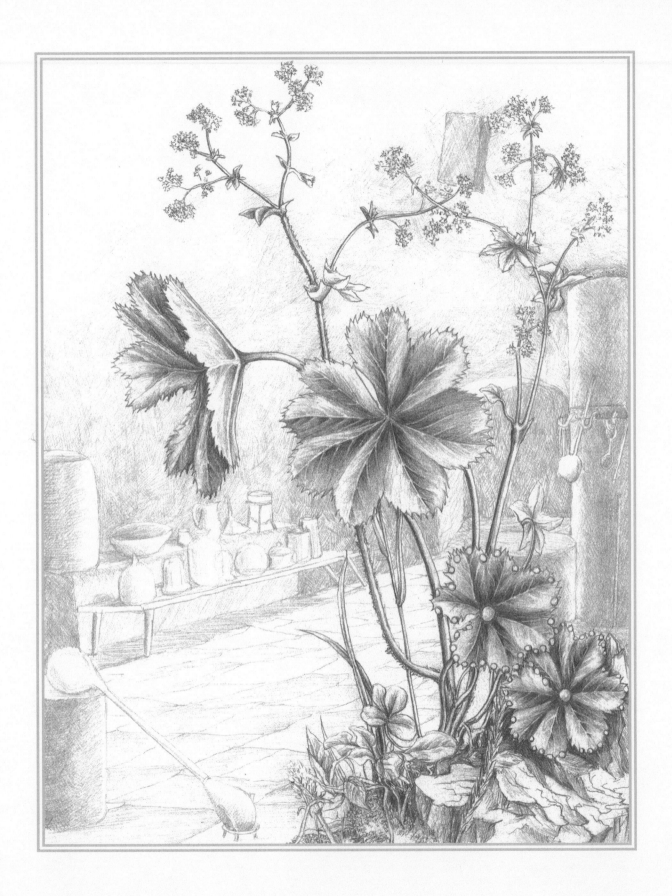

LADY'S MANTLE

Alchemilla vulgaris / Alchemilla xanthochlora

Lion's Foot, Bear's Foot

Rose family—Rosaceae

LADY'S MANTLE APPEARS as from a fairy tale. The leaf, exquisitely folded into a basin, seems to await a gift. And, indeed, the morning dew leaves a glistening magic pearl lying in this green chalice. Medieval alchemists called it "Heaven's water" and, assigning it special powers, gathered these drops at sunrise. As part of a well-kept secret, we know that from this heavenly elixir they sought to manufacture the mythical philosophers' stone that would transmute baser metals into gold. They thought of Lady's Mantle as a little alchemist (hence her Latin name of *alchemilla*) who could soak up the Earth's water, purge it of impurities, and offer it back to Heaven in surrender to the last stage of transformation. This they felt was a metaphor for the path of humankind.

Our modern botanists, of course, offer an alternate explanation for these drops from Heaven. They say that Lady's Mantle precipitates small water droplets at the tips of her saw-toothed leaves that accumulate as one large drop in each leafy basin. By noon, except in humid weather, these dewdrops have usually evaporated.

Many of her old German names refer to this phenomenon: "Fair with Tears," "Dew Cup," "Water Carrier," "Water Chalice Flower." In the old herbals, we find Lady's Mantle under the names *Sinau* or *Sintau* meaning "Ever-Dew" in Old High German.

And, oh, her beauty! In my mind, no plant has more harmoniously designed leaves than Lady's Mantle. In the tradition of the noble Rose family to which she belongs, her proportions are excellent—subtle, elegant, graceful, fair. In her particular case, however, such qualities are reserved for her lovely leaves. Her flowers, sadly, are neglected, it being a peculiar feature of Lady's Mantle that her egg cells do not require fertilization to form embryos. When I discuss Lady's Mantle in my herb seminars, over and over I hear expressions such as "But what do her flowers actually look like?" or "Is that really her flower—I imagined it differently!" This is because the flowers are very small and inconspicuous with a greenish yellow color and a sweet yet slightly musty scent.

Lady's Mantle has always belonged to

women. The old herbalists recognized in her the sign and power of Venus—the scented flowers reflecting the green of Mother Earth and the comely leaf opening in a gesture of receiving. This highly regarded women's remedy has always been under the patronage of a woman deity. For my ancestors this was Freya, goddess of love and fertility. Early Germanic women knowledgeable in herbology gathered the herb during the waning moon to staunch the blood flow of women and to heal wounds. In the Christian era, she was placed under the protection of the new goddess Mary and permitted to bear her name ("Mary's Mantle" or "Mantle of Our Dear Lady"), her round, pleated leaves reminiscent of the mantles worn then by women.

HEALING PROPERTIES

Lady's Mantle is first and foremost a women's remedy. The combination of its active ingredients, primarily the tannins and bitter compounds discovered so far in laboratory testing, heals and strengthens both large and small pelvic organs. In general, it has a balancing and regulating effect on the entire female organism.

Excellent for pregnant women, teas made from the herb strengthen the uterus and can prepare one for a good delivery. Its simultaneous hemostatic and healing effects can also heal possible contracted injuries and cleanse the uterus. In addition, it promotes lactation. About six weeks before delivery, I recommend that a woman begin a course of treatment of Lady's Mantle tea by drinking three cups daily. Following the birth, for about three weeks she can drink one or two cups daily.

Several female complaints are helped with herbal care. I have successfully treated cases of vaginal discharge that lack apparent cause (for example, constitutional leukorrhea or after exposure to cold) with tea and sitz baths. In specific cases of leukorrhea, I have found that Lady's Mantle can help when taken internally as a tea and used externally as a vaginal douche. You can also use it following antibiotic treatment for trichomonas and yeast (candida) infections when the healthy vaginal flora has been disturbed and requires strengthening to keep pathogens at bay. To restore the normal acid-base ratio, I recommend that every day for a week you insert one teaspoon of yogurt and a suppository from an herbal pharmacy (or one lactic acid stick) into the vagina. Concurrently, follow a course of treatment with the following "Restorative Tea" for a month and take a therapeutic sitz bath twice a week.

Lady's Mantle tea is also used as an adjunct treatment for ovarian failure or inflammation, irregular menstruation, prolapsed uterus, constitutional miscarriage, and menopausal difficulties. *Note:* In leukorrhea, as in all gynecological conditions, always keep your feet warm. If necessary take hot foot baths with Mugwort (*Artemisia vulgaris*).

High in the alpine mountains grows Silvery Lady's Mantle (*Alchemilla alpina*), a cousin with especially strong healing powers. Used exactly like our *A. vulgaris*, it is also recommended as a slimming tea. And used as an eye wash, a decoction made from Silvery Lady's Mantle can heal inflamed eyes.

For men and women alike, Lady's Mantle is a great wound herb mostly due to her high tannin content. Our old friend Paracelsus, the early sixteenth century Swiss-born alchemist and physician, praises her ability to heal any wound and benefit any sore when drunk as a tea and applied externally as freshly pressed juice and mashed herb. For surface ulcers, saturate a fresh gauze compress with the fresh juice of Lady's Mantle (extracted in a juicer) and apply it as a dressing. For wounds that are slow to heal, bathe the area in a strong tea made from the herb.

Lady's Mantle tea is available in herb stores as "Herba Alchemillae." The homeopathic mother tincture "Alchemilla vulgaris" is prepared from the juice of the fresh plant. You may find the even more efficient Silvery Lady's Mantle in herb stores as "Herba Alchemillae alpinae."

℘ Tea Blend to Promote Lactation

> 30 grams lady's mantle
> (*Alchemilla vulgaris*)
> 20 grams goats rue (*Galega officinalis*)
> 20 grams fennel (*Foeniculum vulgare*)
> 15 grams vervain (*Verbena officinalis*)
> 15 grams dwarf milkroot
> (*Polygala amara*)

Soak 1 teaspoon of the herbal blend in 1 cup of cold water; bring it to a quick boil and let it steep for 5 minutes. Drink 2 cups daily.

℘ Tea Blend for Weaning

> 20 grams sage (*Salvia officinalis*)
> 20 grams walnut leaves (*Juglans* spp.)
> 10 grams hops fruit (*Humulus lupulus*)

Pour 1 cup of boiling water over 1 teaspoon of the herbal blend and let it steep for 5 minutes. Drink 2 to 3 cups daily.

℘ Restorative Tea

> 35 grams lady's mantle
> (*Alchemilla vulgaris*)
> 15 grams deadnettle flowers
> (*Lamium album*)

Pour 1 cup of boiling water over 1 teaspoon of the mixture and let it steep for 5 minutes. Drink 3 cups daily.

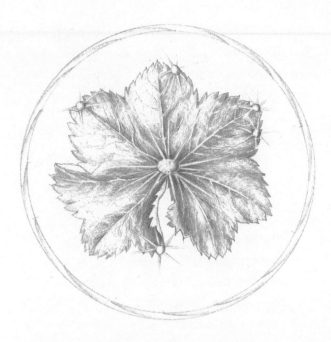

10 grams yellow gentian root
(*Gentiana lutea*)

In a small pan, pour 1 cup of cold water over 1 teaspoon of the mixture, heat it slowly, and let it simmer covered for 20 minutes. Drink 2 cups daily unsweetened. Remember: Bitter teas take their effect through their bitter compounds and should not be weakened by sugar or honey. All other teas are best sweetened with honey.

❧ A Therapeutic Sitz Bath

lady's mantle (*Alchemilla vulgaris*)

horsetail (*Equisetum arvense*)

wild marjoram (*Origanum vulgare*)

oak bark (*Quercus* spp.)

oat straw (*Avena* spp.)

hay flowers

Prepare a blend of these dried herbs or use them singly.

Prepare a large quantity of tea from 500 grams (about 1 pound) of the fresh or dried herbs. Add the strained mixture to the water for a sitz bath. Sitz baths are especially practical for women because they concentrate on the pelvic region and strengthen the pelvic organs. Sitz tubs are available at medical supply stores.

Drink the following two teas for leukorrhea, alternating them daily for 6 weeks:

❧ Tea for Leukorrhea

20 grams lady's mantle
(*Alchemilla vulgaris*)

20 grams sage (*Salvia officinalis*)

10 grams deadnettle flowers
(*Lamium album*)

Pour 1 cup of boiling water over 1 teaspoon of the mixture and let it steep for 5 minutes. Drink 2 cups daily.

❧ Tea to Strengthen the Constitution for Leukorrhea

50 grams horsetail (*Equisetum arvense*)

20 grams sandalwood
(*Santalum album*)

Hay flowers are a mixture of different dried flowering grasses that are very popular in Germany. A traditional folk remedy, they are used for warming, therapeutic baths and compresses for rheumatism and chronic conditions. Gathered on hay farms, they can contain sweet vernalgrass (*Anthoxanthum odoratum*), wild rye (*Elymnus repens*), quackgrass (*Agropyron repens*), orchard grass (*Dactylis* spp.), and foxtail (*Alopecurus* spp.).

COSMETICS

An old beauty secret for a firmer bust—mash the leaves of Lady's Mantle and apply them in a compress soaked in the herbal tea. The tea also makes an effective facial astringent and cleanser and can be used as a skin lotion for enlarged pores and freckles.

CULTIVATION

While Lady's Mantle is available both as seeds or starter plants, it is better to propagate her by dividing older rootstock in the fall or spring. Her natural habitat is wet meadows. Loving humus-rich, moist soil and sunny places, she can thrive in well-tended lawns and gardens where she will reward you with abundant growth. Lady's Mantle also makes a good ground cover.

Several decorative species for the garden include: *Alchemilla hoppeana*, with light yellow flower panicles and a tolerance for shade; *A. hybrida* with yellow-green flowers; and *A. mollis*, who grows up to one foot and makes a good yellow-flowering ground cover.

BOTANICAL CHARACTERISTICS

Name: *Alchemilla vulgaris* — Lady's Mantle

Distribution: Abundant in Europe and Asia

Habitat: Wet meadows, along brooks

Description: Grows to 1 feet 7 inches tall; very particular shaped leaves with 7 to 11 lobes, regularly dentate, almost circular shaped; tiny yellow-green flowers in umbel-shaped panicles.

Confusion with similar plants: None because of its specific leaf shape

Collecting season: Flowers from May to September

Active ingredients: Tannins, bitter compounds, phytosterin, glycosides

Astrological association: Venus

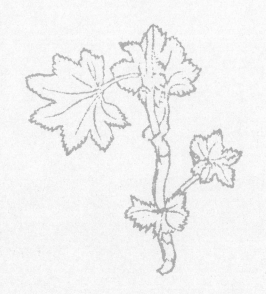

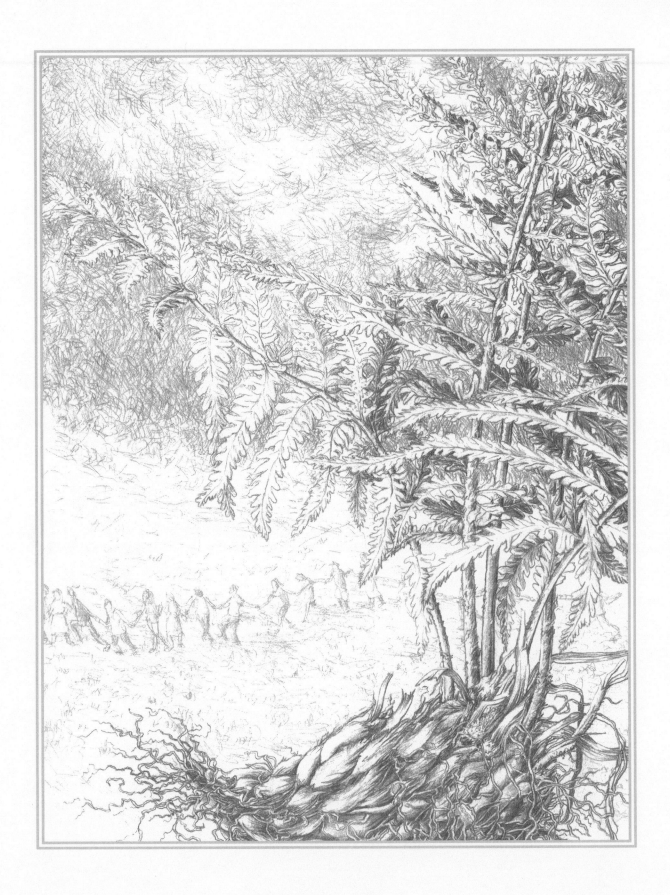

Male Fern

Dryopteris filix-mas (originally *Aspidium filix-mas*)
Aspidium, Bear's Paw Root, Knotty Brake, Sweet Brake
Shieldfern family — Aspidiaceae

IT WOULD BE EASIER to write a whole book on Ferns than to summarize their history on a few pages—but I will try. On Earth the story begins 395 million years ago in the Devonian period of the Paleozoic era. Fifty million years later in the Carbon period, they had developed so magnificently that, had human beings been around, we would have walked under huge Fern trees. Primitive amphibians only then developing from fishes were the ones to enjoy life in the vast Fern and Horsetail forests—as well as spiders, insects, and centipedes. The mild climate produced conditions favorable for luxuriant plant growth and, as these Fern and Horsetail giants fell to the ground, layer upon layer, time converted them into coal that we use today.

Ferns represent a basic step in the evolution of plants, linking the mosses and the higher developed seed-bearing plants. During the Carbon period, however, they were a far advanced plant species whose population declined in the course of millions of years. Today we see stunted remains of their former splendor only in the tropical forests where small Fern trees survive. In our time Ferns still represent the developmental stage between mosses and flowering plants, each forest Fern a reminder of the huge marshy woodlands that existed at Earth's beginning.

Ferns are mysterious. Since ancient times people pondered the secret of their reproduction. How can a plant as substantial as the Male Fern, for example, propagate without flowers and seeds? Today we know the botanical solution to this riddle. We know that prior to flowering plants there was another method of reproduction. In summertime we can see strange signs on the underside of their fronds—many tiny brown dots arranged in pairs and covered by fine veils (indusium) reminiscent of control panels of technical instruments or a secret code. From these "control buttons" (sori) a very fine light yellow dust trickles—spores. By late summer, if we look, we will find small plants growing beneath the Ferns, tender and inconspicuous plants that appear entirely different. Resembling small algae, these little plants have grown from the spore dust. Male and female gametes develop on their leaves. From the fertilization of their eggs another spore-producing asexual Fern will develop. He needs no flowers, surrendering all of his energy to the formation of beautiful leaves. And truly his leaves are a jewel in our forests.

With his tall fronds, the Male Fern is the most commonly recognized member of the family. The spore-producing generation is used for medicinal purposes. Both leaves and root contain many substances missing in the small sexual Fern plant, such as aluminum and potash. For healing, it is best to gather Fern leaves at midsummer when the round clusters of spores (sori) are developed.

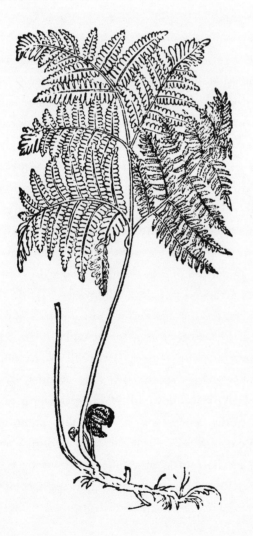

While many Fern species live in our forests, the Male Fern is one generally used in herbal medicine. Distinguished easily from the others, the Male Fern was sometimes called "the little Fern man" because of his stocky rhizome and sturdy, pinnate leaves or fronds springing directly from the root. His sori are shaped like kidneys. The Lady Fern (*Athyrium filix-femina*) has elongated sori often shaped like horse shoes. In her everything appears more graceful and gentler. If you still cannot distinguish the two, cut through a leaf stalk (stipes) and count the vascular bundles. If there are two, it is Lady Fern; if seven, it is Male Fern. Lady Fern's healing properties are similar but slightly weaker than her counterpart's. For this reason, Male Fern was once used for treating men and Lady Fern for treating women.

The vascular tissue test also distinguishes the Toothed Wood Fern (*Dryopteris spinulosa*) with its five vascular bundles. The fronds of this Fern are decompound pinnate, the individual pinnules as sharp as little thorns. This Fern is not used medicinally.

The king of all Ferns—and the largest—is Bracken (*Pteridium aquilinum*), or "Eagle Fern" in Latin. Proudly he stands on a long stipe, spreading his wide fronds like wings. He grows abundantly and was used in the past for fertilizer and as bedding for animals.

Hart's Tongue Fern (*Phyllitis scolopendrium*) is a smaller cousin, his undivided leaves resembling a smooth tongue. He is a rare breed and has protected status in Germany. Native to Europe and eastern North America, he is an old-time remedy for diseases of the lungs and the spleen. Commercially available in shrub nurseries, when given a shady, nutrient-rich place in the garden, he will thrive magnificently.

The tender fronds of the Southern Maidenhair Fern (*Adiantum capillus-veneris*) are the most beautiful in the Fern family. Divided into many filigree-like pinnules, her individual stipes are as fine as hair. Her botanical name derives from the fact that water glides off of her leaves (Latin *a-* meaning "not"; Greek *diainein* meaning "to moisten, to sprinkle"). In Germany we consider her a decorative plant although she is native to the Southern Alps, the Tessin region between Italy and Switzerland, and North America. She is recognized as a lung remedy.

Ferns, however, were not only sought for healing purposes. For millennia, Male Fern in particular was known for magical powers. These qualities were pursued by many cultures through various rituals and countless legends, fairy tales, and songs tell how our ancestors once beheld this character of Nature.

Humans saw in this plant a deep metaphor, an inner image that is barely comprehended today. Sometimes we may still sense something of this plant's magic when in the forest we unexpectedly come across a nest of young Fern fronds uncurling in beautiful spirals. It was this spiral shape that attracted people to Ferns. The spiral is one of the oldest symbols of humanity. From early Paleolithic rock art to decorative vases and wall paintings in all cultures well into modern times we find spirals wherever people have wanted to symbolically portray the path of spiritual development—moving in circles yet always ascending to higher levels. We see this universal symbol in the huge spiral nebulas of galaxies, in the spirals of our fingertips, in the whirl-shaped hair growth of our bodies, and in the whirl-shaped muscle fibers of our hearts. People once imagined the sun's course in the sky as a spiral. They imitated in spiral dances this movement to integrate themselves into the cosmic energies, dances performed especially on the two Solstice days. And so, traditionally, those wishing to gather Ferns for purposes of magic did so—and still do—only on Solstice and Christmas.

The spiral is an ancient symbol of good luck and healing, and Fern fronds, especially when still curled into a spiral, have long been incorporated into feasts and ceremonies. In his book *The Spiritual Earth*, P. Cyrill von Crasinski identifies one such custom that survives today. The squeaking, unfurling, paper-spiral noisemakers that enrapture children and adults alike at carnivals and birthday parties, he says, are really stylized Fern spirals. During the ancient Roman festivals called Saturnalia, in parades similar to our modern Mardi Gras, party-goers threw Fern fronds at one another to bring good luck. They also sprinkled Fern spores—today's confetti—on each other to bring love and fertility. Called the "flower of lovers," these Fern "seeds" were a potent sexual charm throughout the Middle Ages and beyond. Every child knew that Fern seeds could make those who possessed them happy, wealthy, and able to find treasures and understand the language of animals. In fact, the Latin botanical name for Male Fern derives from "happy" (*filix*) and "little man" (*mas*), a reminder of his power over Earth and Water. Also, like the following one, numerous stories tell of mortals using a gift of Fern seed to become invisible.

Once upon a time a farmer was searching for a missing foal during Midsummer night. He wandered through meadows and came upon a forest where, brushing against a large Fern, he walked away with some of its seed in his shoes. Empty handed, he returned home—where nobody paid attention to him. "I couldn't find my foal," he finally said loudly. Startled, people could hear but not see him. And thus he remained until removing his shoes, when the Fern seeds lost their effect and he became visible again.

That the Fern's spore dust was not true seed, that much people knew—but where were the seeds of this plant, they wondered? Our forebears believed that only on Solstice and Christmas would Ferns bear seeds, and only following a complicated ritual could they then find them. Sometimes a frenzy would break out among people wanting to find Fern seed, causing their Christianized lords to fear a reemergence of the old faiths. In many areas the gathering of Fern seed was therefore forbidden. In 1611 Duke Maximilian so decreed, and the synod of Ferrara followed suit the next year.

People gathered Fern fronds from the forest to work their magic. They hung them in stables to protect animals from disease and, in hopes of bearing a child, women hung them by their beds. Interestingly, I have observed that the cervical mucus of women at the time of ovulation exhibits a frond-like pattern when observed under a microscope.

The Fern's root was considered a means to banish evil. From the root, small child-like hands were carved—the so-called "St. John's hand"—and worn as an amulet around the neck. It was supposed to strengthen and protect the wearer

from disease. However, the power of Fern roots could be dangerous. Called "Err Roots," some of them, when stepped upon, caused wanderers to lose their way forever in the forest. Some Germans still use the expression "he must have stepped on an Err Root" when speaking of someone who lost his way.

Finally, Hildegard von Bingen summarized the knowledge of her time about the Fern in this passage from her handbook on Nature (*Physica*):

> Fern is warm and dry and has a medium measure of juice. The Devil shuns the plant, and it has certain powers that remind one of the sun, for like the sun it illuminates the darkness. Thus it chases away hallucinations and fantasias and therefore the evil spirits do not like it. On a place where it grows the Devil will rarely practice his trickery, and the plant in turn will avoid and despise the house where the Devil is. Lightning and thunder will rarely strike there, and on the field where it grows, it will rarely hail. Whoever carries Fern with him is safe from the Devil's snares and from evil attacks on life and limb. Just as a sense of good and evil is innate to human beings, so good and bad herbs are grown for them . . .

HEALING PROPERTIES

Frederick the Great paid an impressive annuity to a pharmacist, on whom he conferred the title of Privy Counsellor, for a secret remedy against tapeworms. This secret remedy contained, as we know today, a large portion of powdered Fern seed.

Male Fern is among the best-known tapeworm remedies from our herbal pharmacy. Active ingredients immobilize tapeworms and prevent them from clinging to the intestinal wall. Following the patient's ingestion of a laxative, they are then eliminated. Unfortunately, however, while the plant's powdered root (or root extract) is useful for treating tapeworms, it is highly toxic when taken in overdose. At the same time, an application of insufficient dosage is ineffectual. Symptoms of poisoning usually start with headache and dizziness and are followed by fainting, unconsciousness, and cramps. Fern's toxicity severely damages the liver and kidneys and death occurs due to cramps and respiratory paralysis. *Note: Again I warn against the improper use of Male Fern. Use it only under the supervision and care of an experienced healthcare practitioner.*

Happily, there is less danger in the treatment of small white pinworms or threadworms. They usually occur in children but occasionally attack adults. These little tormentors colonize the large intestine and rectum, thereby ensuring an annoying itch. Abdominal pain, teeth grinding during sleep, and dark rings under the eyes are further signs of worms. A stool analysis will ascertain their presence.

In most cases dietary measures can be employed to expel pinworms. People who eat quantities of raw and unprocessed natural foods are less likely to get worms. Therefore, if so afflicted, it is advisable to eat raw vegetables, particularly salads of grated carrots, celery, and, season permitting, Ramsons salad. (See the chapter on Ramsons.) Other appropriate foods are uncooked sauerkraut, onions, pumpkin seeds, and abundant amounts of garlic. Beverages should include carrot juice, sauerkraut juice, and teas prepared from the following: Hyssop (*Hyssopus officinalis*), Wormwood (*Artemisia absinthium*), Pineapple Weed (*Matricaria matricarioides / Chamomilla suaveolens*), or Centaury (*Centaurium minus*).

This dietary course of treatment is supported by taking enemas using garlic water. For this, simmer two garlic cloves in one cup of water with the pot covered. Use the broth, cooled to body temperature, two or three times a week.

For external purposes, Male Fern can be used without danger of side effects. Use the tincture for liniment rubs and compresses. It is helpful for a variety of ills: lumbar pain, sciatica, rheumatic pain, gout's aches and twinges,

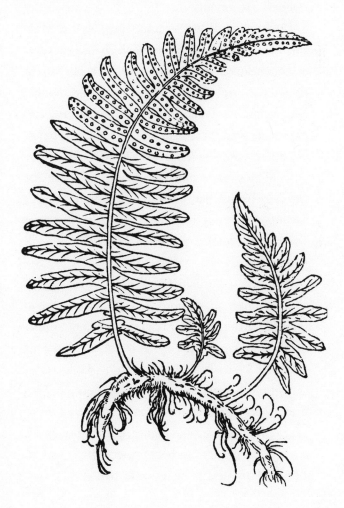

neuralgias, pain due to cold and draught, toothache, calf spasms, writer's cramp, and varicose veins. Soak a compress (such as a washcloth or cloth diaper) in Fern tincture and apply it to the painful area. Cover it first with a towel and then a wool blanket, a hot water bottle slipped in between.

To treat calf spasms and writer's cramp, I recommend hot baths for feet or hands with a decoction of the root. Boil two cups of fresh or dried roots in five quarts of water, strain it, and use when the temperature is comfortable. This footbath also aids in cases of cramping headaches. (For the latter I suggest more frequent treatments.)

When digging up a large root of the Male Fern, I am always impressed by its natural artistic beauty. Many small root branches weave themselves into a thick braid that I disassemble and clean. As I cut them into small pieces, I notice a wild and aromatic odor and pause to admire how the formerly whitish color now shines in a phosphorescent green inside the dark brown hair pelts. I look within the root to find the "St. John's hand" that people once wore as an amulet. To me, it looks like a small hedgehog.

To make a tincture, I place the freshly chopped root pieces into a wide-mouth mason jar and cover them with grain spirit or vodka (approximately ¾ liter per root). Closing the jar tightly, I let it sit for three or four weeks, later straining the tincture into dark bottles. Fern tincture should be prepared in new batches every year. My personal experience is that the root's healing properties are best preserved in alcohol. I find oil extracts to be less effective.

Note: Always label bottles containing Fern tincture or Fern oil with the caution "EXTERNAL USE ONLY" to avoid accidental ingestion. Remember that it is poisonous!

The fronds' pinnate leaves hold healing powers as well, their effect best taken overnight. Herbalist-clergymen Künzle and Kneipp both recommend the use of pillows and mattresses stuffed with Fern leaves to patients suffering from rheumatism and gout. Fern leaves for this purpose should be gathered during the height of summer when the spores are mature—and at midday when they are not damp. Strip the little pinnules from their stalks and stuff them into a pillow one or two inches thick to place under a patient's painful body parts.

As an aside, the Fern fragrance "Fougère" found in many European-style soaps, perfumes, and bath waters is not actually Fern. It comes from a distillate of Oak Moss (*Evernia prunastri*).

Male Fern is no longer used for tapeworm remedies. (Even in the past, only the root's oil was used.) In Germany, England, and elsewhere the root of Male Fern and its preparations are strictly controlled and available only by prescription. The root is known as "Rhizoma filicis" and the root extract as "Extractum filicis."

VETERINARY MEDICINE

Folk wisdom says that evil spirits flee from Fern —especially those with many legs who torture people and animals. Therefore, to protect your dog and chickens from their respective fleas, you should put Fern leaves into their bedding. The old herbals also praise Fern as a remedy for horses. Although I have no experience in that area, old Hieronymus Bock notes in his 1577 herbal:

> Of this root lay a piece under the tongue of a horse that has fallen and one cannot know what kind of ailment will be healed . . . soon [the beast] will begin to make dung and stand up again. This I have truly found for myself.

CULTIVATION

Starter plants for various Fern species are commercially available. Male Fern prefers humus-rich soil and shady places. It is a perennial plant whose fronds die in late fall and reemerge the following spring. Male Fern likes to grow about 15 to 20 inches apart in the shade of trees. A beautiful, graceful plant, Bracken Ferns (*Pteriddium aquilinum*) can grow almost 6 feet high. Its roots can be used like those of Male Fern although their effect is somewhat weaker.

Fern leaves contain potash, making them an excellent mulch for potato plants. For this purpose, cover the soil between the plants with Fern fronds and put Fern leaves into the hole before planting. Placed beneath strawberries plants, Fern will prevent the fruit from rotting too soon. Also, fruits and vegetables keep longer on storage shelves spread with Fern leaves— as will hard and soft cheeses wrapped in Fern leaves.

This is because Fern is strongly antiseptic. Unfortunately, the preserving properties of Ferns and other plants are nearly forgotten. If we knew more about such properties, we could eliminate many new and toxic methods of preservation.

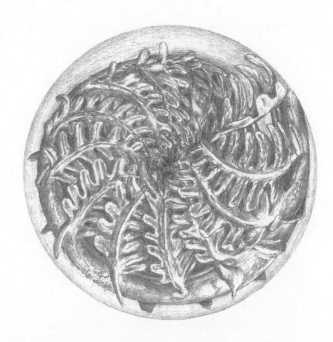

Dr. Ferdinand Müller wrote extensively about this in his 1874 herbal:

> On our last visit to London we observed that fruit offered for sale, especially the more valuable varieties, was packed in Fern leaves. Initially we paid little attention to this fact, thinking that this was done because of a lack of wine leaves. However, a friend and famous botanist L. pointed out to us that Fern leaves possess the quality to keep substances of animal or plant origin surrounded by them fresh for a longer time period and preserve them from rotting. This we noted on the Isle of Man where fresh herrings were packed in Fern leaves for shipping. Later we performed our own experiment: In a storage pit, we surrounded half of the potatoes with straw and the remaining half with Fern leaves. By spring most of the former were rotten while the latter were perfectly preserved.

BOTANICAL CHARACTERISTICS

Name: Dryopteris filix-mas (the old botanical name is *Aspidium filix-mas*) — Male Fern

Distribution: Nearly everywhere in Europe, northern Africa, Asia, and North America

Habitat: In forests, on humus-rich soils

Description: Green fronds up to 3 feet high in a funnel-shaped arrangement; pinnate to bipinnate, opposite leaflets (pinnate); spore cases (sori) in double rows on the underside of leaves.

Confusion with similar plants: Several other Fern species are distinguishable by vascular tissue test: Male Fern has 7 vascular bundles visible in a cross-section of the leaf; Lady Fern has only 2 bundles; Toothed Wood Fern has 5.

Collecting season:
    Root – August to September
    Leaves – June to September

Active ingredients: Filmaron, filicin, phloroglucine, essential oils

Astrological association: Saturn / Mercury

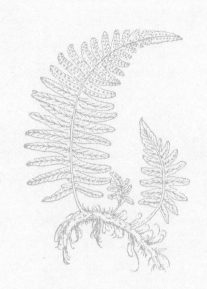

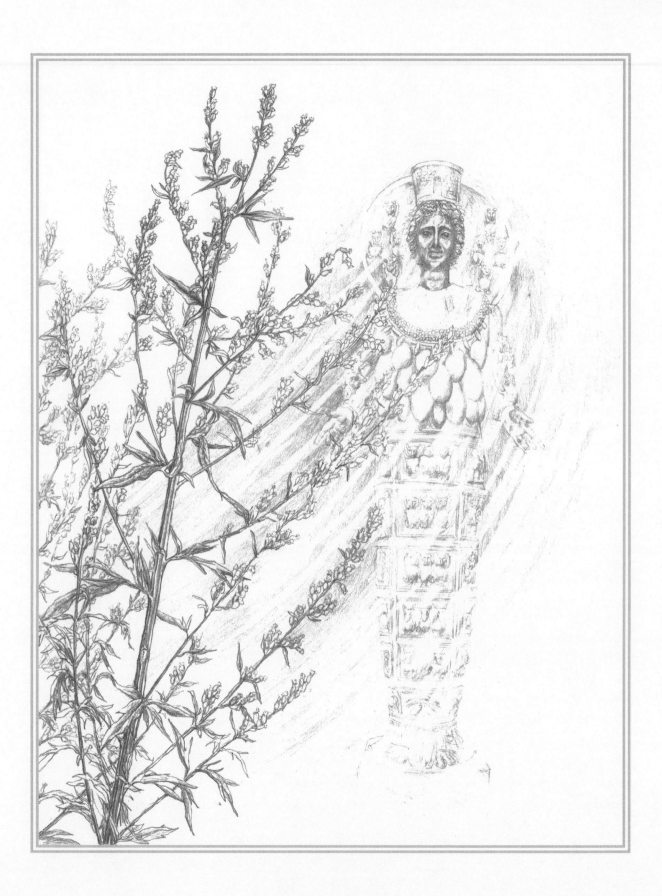

Mugwort

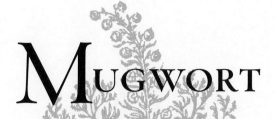

Artemisia vulgaris

Common Mugwort

Artemisia, Sagebrush, Sailor's Tobacco, Felon Herb

Daisy family—Compositae

Do you remember, Mugwort, what you
   make known,
What you decree in solemn proclamation?
Una is your name, the oldest of herbs;
You have power against three and
   against thirty,
You have power against poison and
   against contagion,
You have power against the ailment
   that passes across the land.

from an eleventh century
Anglo-Saxon nine-herb blessing

INCONSPICUOUS IN APPEARANCE is Mugwort, her flowers among the humblest of the
plants described in my book. Therefore, it is
initially strange to discover that she was once
worshipped as the "Mother of All Plants," her
medicinal powers praised since ancient times. We
of this era can barely comprehend which powers
our forebearers beheld in Mugwort, what relationships they perceived among Creation's things
when they worshipped her as a gift of the
Goddess. We can only follow the blurred and
centuries-old trails of her history.

The earliest path leads us to Persia in the
fourth century B.C. to meet Artemisia, the wife of
King Mausolus whose tomb (or mausoleum) was
one of the seven wonders of the ancient world.
Artemisia was skilled in the healing arts and
indeed Mugwort's botanical name to this day is
Artemisia vulgaris. However, our healer-queen
was named for Artemis, the Great Mother
Goddess, worshipped by both Persians and
Greeks and whose most famous image stood in
Ephesus in Asia Minor. Two plants sacred to
Artemis were Spruce and Artemisia, the latter's
healing powers considered helpful for all
women's complaints, especially birth related.

The ancient Greeks called her "the herb of the
virgin" (*parthenis*), again dedicated to the goddess Artemis. The ancient Egyptians dedicated
her to Isis, whose priestesses during processions
carried Mugwort plants. And the ancient
Romans, changing the name of Artemis to Diana,
called the sacred herb "Diania." The ancient
physicians—Hippocrates, Pliny, Dioscurides,
and Galen—all praised Mugwort as a great
women's remedy.

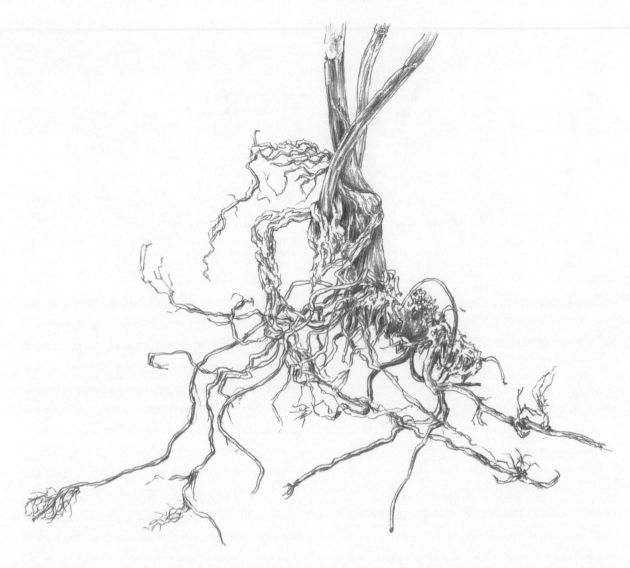

Our path now leads to Europe where the herb of the Goddess Who is Mother of All Things bore the title "Mother of All Plants." Throughout the Middle Ages, the Renaissance, and into modern times, European practitioners of the healing arts used Mugwort almost exclusively as a woman's remedy. A few who describe her healing properties are Hildegard of Bingen, Paracelsus, Tabernaemontanus, Bock, and Lonicerus. Nicholas Culpepper in his seventeenth century herbal called her an herb of Venus whose aromatic tops, leaves, and flowers are full of virtue and "most safe and excellent in female disorders."

We can gather from the old herbals that Mugwort was used to increase fertility, ease birth, stimulate the afterbirth, alleviate menstrual pains, and balance menstrual irregularities. In addition, it was used to treat all conditions with cramping, especially those of women. Mugwort is described as a plant with particularly strong dry and warming energy. Women called it

"Womb's Wort" (*wort* meaning root, plant, or herb) and tied it around their wombs to stimulate labor when giving birth.

Like many other plants originally dedicated to a goddess, Mugwort is included in the bunch of herbs offered for Mary's blessing on the Day of the Assumption of the Blessed Virgin (August 15) in the southern Catholic regions of Germany. At that time, women bring ritually arranged bundles of herbs to the church after which they place them in a conspicuous place in the home or stable. Some people burn Mugwort as incense in the stables on Assumption Day to protect the animals from disease.

Archaic German names like "Mugwurz," "Powerwort," "Solstice Girdle," and "Thorwort" lead us to the Germanic and Celtic pasts, revealing Mugwort's important role in these cultures. We know from shamanistic religions still practiced today that people strongly connected with nature are believed to recognize places of power, animals of power, and plants of power. For instance, a plant of power can bestow strength and power on someone, if he or she knows how to approach it. Mistletoe was a powerful plant for the Celts. Using golden sickles, druid priests would cut it from oak trees on a certain day to distribute among their followers. When worn as an amulet, this mistle "toe" was believed to give yearlong strength and protection from illness. Mugwort was another magical plant of power, her name derived from the Celtic for "to warm or strengthen."

Even the Gods made use of Mugwort's power. Thor, the Thunder God, possessed the magical girdle Megingjardr that, when worn, doubled his strength and endurance for journeys and battles.

It was said that even mortal humans could gain strength by wearing girdles braided from the "Girdle Herb" on the year's most powerful day—the Summer Solstice when the life-giving sun has its greatest strength. Solstice celebrations can be traced back over many millennia. Tradition has it that, at the end of the feast, the solstice girdle was thrown into the fire with all the evil that one wanted to banish. Or a person could keep the girdle to wear for protection and strength, to burn as incense, or to hang in the stable to protect animals from disease and enchantment.

Worn as an amulet, the herb's root bestowed strength and health, said a fifteenth century manuscript:

> Artemisia is mighty among herbs!
> If you fear magic, hang four bundles
> in your rooms, and demons or
> other bad things will not harm you,
> your children, or the cattle . . .

In 1731 Tabernaemontanus wrote that Mugwort root worn around the neck could heal diseases caused by demons and epilepsy. Later, the physician Rademacher described in *Empirical Medicine*, published in 1848, how he used Mugwort to heal epilepsy. And in this century Dr. W. Bohn, after studying the herb, also cited it as a remedy for epilepsy.

Today Mugwort is rarely used. Only in the practice of homeopathic medicine do we find the root prepared and used for epilepsy, St. Vitus' dance, and hysteria. Some contemporary herbal books fail to even mention Mugwort—hardly proper for the "Mother of All Herbs"!

I am now left to explain the modern German name for Mugwort—*Beifuß*, or "By Foot."

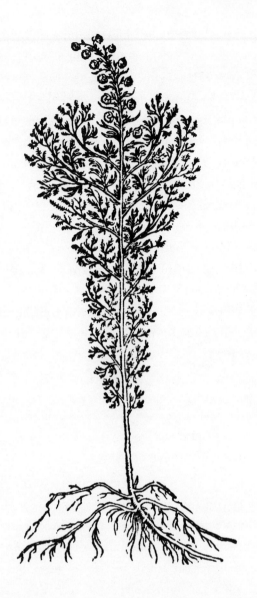

Leonhard Fuchs writes in his 1588 herbal that "when one who travels across the country carries 'By Foot' with him, it will chase away fatigue." Like the Broad-leaved Plantain whose German name means "Way Ruler," so Mugwort, too, is a companion for travelers on foot. It prefers to grow along waysides, offering aid to those with tired feet. Herbalists as far back as Pliny praise Mugwort as a remedy that refreshes tired travelers who wear it in their shoes or tied to their legs.

However, there were skeptics, even then. Konrad von Megenberg expressed his doubts about this property of Mugwort in his fourteenth century *Book of Nature*:

> Artemisia is called "By Foot." The herb is hot and dry and benefits those who are infertile . . . Master healers also say that when bound to the legs, it takes away the tiredness of travelers. Failing to believe this, I tried it, and so say: if it had worked, I would have called it enchantment!

Clearly, this gentleman never experienced the comfort of a Mugwort footbath after an exhausting day spent on his feet. I wish I could have recommended it to him.

Of course, how can we perceive Mugwort's powers from appearance alone? We can read a thousand books but without direct experience her attributes will never come alive for us. In my case, only when I felt her strength in my own body did I finally understand what the ancients meant about Mugwort being "hot to the third degree." Today I consistently prescribe Mugwort for strengthening and warming, and for illnesses (especially of women) that originate after exposure to cold and from tension. It has proved helpful often.

I always hate to send friends and patients to an herb store for Mugwort. I would rather say, "Go out and pick the plant" but, unfortunately, few people know it by sight. Full of strength and warmth, our "Mother of All Plants" is easily overlooked. To find her, we must check around paths, gravel pits, and quarries—even along railway embankments. Mugwort appears so light and airy from afar that one sees right through it. However, the firm, erect, often reddish brown stem from which many side branches originate can rise five feet above the ground. The bipinnate leaves end in a pointed tip and are matte green on top and covered with white hairs (tomentum) underneath. Flowers appear only in late August and September in panicles on top of the branches. The small, gray, felt-like flower heads carry tiny, inconspicuous yellow or reddish brown flowers. Containing no nectar, they are pollinated by the wind.

Mugwort is closely related to Common Wormwood (*Artemisia absinthum*, or absinthe). While the two plants look similar, they are easily distinguished. Wormwood's leaves are covered with thick, fluffy hairs that make the plant shimmer in a silky gray-green hue. The flower heads are surrounded by silvery gray bracts with light yellow flowers. Wormwood contains a lot of essential oil making it intensely aromatic. It grows throughout Europe, except in the far northern and some southern regions, and in North America. It is a well-known medicinal plant with a high content of bitter compounds. This marks its use as a stomachic, appetizer, or digestive, for loss of appetite and nutritional disorders; it also stimulates bile secretion. However, it is highly toxic in concentrated form and should be utilized in home remedies with caution. Once used in the preparation of vermouth, absinthe, and other liquors, Wormwood is now prohibited in many countries (including Germany, England, and the United States) because its neurotoxic substances can cause brain damage when ingested over time.

Another—and safer—relative is Southernwood (*Artemisia abrotanum*)—also called Old Man or "Lad's Love." Originally native to southeastern Europe and western Asia, it has spread by cultivation throughout Europe and the Americas—although in cooler climates the seeds may fail to mature. It was known in Europe as early as the ninth and tenth centuries. The Southernwood in my garden has survived the cold winters of the German Alps pretty well so far, and every year I enjoy its tender filigreed leaves and subtle lemon fragrance. It is said that peasant women would wear a twig of Southernwood to church so that its fresh scent would keep them awake during sermons. Fresh or dried, the twigs of Southernwood make a pleasant-tasting medicinal tea. In fact, Costmary (*Chrysanthemum majus*) and Southernwood in equal parts is one of my favorite tea blends. Southernwood tea stimulates and invigorates and is helpful for anemia, lack of appetite, fever, and gout. In the past, it was used to treat tuberculosis. I could not praise Southernwood more beautifully than did Abbot Walahfried Strabo over ten centuries ago in these excerpted lines:

> It is easy to praise the high growth
>   of your shrub,
> Southernwood, admiring your foliage,
>   amply unfolding,
> Luxuriantly divided into branches,
>   comparable to delicate hair.
> This fragrant tuft of hair, together with
>   your pliable twigs
> Mingled with medicinal remedies,
>   makes a useful mixture.
> Fevers she wards off, chases away a
>   stitch in the side, brings help
> When the insidious gout troubles us
>   with a sudden attack.
> But more: She has as many powers as
>   she has delicate leaves.

> from *The Hortulus*
> of *Walahfrid Strabo*

HEALING PROPERTIES

Once familiar to all, Mugwort today is nearly forgotten as a medicinal herb. Only in homeopathy does she still play a modest role, which I find surprising because my experience shows Mugwort to be a very potent and reliable remedy. As is the case with most medicinal plants, correct dosage and application is crucial for treatment success. An overdose can cause unpleasant side effects attributed to the cineole content in its essential oil. *Note: Do not use Mugwort during either acute febrile diseases or pregnancy. (It can induce an abortion.)*

Having repeatedly mentioned its connection with the Great Goddess, I will begin with the herb's use as a woman's remedy. Mugwort is an emmenagogue that promotes menstruation, thereby helping in cases of late or scanty menstrual periods. A woman's monthly period cleanses and balances function in the female organism and there is a strong connection between a missing or weak menstruation and psychological problems. Therefore, it is important to ensure a regular menstrual cycle. Additional remedies that promote menstruation include:

- Rosemary (*Rosmarinus officinalis*): as an infusion or wine
- Chaste Tree (*Vitex agnus-castus*): as a homeopathic mother tincture from an herbal pharmacy; 15 drops, 3 times daily
- Rue (*Ruta graveolens*): as an infusion or a spice
- Lady's Mantle (*Alchemilla vulgaris*): as an infusion

- German Chamomile (*Matricaria chamomilla*): as an infusion
- Calendula (*Calendula officinalis*): as an infusion
- Vervain (*Verbena officinalis*): as an infusion
- Saffron (*Crocus sativus*): as a spice
- Cinnamon (*Cinnamomum cassia*): as a spice

Mugwort also has an antispasmodic effect on the female reproductive organs. Therefore, like Silverweed (*Potentilla anserina*), it is used for painful menstruation. A course of treatment consisting of teas of both plants is enhanced when accompanied with footbaths and sitz baths of Mugwort. (See the chapter on Silverweed.)

For weak or painful menstruation, I recommend taking Mugwort internally as an infusion (tea). A dose is one cup taken three times daily. If you prefer a tincture, you can take five drops of tincture three times a day while externally adding it to the warm water of a footbath or sitz bath.

Mugwort is especially helpful for all illnesses of the abdominal and pelvic organs caused by exposure to cold. (Remember that Mugwort was described in the old herbals as one of the "hottest" plants.) In cases of weak or painful menses after exposure to cold, chronic cystitis, vaginal discharge, or a chronically cold lumbar region, Mugwort soothes women with its comforting warmth. Indeed, most diseases of the female reproductive organs are accompanied by symptoms of cold feet—and until they are treated, all else will fail! Addressing this reflexological connection between a patient's pelvic organs and feet greatly enhances the treatment. As a basis for treating these illnesses as well as chronic ovaritis (inflammation of the ovaries) and weak ovarian function, I usually prescribe a Mugwort footbath before going to bed as well as a steam sitz bath once a week. (For a description see the chapter on Horsetail.)

Always use it concurrently, internally and externally, as a tea, wine, powder, tincture, foot-bath, or sitz bath. Mugwort stimulates labor and a tea was once administered to birthing women by their midwives. Later it was given to the mother to stimulates afterpains, thereby promoting passage of the placenta.

After a strenuous hike or a long day on one's feet, a Mugwort footbath will relax and invigorate tired legs and feet. Likewise, the tincture rubbed into sore muscles and weak limbs refreshes and strengthens.

Because Mugwort relaxes the central nervous system, it was once used as a basic remedy for all diseases connected with tension—whether physical or emotional. Often a patient's pillow was stuffed with the dried herb to calm the nerves and promote sleep.

Mugwort was used not only for "minor" sleep disturbances but also for severe nervous disorders such as epilepsy. This has a long history. More recently, we have access to empirical accounts (Schulz and Bohn, 1927). In his book *Medicinal Values of Native Plants*, Dr. W. Bohn reports on his proved application of Mugwort for epilepsy: On feeling an approaching attack, the person should take a teaspoon of freshly powdered Mugwort root in a cup of hot grain coffee substitute, go to bed, bundle up, and sweat. If not done before, the person should do

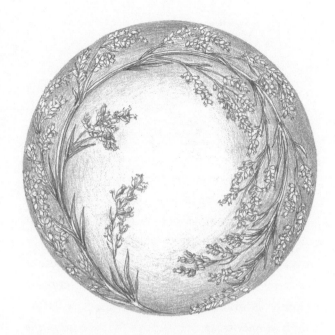

so following the attack, repeating the procedure on the third and sixth day after. For a long-term epilepsy treatment, the person should ingest a pinch of the freshly ground root three times daily.

What does Mugwort have to do with the traditional Christmas goose or turkey? Why, it helps us digest it easier. Mugwort is a traditional spice for roast goose and other fatty meats. Remember: Mugwort stimulates digestion, strengthens the stomach, stimulates the appetite, and helps with flatulence. For this purpose, it can be ingested as a spice, wine, or tea.

From oriental medicine we learn yet another way to experience Mugwort's comforting strength. Traditionally, the fine fibers (moxa) of the local Mugwort plant are dried and pressed into small cones or sticks. When lit, they burn for a long time with a pleasant smell. They are placed on acupuncture points related to the disease being treated so that the warmth of the burning moxa affects the point and the meridian.

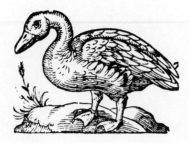

The cone is removed before it can burn the skin. Personally, I prefer to use moxa sticks, which are lit and held about an inch away from the area of the body being treated. Moxa's warmth penetrates deeply to relax and release all kinds of tension—headaches, low back pain, chronic sinus conditions, and stomach cramps. *Note: As with Mugwort tea and powder, it is not advisable to use moxa in cases of acute inflammatory illnesses.*

The right time to gather moxa is from July to September when Mugwort is flowering. I cut the plants a little above the ground and hang them singly upside down to dry in an airy, shaded spot. They are sufficiently dried when they rustle when rubbed together. I then strip the leaves and flowers from the stems.

Mugwort root is best dug up in November. Do not wash it with water. Instead clean it carefully with a brush before hanging it to dry in a protected place. Prepare only the amount of powder needed at a time so that it retains its strength. (I use a mortar and pestle.) Taken internally a pinch at a time, a daily dose is two or three pinches. *Note: Because the powdered root is stronger than tea prepared from the herb, be careful not to overdose.*

Mugwort tea is available in herb stores as "Herba artemisiae." If you would rather not make your own tincture, use the homeopathic mother tincture "Artemisia vulgaris."

ﻬ Mugwort Tea

> 1 teaspoon dried mugwort herb
> 1 cup boiling water

Pour the boiling water over the dried herb, letting it steep for 10 minutes. A daily dose is 2 or 3 cups. Do not sweeten the tea.

ﻬ Mugwort Footbath

> 2 handfuls mugwort herb, dried or fresh
> 3 quarts cold water

Bring the herbs and the cold water to a boil in a covered pot, reduce the heat, and let it simmer for 5 minutes. Strain the liquid into a bucket or large bowl, adding more hot water as needed. Administer hot mugwort footbaths for disorders of the pelvic organs, tension, cold feet, and headaches. Cold footbaths are used for swollen and tired feet. For this purpose, let the brew cool before adding cold water.

ﻬ Mugwort Oil

> fresh mugwort
> cold-pressed sunflower oil
> essential oil of Scots pine
> (*Oleum Pini sylvestris*)

Fill a mason jar with chopped mugwort leaves, flowers, and roots. Add sunflower oil to cover and close the jar. Place it in a warm, sunny spot for 2 or 3 weeks. Strain the oil into another jar, adding 15 drops of essential oil of Scots pine for every pint of oil. Shake the mixture well before transferring it to dark bottles.

This oil makes an excellent rub for swollen, tired feet and for sore or tense muscles.

৬৯ Mugwort Tincture

> mugwort root
>
> grain spirit or vodka

Fill a small dark mason jar halfway with freshly crushed mugwort root. Cover the root with the alcohol, close the jar, and let it steep for 2 or 3 weeks; shake it occasionally. Strain the tincture into dark dropper bottles. A daily dose is 3 to 5 drops administered 3 times daily. Mugwort tincture is a good liniment for tired feet, sore muscles, and neuralgias.

৬৯ Mugwort Sleeping Pillow

Make a pillow of dried mugwort flowers and leaves to use for insomnia and muscle cramps. In a child's pillow use one-third dried chamomile flowers.

৬৯ Moth Sachet

Mugwort keeps moths away. In the past, people placed mugwort twigs in dressers and closets or sewed the herb into sachets for placing between the linens. Use mugwort by itself or mix it with other moth-repelling herbs. (I add fragrant herbs to mugwort to give a fresh scent to my clothes.) Choose from this list of moth-repelling herbs: sweetclover (*Melilotus officinalis*), sweet woodruff (*Asperula odorata*), southernwood (*Artemisia abrotanum*), mint (*Mentha piperita*), tansy (*Tanacetum vulgare*), cypress (*Cupressus sempervirens*), rose pelargonium (*Pelargonium graveolens*), clove (*Eugenia caryophyllata*, *Syzygium aromaticum*), thyme (*Thymus vulgaris*), lavender (*Lavandula* spp.).

Culinary Use

In times past Mugwort was never missing from any fatty dish—roast goose, for instance. Like all traditional spices, its function was to aid the stomach with digestion, especially of fatty foods. For this purpose, use only the uppermost panicles of flowers just before the flowers open—and they can be used fresh or dried. Mugwort is a welcome addition to potato soup, bean stew, cabbage dishes, sauces and gravy, meat, fish, and mushrooms.

Cultivation

Mugwort can grow into a shrub reaching five feet in height. Her preferred soil is limy, sandy, gravelly, and loamy. Seeds can be sown in pots from April to June and will germinate in about one week. However, because Mugwort needs light to germinate, press the seeds gently into the soil—do not bury them. Later, transplant the seedlings 10 to 15 inches apart. Older plants are easily divided. Mugwort will begin to self-seed as early as the following year. Around a single Mugwort plant in your garden, you will soon see many small seedlings sprout. In the fall, cut back the plants to 5 or 6 inches above the ground. Being very robust, they will need no special protection over the winter. Seeds and starter plants are commercially available.

BOTANICAL CHARACTERISTICS

Name: *Artemisia vulgaris* — Mugwort

Distribution: Europe, Asia, and the Americas

Habitat: Waysides, quarries, railway embankments, thickets

Description: Plants grow 3 to 5 feet tall; firm, erect stem with spreading side branches; stem often a dark reddish brown; underside of leaves covered by white tomentum, top is glabrous and dark green, pinnate or bipinnate with pointed tip; gray, felt-like flower heads are oval or elongated; tiny yellow or reddish brown flowers bloom from July to September.

Confusion with similar plants: Wormwood (*Artemisia absinthum*) has leaves with a silvery white tomentum on both sides; leaf tips are rounded; petiole and stem are not dark red like Mugwort's. Wormwood is strongly aromatic.

Collecting season:
    Herb – July to September
    Root – November

Active ingredients: Bitter compounds, tannins, essential oil with cineole and thujone

Astrological association: Venus / Mercury

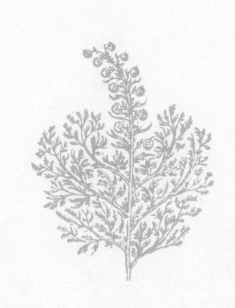

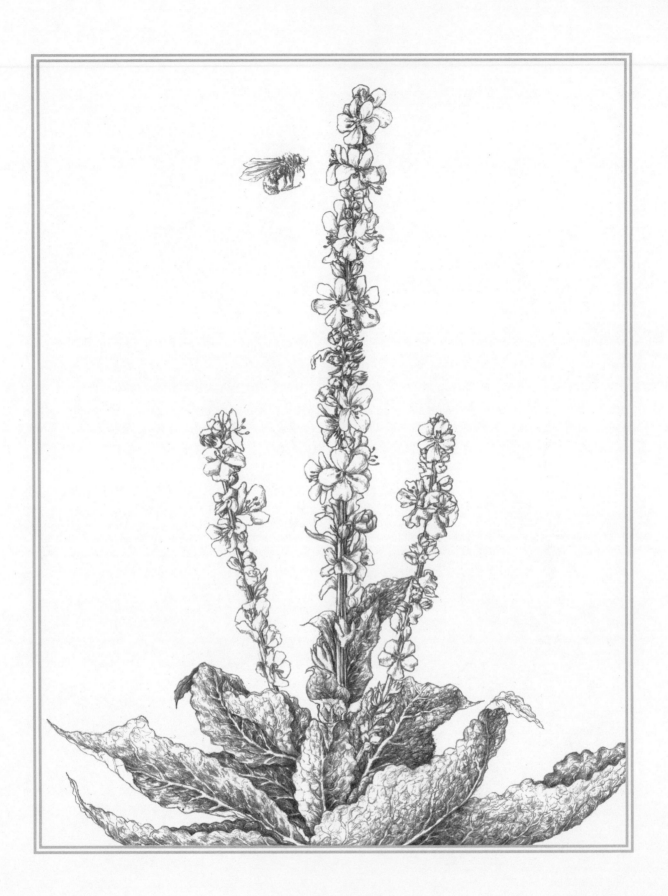

MULLEIN

Verbascum thapsiforme (*V. densiflorum*) – Wool Mullein, Large-Flowered Mullein
V. thapsus – Common Mullein, Great Mullein, Flannel Mullein
V. phlomoides – Clasping Mullein, Orange Mullein
Snapdragon or Figwort family — Scrophulariaceae

AN ALPINE HIKER MIGHT FIND some medicinal plants too inconspicuous to warrant a glance—but never Mullein! Straight as a candle rises this stately plant, high above the foliage of other plants and sometimes taller than a person. A closer look reveals single, golden yellow flowers radiating toward us like twinkling lights arranged one above the other around the tall stem. They bloom one after the other, one opening as soon as another little light goes out. Personally, I find no yellow friendlier or warmer than that of Mullein flowers. And I am not the first to find a good companion in this herbal plant. In the twelfth century, Hildegard von Bingen prescribed Mullein to those with "sad hearts:"

> Let those people who have weak and sad hearts cook and eat Mullein together with meat and fish or cake so that their hearts will become strong and joyful again.

Mullein's flowers have a fragrance like that of delicate yellow roses on a summer morning. Within the petals are five stamens bearing orange pollen, three of which are smaller and sport thick, white beards. Indeed, their botanical name *Verbascum* refers to these amusing beards and is derived from the Latin word *barbascum* (*barba* or "beard").

Before extending its elegant flowering candlesticks skyward, Mullein requires a year to develop. I can still remember first noticing Mullein leaves hanging in large rosettes on a steep slope, arranged as beautifully as a lotus mandala, with a touch as soft and velvety as rabbit ears. Moving closer, I noticed a pelt of woolly hair enclosing the leaf—giving to Mullein common names like "Woolherb" in German and "Flannelflower," "Feltwort," and "Velvet Plant" in English. This felt-like hair is a protective layer that allows the plant to survive in the hot, sunny, arid habitats it loves—gravel pits, mountain slopes, and waysides. In the old days the furry leaves were dried, cut into strips, and used as candlewicks. And the plant's stem dipped in oil, resin, pitch, or wax would burn for a long time as a candle or torch. Crushed, the leaves made a good tinder because the fine hairs ignited easily. Hence, Mullein bore practical, descriptive names

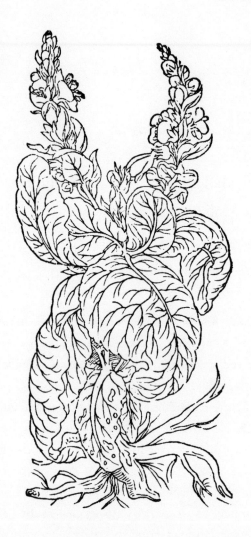

instructions on how to make such an amulet as well as revealing something about medieval birth control:

> It aids all kinds of catarrh as a strong amulet, especially when made from a root that has not yet flowered in the summer that it is gathered. Instead, dig it up on the last Friday of the waning moon before sunrise between the 15th of August and the 8th of September. Dry the cleaned root in a shady place. When one wraps pieces of it in gold to hang around the neck, it has miraculous powers against all flows of the body. However, it is not appropriate for women wishing to conceive a child as it hinders conception as long as she wears it.

An old belief in a mysterious connection between Mullein and the weather survives today. In rural areas, some farmers still grow Mullein beside their houses and outbuildings claiming that it keeps lightning away. These so-called "Weathercandles" are never brought into the house for fear that lightning will strike.

The deep roots of Mullein's magic reach far back in history, touching upon ancient spiritual beliefs. It plays a primary role in the ancient practice of Herb Blessing, one of humankind's original mysteries and a custom still found in rural areas of southern Germany. The period between August 15th (Mary's ascension into Heaven) and September 8th (the birth of Mary) was referred to as "the 30 days of women," long considered an auspicious time for herb gathering. This period began with the church blessing of a ritual bunch of herbs on August 15th. The number of herbs was precisely dictated, indicating its probable origins as a pagan magical ritual. The magic number of herbs was—and is today—always 9, 15, 77, or 99, ritual numbers that can

such as "Candlewick," *Königskerze* or "King's Candle," and *Herba lucernaria* or "lamp herb."

Many readers recognize Mullein but few are familiar with its history. My ancestors saw in Mullein a benevolent, magical spirit that could help them in times of danger and distress. One old German name "Demon Plant" (*Unholden-pflanze*) refers to these powers. People believed that Mullein could banish demons and ward off harmful magic spells and diseases. When worn as an amulet, the root had to be dug up on a certain day to align its powers with those of the Planets. In his *Most Precious Medicinal Treasure* of 1685, Johann Schröder wrote very detailed

be traced to ancient Babylonian and Assyrian civilizations.

Not just any plants grace the ritual bunch—the herbs were prescribed as well. It is striking that the choices were always old magical plants. The stately and beautiful Mullein took the throne at the center of this bunch of nine. The plants grouped around it were St. John's Wort (*Hypericum perforatum*), Centaury (*Centaurium erythraea*), Yarrow (*Achillea millefolium*), German Chamomile (*Matricaria chamomilla*), Wormwood (*Artemisia absinthium*), Valerian (*Valeriana officinalis*), Peppermint (*Mentha piperita*), and Arnica (*Arnica montana*)—all strong medicinal herbs with which one could equip a good herbal pharmacy! The composition of the 99 herbs used is not so well known although I can list some of them: Hemp Agrimony (*Eupatorium cannabinum*), Southernwood (*Artemisia abrotanum*), Elecampane (*Inula helenium*), Yellow Bedstraw (*Galium verum*), Tansy (*Tanacetum vulgare*), Bitter Nightshade (*Solanum dulcamara*), Wild Marjoram (*Origanum vulgare*), Rue (*Ruta graveolens*), Agrimony (*Agrimonia eupatoria*), Martagon Lily (*Lilium martagon*), Male Fern (*Dryopteris filix-mas*), and Spiny Restharrow (*Ononis spinosa*).

The bunch of ritual herbs retains a special place in the living area of southern German farmhouses. In the old days, a pinch of it was thrown into the hearth fire whenever thunder and lightning threatened. On Epiphany, the herbs were burned in a metal pan to smudge the house with its sacred smoke. Our ancestors expressed their gratitude for these healing plants in the custom of the "Herb Blessing," asking the blessing of the Goddess under whose protection the herbs were placed. Christian lore placed

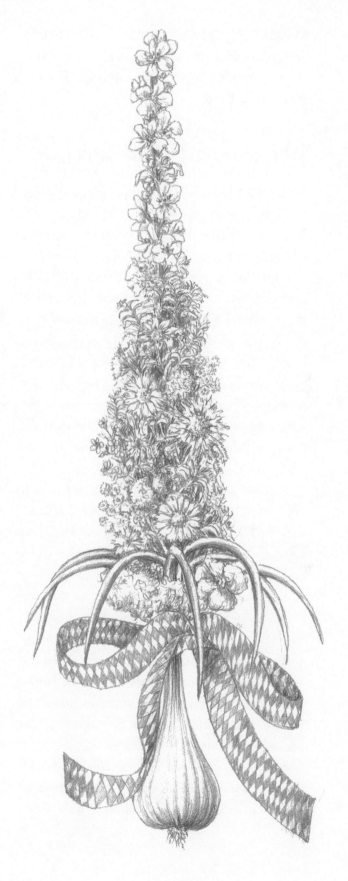

Mullein (or "Heaven's Blaze") under Mary's protection, as illustrated in this old saying: "Our Dear Lady travels the land, carrying Heaven's Blaze in her hand."

HEALING PROPERTIES

When Winter confines us to bed with a cold or bad cough, we should remember Summer's sunny Mullein flowers. For all respiratory diseases, especially for irritations and inflammations but also for chronic conditions in this area, Mullein can work small miracles. Long considered one of the "pectoral herbs" ("species pectorales"), it can be trusted to help the following conditions: cough (including an irritating or tickling cough), hoarseness, a scratchy voice (along with the root of Burnet Saxifrage), bronchitis, phlegm in the lungs, the common cold (due to Mullein's slight diaphoretic properties), and asthma (as an adjunct with other plants).

Mullein tea requires only the flowers, which you can pick yourself. However, they are delicate and turn a moldy black easily when dried improperly. I like to gather them at midday when it is dry and sunny. Immediately I pluck them from the calyx and spread them out on a screen to dry in an airy place away from any moisture. To prepare the tea, pour a cup of boiling water over one teaspoon of the dried flowers, cover the cup, and let the mixture steep for several minutes. Strain it carefully because the fine hairs can irritate the patient's mucous membranes. This tea can be sweetened with honey.

Mullein flowers can also be combined with other pectoral herbs to make a tea designed to treat a specific respiratory illness. I have listed some other medicinal herbs you can choose from when preparing an individual blend:

- Garden Angelica (*Angelica archangelica*) promotes expectoration in cough and bronchitis; calming. It is less suitable as a children's remedy due to its bitterness.
- Burnet Saxifrage root (*Pimpinella saxifraga*) makes a good single-herb tea for gargling; boil 1 teaspoon root in 1 cup water. This is helpful for sore throat, tonsillitis, pharyngitis, pain with swallowing. Combined with Mullein and Coltsfoot, it makes a good tea for chronic smoker's cough.
- Coltsfoot (*Tussilago farfara*) protects the mucous membranes in acute and chronic cough and promotes expectoration.
- Common Mallow (*Malva sylvestris*) protects irritated mucous membranes; helps painful cough and pain with swallowing. It works well as a gargle.
- Corn Poppy (*Papaver rhoeas*) soothes spasmodic cough in children who prefer it as a sweet syrup (homemade or from the pharmacy).
- Cowslip (*Primula veris*) dissolves phlegm in cough and congestion.
- Elecampane root (*Inula helenicum*) is for chronic cough, irritating and tickling cough, asthma, and bronchitis.
- Greater Celandine (*Chelidonium majus*) soothes the cramping of spasmodic cough. It is not recommended for children.
- Iceland Moss (*Cetraria islandica*) protects irritated mucous membranes from painful cough and dissolves phlegm from

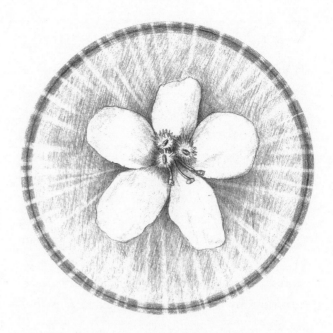

cough with congestion. It is especially suited for chronic catarrh and long-standing cough.

- Lungwort (*Pulmonaria officinalis*) promotes expectoration, protects mucous membranes; helps cough, hoarseness, and phlegm retention in the respiratory tract. It is well suited for treating chronic conditions. It is a good tea for heavy smokers and as adjunct therapy for pulmonary tuberculosis.
- Marshmallow (*Althaea officinalis*) dissolves phlegm and promotes expectoration. It is especially good for cough and acute bronchitis.
- Ribwort Plantain (*Plantago lanceolata*) as a syrup or tea is used to treat lung diseases.
- Sage (*Salvia officinalis*) is a good gargle for sore throat. It heals irritated mucous membranes and is antibacterial. For a long-standing cough, a blend of 1 part Sage and 2 parts Mullein can be inhaled like snuff. For inhaling during acute rhinitis, mix Sage, Thyme, and Eucalyptus in equal parts.
- Round-leaved Sundew (*Drosera rotundifolia*) soothes the cramps of spasmodic cough. It is not recommended for children.
- Thyme (*Thymus vulgaris*) dissolves mucous and soothes cramping cough. Antibacterial properties make it an effective herb to inhale.

Lastly, I can recommend a remedy from Mullein flowers that is quite effective for earaches, hearing problems, and the early stages of middle ear infection (otitis media). And it is another medicinal preparation easily made at home. To do so, fill a small jar with fresh Mullein flowers; close it tightly and place it in the sun for several days. Soon a slimy, watery substance will be exuded that can be carefully strained into a dark bottle. Put a few drops of it into the ear when needed.

Mullein flowers are available in natural food stores or herbal pharmacies as "Flores Verbasci."

VETERINARY MEDICINE

A well-strained tea of Mullein flowers can help alleviate the irritation of cough and catarrh in animals. The oil also works well against infection, especially in dogs.

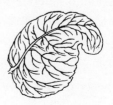

CULTIVATION

Truly a royal plant, Mullein is an eye-catcher anywhere—and a traditional plant in rural gardens. It is especially suitable as a backdrop for perennial borders when smaller plants (for example, blue Petunias) are planted in front of it.

For a plot to use for medicinal teas, I plant Large-Flowered Mullein (*Verbascum thapsiforme*) or even Great Mullein (*V. thapsus*). Some people use the flowers of Orange Mullein (*V. phlomoides*). Perennial nurseries and seed stores offer a wide variety of Mulleins, each attractive in its own way. I include a partial list here:

- 'Arctic Summer' (*Verbascum bombyciferum*) is a biennial with sulfur yellow flowers and silvery white leaves. It can grow 6 feet tall and has a long flowering time. Hybrids are 'Cotswold' and 'Queen' with amber flowers (grows to 5 feet), Densiflorum with copper flowers, and 'Hartleyi' with lemon-colored flowers with a dark center (grows to 3 feet).
- Long-leaf Mullein (*V. longifolium*) has a single, unbranched flowering stem.
- 'Olympic Mullein' (*V. olympicum*), a perennial, is the the tallest of all, growing 6½ feet, crowned with many long, bright yellow flower spikes.
- Purple Mullein (*V. phoeniceum*), a perennial with purple flowers, grows 2 feet tall and is suitable for dry meadows. A 3-foot hybrid is 'Pink Domingo' with pink flowers.
- Black Mullein (*V. nigrum*) has pale yellow flowers and grows 3 feet tall.

The modest Mullein biennials or perennials like a loamy, sandy, dry habitat, needing a sunny place more than anything else. Plant them in nutrient-rich earth and fertilize them if you want them to grow tall and strong. They seed themselves.

Starters and seeds are commercially available. Start seeds indoors in March or sow them outside in April or May. In fall, thin them to 20 inches apart. *Note:* The flowers can be harvested as soon as they open.

BOTANICAL CHARACTERISTICS

Name: *Verbascum thapsiforme* — Mullein

Distribution: Europe, western Asia, and the Americas

Habitat: Sunny dry places, railway embankments, waysides

Description: Grows to 6 feet; the first year forms a basal rosette of up to 15 inches with long, pointed leaves with woolly hairs. The second year an unbranched (usually), tall, flowering stem grows with lemon yellow flowers and with stem leaves whose bases extend downward. Flowers sit mostly in clusters of 4 in the upper leaf axils.

Confusion with similar plants: With other Mullein species. My experience is that none are poisonous although some herbalists disagree. Possibly confused with Agrimony (*Agrimonia eupatoria*), which appears much smaller and more delicate than Mullein; it has even-pinnate leaves and yellow flowers that grow in racemes; leaves are not hairy.

Collecting season: Flowers – July to August

Active ingredients: Mucilage about 3%, flavonoids, inverted sugar about 11%, essential oils, steroids, digiprolacto.

Astrological association: Sun / Mercury

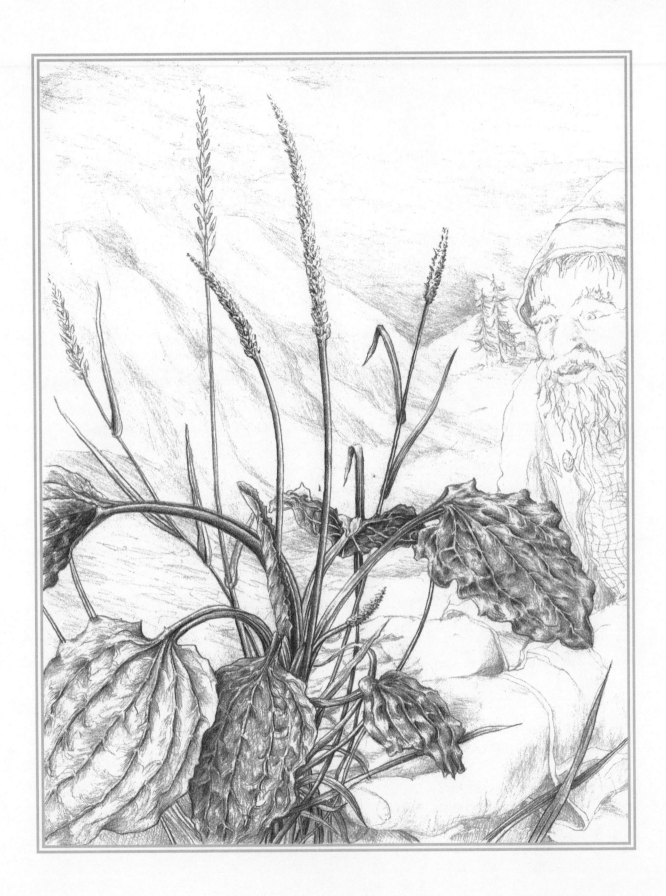

PLANTAIN

Plantago major – Common Plantain, Broad-leaved Plantain
Plantago lanceolata – Ribwort Plantain, Lance-leaf Plantain
Plantago media – Hoary Plantain, Sweet Plantain
Plantain family – Plantaginaceae

O, Plantain, mother of plants,
open to the East, powerful inside:
Carts creaked over you, women rode
   over you,
brides cried over you, bulls snorted over you.
All you have withstood and
   set yourself against.
So may you resist, too, the poison, contagion,
and evil that spreads across the land.

from an old English spell to
bless the nine sacred herbs

PLANTAIN'S HISTORY LEADS US far back into ages long past. It leads us to the Underworld to encounter Orcus, King of the Dead, sorcerers with their apprentices, and plant fairies and root diggers. We enter medieval birthing rooms or meet secretly at a crossroads in the night. In all of these stories Plantain plays the featured role: a powerful supernatural plant spirit, the vanquisher of deadly diseases, arising from the Underworld. In German we call him *Wegerich* or "Ruler of the Way." This is because he controls the way, especially the path leading directly to the realm of the dead. My ancient forebearers often buried their dead on grassy paths and waysides and thought that plants who grew there embodied the souls of the departed.

Tribal peoples have always considered the dead to have a role in life. Souls restless in death might bring misfortune—but they might also aid the living. They might choose to enter plants whose form thereby took that of medicinal or magical herbs. Plantain always attracted attention because he grew along their paths. Seeming to follow human footsteps, he made his presence everywhere apparent. In fact, I only have to get up from my desk and walk down the lane in front of my house to find him, skirting the way with his thick, round leaves.

For the old Germans, this small, troublesome companion embodied those souls who still sought the light after entering the Underworld. The ancient Greeks and Romans also believed in Plantain's connection to these powers. The following spell has been preserved from the eleventh century, marking Plantain's position as a plant of the Roman god Orcus (the Greek Hades or Pluto) and Ruler of the Underworld,

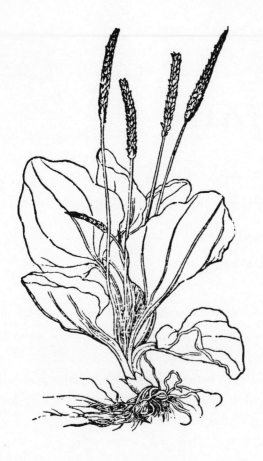

The best time of year to gather plants for amulets and remedies is between August 15th and September 8th ("Women's Thirty Days"), the time between the Blessed Mary's ascension and her birth. This is a period long valued as especially favorable for herb gathering.

To observe a medieval root digger—then a common profession—we must travel back many centuries and arrange to meet him at a crossroads an hour before sunrise. This is the time when spirits of the dead still swarm and when Plantain's powers are considered strongest. Only specific magic spells can protect a root digger from attack by the spirits, including packs of Orcs. (Readers will recognize these beings who were more recently revived by J.R.R. Tolkien in his Lord of the Rings trilogy.)

Our root digger pays attention to everything—time, incantations, place. He follows his instructions, yet every noise startles him. Maybe he can calm himself with thoughts of the root's great healing power that are said to bestow supernatural powers on him and to heal life-threatening diseases—even the plague. It is supposed to save women from bleeding to death. (And here we can leave our root digger alone for a while. It will take him some time to get the root out of the ground because, according to rules of the trade, he must not employ a metal tool but must use his bare hands. And since it grows in hard-packed stony soil, it will be safe for us to stop and consider more about Plantain's healing powers.)

The earliest written accounts about Plantain originate in classical antiquity with the Greek and Roman physicians who praised and prescribed it. Ruling the waysides, he grows exactly

and his daughter Proserpina (the Greek Persephone) and Goddess of Death.

> Plantain, herb of Proserpina, Daughter of
>   King Orcus!
> As you have made infertile the mule,
> So may you also shut the wave of blood
>   from this woman's womb!

To conjure up the spirits of this realm in order to gain control over their supernatural powers was to venture into grave danger. Indeed, many sorcerers' apprentices attempted it without their masters—and failed. There were certain rules to follow when digging out a magical Plantain root to use for healing. Surviving still in modern times, many such ancient incantations have their sources in Assyrian, Egyptian, Celtic, or Germanic lore.

where he is needed—because things happen to travelers. Things such as accidents, robberies, injuries, bites, punctures, bleeding, leg injuries. A traveler afoot suffers from legs that feel heavy, sore, and tight, all ailments for which the old doctors recommended Common Plantain. Around 50 A.D. Dioscurides recommended Plantain for bleeding and hemorrhaging, for dog bites, and for burn wounds. Pliny, his contemporary, called him an infallible remedy for wild animal bites. Tidings of Plantain's healing power even found their way into world literature with Shakespeare recommending Plantain as a remedy for skin injuries in "Romeo and Juliet." And Hieronymus Bock claimed in his 1577 herbal:

> I need not mention that there is hardly a person who does not know what Plantain is good for. This we see in daily practice and experience.

At the time of the vast European emigration to the Americas, Plantain received yet another way-related name. Everywhere the Europeans went in this new land, Plantain followed. He stuck to the heels of people, attached himself to wagon wheels, pressed himself into the hooves of horses. Sticking by way of a slimy outer film, the seeds spread for miles along trails. Observing this, the Native Americans called Plantain "White Man's Foot."

HEALING PROPERTIES

There are three easily distinguished Plantain brothers, each with his particular healing applications. Common Plantain (*Plantago major*) is also known as Broad-leaved or Rippleseed Plantain. He has very broad ovate leaves—looking like huge ears—that surround the stem in a basal rosette laying flat on the ground. He likes to grow along waysides and in arid wastelands.

Ribwort Plantain (*Plantago lanceolata*) is sometimes called Lance-leaf or Buckhorn Plantain. Stretching narrow lanceolate leaves upward in a graceful manner, he prefers meadows and a moister habitat than his large-eared brother.

The third brother seems unable to make up his mind. With leaves narrower than Common Plantain's yet broader than Ribwort Plantain's, he sports a Latin name that means "in between" —*Plantago media*. In English he is commonly

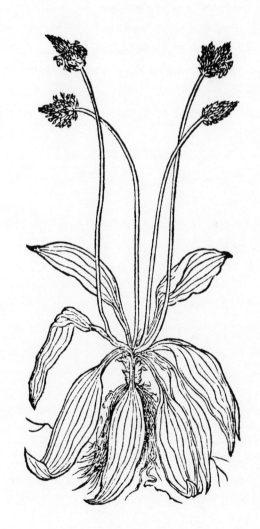

called Hoary Plantain (or Sweet or Gray Plantain). However, we will leave him and return to his two brothers.

In recognizing Plantain's particular healing powers, people doubtlessly followed Paracelsus' "Doctrine of Signatures" in which the sixteenth century Swiss-born physician-alchemist said that signs such as color, shape, and chosen environment revealed a plant's God-given destiny to those who could interpret them.

For example, Common Plantain's broad leaf resembled a footprint. His corresponding Latin genus name *planta* meant "sole of the foot"— and he was long prescribed for healing and strengthening tired and sore blistered feet. Indeed, a fresh Plantain leaf placed in each shoe strengthened many a tired wayfarer (although Mugwort *Artemisia vulgaris*, whose German name means "By Foot," was also used for this purpose).

In the third volume of his complete works, Paracelsus gives us even more detailed instructions:

> When one has developed blisters on the feet from walking, Plantain should be crushed with salt and a small amount of it should be applied overnight. In the morning, fill the shoes with it to help chase away the pain.

Common or Broad-leaved Plantain, by shape alone, offers itself as a wound plaster. Again, listen to Paracelsus:

> No plant dries up and at the same time astringes as well as Plantago. For a wound, Plantago should be crushed with Chelidonia [Greater Celandine] and mixed with the juice of either plant. A cloth subsequently should be dipped into this mixture and applied to the wound.

Its traditional application as a wound compress is confirmed. Modern scientists have proved that Common Plantain contains chemical constituents that disinfect wounds, kill pathological germs, prevent inflammation, and speed the healing process in wounds, ulcers, inflamed nipples, insect bites, and infections. The fresh leaves are the most effective. For this purpose: clean the leaf, mash it slightly, and apply it fresh as a dressing. Change it frequently.

You can also prepare a medicinal oil to alleviate itchy skin by finely chopping fresh leaves of both Common and Ribwort Plantain in equal parts and then steeping them in cold-pressed sunflower oil (prepared like St. John's Wort oil). When enriched with essential oil of Thyme (10 drops for 50 milliliters of the oil), it makes a good liniment for cough and bronchitis in children.

Different qualities make Ribwort Plantain an effective lung remedy. Its leaves contain a successful combination of active ingredients that affect the lungs in many ways. Silicic acid firms lung tissue, mucilage protects irritated mucous membranes and alleviates pain with coughing and respiration, tannins firm the mucous membranes, and antibacterial constituents fight pathological bacteria without weakening the body. It also contains vitamin C—and probably other ingredients that are not yet discovered in the laboratory. Together these make Ribwort Plantain a remedy for all lung and bronchial conditions (such as cough, bronchitis, pneumonia, and asthma). As an adjunct remedy for pulmonary tuberculosis, he strengthens the lung tissue. Finally, heavy smokers and those who have broken the habit can use Ribwort Plantain to strengthen their lungs.

We can gather Ribwort Plantain's leaves from May through August. However, they must be dried with care because they mold and turn black easily. My method is to place them loosely on an elevated mesh screen in an airy location. And you can make absolutely certain that the goods of your wildcrafting do not turn bad by stringing freshly gathered leaves on twine and hanging them up to dry like clothes on a line. Once dried, cut the leaves into small pieces and store them in a tightly lidded container to use for tea.

However, even more effective than Plantain tea is a sweet syrup made from the fresh leaves. Traditionally called "Earth Chamber Syrup" (see the recipe), its ancient method of preparation extracts the chemical constituents gently without destroying their active ingredients. The slow fermentation process carefully preserves the syrup. For all the diseases mentioned earlier, Ribwort Plantain syrup administered by the teaspoon is highly effective—especially in pediatric medicine because young people naturally prefer the sweetened juice over the tea prepared from the root.

Common Plantain is available in natural food stores or herbal pharmacies as "Herba Plantaginis majoris." The homeopathic mother tincture "Plantago major" is prepared from the fresh plant with its rootstock.

Ribwort Plantain is available as "Herba Plantaginis lanceolatae." The homeopathic mother tincture "Plantago lanceolata" is also prepared from the fresh plant with its rootstock.

❧ PLANTAIN TEA

Pour 1 cup of boiling water over 1 teaspoon of the herb and let it steep for 5 minutes. You may drink several cups of this tea daily when needed, sweetened with honey.

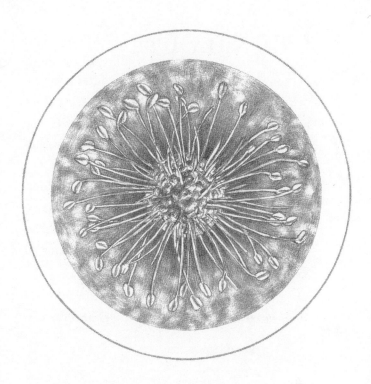

❧ "EARTH CHAMBER SYRUP"

Sterilize a quart mason jar with boiling water. Pack it tightly—about 1 centimeter (³⁄₈ inch) thick—with a layer of fresh but dry leaves of Ribwort Plantain. (Do not gather them in the early morning or after rain). Pour in enough liquid honey to cover the layer completely. Press another layer of leaves on top and again cover it with honey. Repeat the procedure until the jar is full. Let the jar stand for several hours or overnight until things settle—and then top it off with more honey. Be sure the leaves are covered. Cover the jar with several layers of thick parchment paper and wrap the neck tightly with wire. Place the jar in a hole in the ground that is about 20 inches deep. Over it put a small board and then cover it carefully with dirt. Be sure to mark the spot. The jar is now surrounded by an even ground temperature that produces a slow fermentation. After 3 months, dig up the jar, press the syrup from the leaves, and pour it into bottles. Store them tightly lidded in a cool place.

CULINARY USE

Plantain leaves generally have a bitter-pungent taste—although Ribwort Plantain is slightly milder than Common Plantain. The leaves are more tender before the plant flowers. If you harvest them later, be sure to remove the celery-like strings of Common Plantain before cooking them. Prepared as a vegetable, Plantain tastes a little like spinach and cabbage cooked together. The leaves can also be used as wild greens in salads, herbed butter, soups, and sauces.

ℰ RIBWORT PLANTAIN SOUP

> 4 tablespoons butter
> ¼ cup flour
> 2 cups milk
> 2 cups vegetable broth
> sea salt and nutmeg to taste
> 1 cup minced ribwort plantain
> 1 tablespoon minced parsley
> juice of half a lemon

In a saucepan, slowly melt the butter, whisk in the flour, and stir until it bubbles. (Do not let it brown or burn.) Stirring constantly, carefully add the milk and vegetable broth; whisk in the spices. Add the plantain and parsley and simmer the mixture over low heat until the plantain is soft and the soup thickens. Remove the soup from the heat, stir in the lemon juice, and serve with a crusty loaf of fresh bread or toasted croutons.

CULTIVATION

All Plantain species are hardy plants. Ribwort Plantain likes a dry, grassy habitat. On the other hand, Common Plantain does not like to grow in the middle of a meadow but rather along its borders, preferring well-watered and nutrient-rich soil.

Self-propagating by nature (remember the tale of "White Man's Foot") and easy to grow, seeds are available commercially. You can sow the seeds in spring and later thin the young plants six or eight inches apart.

BOTANICAL CHARACTERISTICS

Names: *Plantago major* — Common Plantain
          Plantago lanceolata — Ribwort Plantain
          Plantago media — Hoary Plantain

Distribution: Found in all temperate zones

Habitat: Common Plantain – paths and waysides
         Ribwort Plantain – grassy meadows

Description: Common Plantain reaches 16 inches with broad, ovate, stalked leaves in a basal rosette. Flowers in a long cylindrical spike; round stem; leaves have clearly visible parallel veins.

Ribwort Plantain reaches 20 inches with narrow lanceolate leaves in a basal rosette; leaves are directed more upward. Flowers in a short cylindrical spike; furrowed stem; leaves have clearly visible parallel veins.

Hoary Plantain reaches 16 inches with unstalked elliptical leaves in a basal rosette. Flowers in a spike; round stem; leaves with visible parallel veins.

Confusion with similar plants: None

Collecting season: Leaves – May to August

Active ingredients: Mucilage, tannins, silicic acid, vitamin C, bacteriostatic chemicals, glycoside aucubin, flavonoids, and saponins. The seeds contain a lot of mucilage and fat and make an excellent bird seed.

Astrological association: Common Plantain – Pluto
                       Ribwort Plantain – Mercury

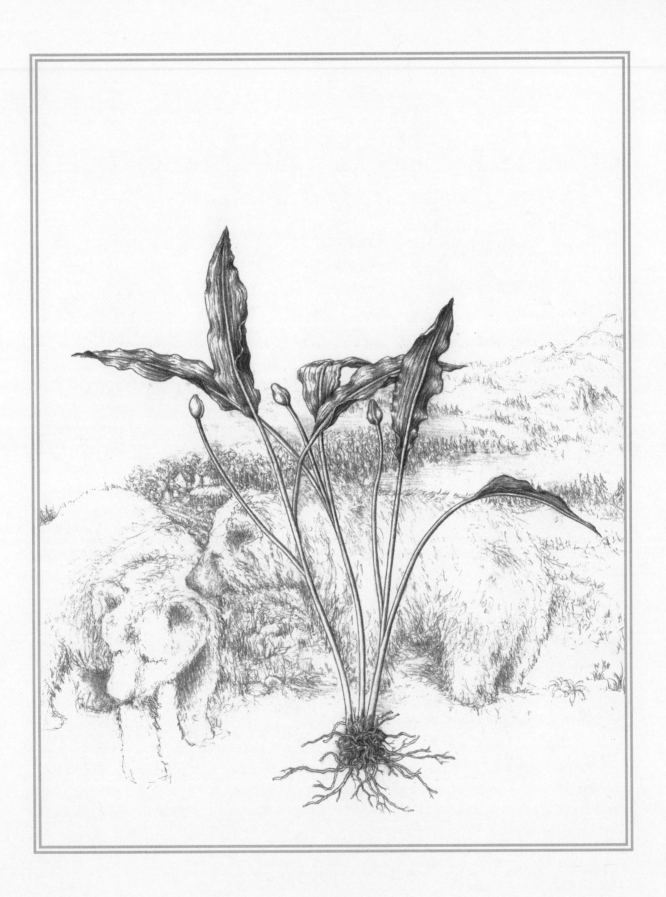

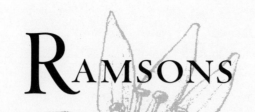

RAMSONS

Allium ursinum

Ramps, Wild Garlic, Bear's Garlic

Lily family — Liliaceae / Alliaceae

THREE ANIMALS—the bear, the wolf, and the fox—impressed and influenced our ancestors. Situated in the middle of the woods, early Germanic settlements and later medieval agricultural communities were like small protected islands in a sea of vast forests, the realm of wild beasts who threatened people and domestic animals. Strongly interwoven in human thought was the magic lore of animals and plants. The bear, the wolf, and the fox were considered soul animals by the ancient Germans in much the same way that certain animals still play important roles as helpers and guides in surviving Native American traditions. It is the totem animal who shows life's purpose to a seeker and grants to him or her special powers. Even now, during times of difficult life situations, such animals can appear to us in dreams as archetypal images. A person who understands their language can follow their advice.

In Germanic tradition, the bear was a vigorous primordial demon whose strength and power could break winter's hold and return fertility to vegetation. He was the bringer of spring who still stomps through the streets in the shape of straw- or fur-clad men during Alemanian Shrovetide carnivals. The bear's fertility symbolism is still retained in the German verb *gebären* ("to give birth") and in the English verb "to bear" (as to bear a child).

Certain plants were believed to embody the soul animals, and a person ate them to incorporate their powers. The old Germans consumed such magical plants, thought to be especially healing, on certain holy days as a ritual meal. Today, many healing plants retain the names of Germanic soul animals: "Wolfberries," "Wolf's Milk," "Wolf's Thistles," "Foxberries," "Fox's Salveherb," "Foxwort," "Bearwort," "Bearlobe," "Bearclaw,"—and "Bear's Leek." This last one is the German name of Ramsons. Similarly, an old English name is Bear's Garlic.

Plants of the bear contain the power of renewal and purification. Specifically, they break up hardenings, warm the body, and make a person "as strong as a bear" (*bärenstark*). Bear's Garlic, one of the mightiest of these plants, is, unfortunately, all but forgotten. Just as his bear-master brings Spring, so is he a spring plant, unfolding his strongest powers in that season. Indeed, this is the time to use the bear's own garlic as a remedy for strengthening and cleansing the body.

Let us stay with his name a little longer because every old plant name holds a story of its purpose and healing power. The English name of this plant is Ramsons, or Ramps. Old German names include *Ramser*, *Räms*, and *Rames*. These names point to the Old English root "hramsa," the Germanic root *hroms*, and Old High German *rämesadr*, a connection found in all European languages for plants of the onion and garlic family.

The Leek family is a medicinal plant family. The healing powers hidden in our ordinary kitchen leeks stimulate the gastric and intestinal juices and inhibit organisms that cause fermentation and putrefaction. My northern German ancestors cultivated leeks for food as well as for medicine in their "leek gardens" (*Lauchgärtlein*). In the Edda, a collection of mythology and heroic poems written in Iceland from the ninth to twelfth centuries, the leek was highly praised and recommended as a test for poisonous food. This Norse epic named the leek as one of the first plants created at the World's beginning:

> Sun from the South fell on the rock,
> and from the ground sprouted the green leek.

Names like "Bear's Leek" and Bear's Garlic remind us that our little Ramsons represents this honorable leek family. In his eighth century "ordinance for rural estates," Emperor Karl decreed that Ramsons should appear with certain other plants in every garden. But the plant, fallen out of fashion, runs wild again even though it is said to surpass garlic's healing powers.

When I saw the first glistening, metallic green Ramsons leaves this spring in the wooded marsh of a small alpine peninsula, I was not surprised. I sensed—or rather smelled—their presence before I even got there. An intense garlic smell permeated the small clearing. And for a member of the Lily family, Ramsons can smell pretty strong!

Ramsons loves company. In favorable habitats—moist, humus-rich, and shady deciduous forests—he makes his appearance en masse. In early spring he thrusts his shiny green, sword-shaped leaves straight up, quite optimistically, toward the sky from long, narrow bulbs similar in appearance to garlic cloves. Now is the time to gather and use the fresh leaves because dried Ramsons is worthless.

From April and well into June, beautiful clusters of white flowers radiate above the green foliage. The flowers occur in multiples of three, forming nectar in three nectaries within a three-chambered ovary to be collected in six stamens. Ramsons offers this sweet juice to a variety of insects—to bees and bumblebees as well as to flies who can reach it with their shorter proboscis. The small, black Ramsons seeds are enclosed in a black capsule that opens in June and July with special admirers all their own. Ants are keen on these oil-containing pellets and carry them everywhere in their industriousness, thereby sowing new plants. But Ramsons himself ensures offspring in his vicinity. When mature, the stem pregnant with seeds collapses and creates a new Ramsons carpet.

With a basketful of Ramsons leaves, I hiked back from the peninsula that spring morning. I had already nibbled on some fresh leaves and their effect was obvious as my steps became faster and faster. I was as hungry as a bear!

HEALING PROPERTIES

Why are the healing powers of Ramsons so little known today? Could it possibly be his strong garlic odor? After all, Ramsons is one of the oldest medicinal plants. Not only did the ancient Germans and Celts consider him a healing plant, but the Romans also used him. They named him *herba salutaris*, the healing herb. The last in a long succession of well-known herbalists to praise Ramsons properly was the German herbalist-cleric Künzle:

> Probably no herb on Earth is as effective for cleansing the stomach, intestines, and blood as the Bear's Garlic. People who are chronically ill and those afflicted with lichens, rashes, scrofula, and chlorosis should worship this plant more than gold. And young people would blossom like a trellis of roses!

And these exuberant words do not exaggerate. I have observed Ramsons' cleansing and strengthening power in many people. It helps those who in spring still have winter stuck in their limbs and spirits. Ramsons accomplishes this through its successful mixture of active ingredients—especially high contents of essential oils and a good shot of vitamin C.

Besides its generally invigorating action, Ramsons has three main points of application in the human body. First, it aids in healing chronic skin rashes and lichens by cleansing the blood, thereby remedying the cause of illness from within. Second, its high content of mustard oil glycosides stimulates the digestive juices. Finally, Ramsons has a bactericidal effect on the intestinal flora without destroying the beneficial intestinal bacteria necessary for digestion. This is why I always recommend Ramsons to patients once they finish a course of treatment with strong drugs like antibiotics and sulfonamides. The herb reestablishes the intestinal balance destroyed by the drugs. In addition, before a person travels to countries where the risk of intestinal infections is high, a preventive course of treatment with Ramsons can strengthen the resistance of the intestinal flora. Like garlic, Ramsons helps treat hardening of the arteries and high blood pressure. For these diseases, a spring-cleansing diet should be high in Ramsons.

A common attribute of all leeks is a high concentration of essential sulfurous oil, which forms the basis for their stimulating, detoxifying, and cleansing effect. Ramsons bursts with it! With its sulfur content, Ramsons can help our body eliminate environmental toxins such as mercury, lindane, or cadmium. Its chemical constituents bind the harmful molecules.

Ramsons is at its strongest in early spring before flowering. This is the time to gather the leaves and use them to spice up a salad, cottage cheese, and such. A course of treatment with Ramsons lasts four to six weeks and consists of eating a handful of the fresh leaves daily.

After its gathering time, Ramsons seemingly withdraws and the leaves wilt. Therefore, to store Ramsons' active ingredients for use in regenerating the intestinal flora, we must prepare

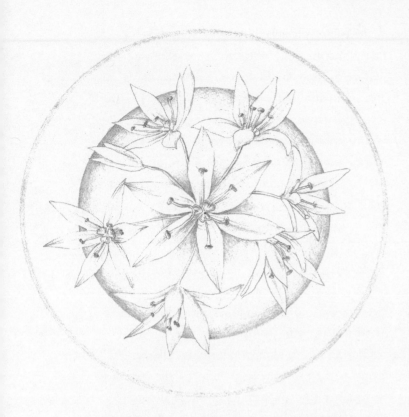

VETERINARY MEDICINE

Garlic and Ramsons are common remedies in veterinary medicine. They help with all intestinal illnesses. For dogs and cats, occasionally mix finely chopped Ramsons (and later in the year, garlic) with their food to prevent intestinal parasites. When mixed with horse fodder, the smell will keep flies away and help prevent the summer eczema to which horses are susceptible.

CULINARY USE

If you want to try out the delicious dishes that can be made with fresh Ramsons leaves in the relatively short period between the herb's sprouting and its flowering, you must hurry! Besides using them in the dishes I include here, Ramsons leaves can be added to salads, cottage cheese, yogurt, sauces, marinades, pasta, herb butter, herb vinegar, and salad dressings. When heated, the leaves lose their characteristic strong flavor and taste agreeably mild. The flowering buds also taste good, especially in béchamel sauce or potato soup.

a tincture from the leaves—again, in spring. To do so, fill a jar with freshly chopped Ramsons leaves and cover them with a 45% grain spirit or fruit liqueur. Let it sit, covered well, for a few weeks before straining the tincture into bottles. A dose is 20 drops taken before meals, three times daily.

The homeopathic pharmacopoeia prescribes a preparation from the fresh plant. If you prefer not to make your own, the homeopathic mother tincture "Allium ursinum" is available commercially from a naturopathic or homeopathic pharmacy. This tincture has proved especially helpful with atherosclerosis. A dose is 10 drops once a day, best taken in the evening.

SPRING ROLLS

    3 onions, diced
    melted butter
    3 ounces bacon or smoked ham
    6 cups ramsons, coarsely chopped
    salt, pepper, and oregano
    1 pound packaged filo dough
    1 egg white

Sauté the onions in melted butter with the bacon or ham. Add the ramsons leaves, sautéing them until they are limp. Season to taste with salt, pepper. and oregano; reserve.

Roll out the filo dough and cut it into rectangles. Place some of the ramsons mixture on top, form into rolls, and brush each with a little egg white. Place the spring rolls on a baking sheet rinsed in cold water and let them sit for 15 minutes. Bake them in a preheated 400° oven for 15 to 20 minutes or until browned.

❧ Egg Salad with Ramsons

> 5 hard-boiled eggs
> 2 pickled cucumbers, diced
> ½ cup ramsons, finely chopped
> 1½ ounces diced cheese

dressing:

> 1 cup yogurt
> 2 teaspoons mustard
> salt, pepper, paprika to taste

Slice the hard-boiled eggs and gently mix with the pickles, ramsons leaves, and cheese. Combine the dressing ingredients and add to the egg mixture. Chill and serve.

❧ Sautéed Ramsons

Here is a vegetable dish that goes very well with mashed potatoes or fish. To prepare, slice some onions into thin rings and sauté them in butter. Add freshly chopped ramsons leaves, stir-cooking until they wilt. Serve seasoned with pepper and salt and garnished with sour cream.

❧ "Beartsiki"

> 6 cups yogurt
> 1 dill pickle, diced

> 1 tablespoon fresh dill, minced
> 1 garlic clove, peeled and crushed
> 1½ cups ramsons leaves, freshly chopped
> salt and white pepper
> 1 cucumber, grated and pressed to
>   remove the juice
> 1 tablespoon olive oil

This is a variation of the Greek garlic dish *tsatsiki*:

Place the yogurt in a piece of cheese cloth to drain overnight in a colander. The following day, mix the remaining ingredients together and combine with the yogurt. Allow the salad to stand for a while before serving with toasted slices of crusty bread.

CULTIVATION

Ramsons loves deep humus-rich soil and shady places under deciduous trees. If you can spare such a spot in your garden, you could plant a patch of this herb there. It is available as both seeds or starter plants. However, because Ramsons' black seeds take 14 months to germinate, most people buy a few starters.

The plants multiply quickly through underground runners (stolons) and through the seeds that are spread by ants. In early June, if you lose sight of the Ramsons you harvested leaves from earlier, do not despair. The plant has just withdrawn after its brief yet intense period of vegetation. Only single stems with the seeds on top remain, and soon they, too, disappear.

BOTANICAL CHARACTERISTICS

Name: *Allium ursinum* — Ramsons

Distribution: Over nearly all of Europe, North Asia, and North America

Habitat: Deciduous and mixed forests, wet woodlands and water meadows, loamy soils rich in humus, and shady places.

Description: Grows 8 to 20 inches tall; juicy green leaves, lanceolate, and slightly darker on top; flowers sit on long three-edged stems as an apparent umbel with white crowns of star-shaped florets on long stalks; a strong garlic smell. Flowering time is April to June.

Confusion with similar plants: With the leaves of the poisonous Lily of the Valley that have no garlic odor

Collecting season: Gather leaves before the plant flowers (from March to May)

Active ingredients: Essential oil with allyl and alkyl-polysulphides, vitamin C, mineral salts, flavonoids, prostaglandins A, B, F.

Astrological association: Mars / Neptune

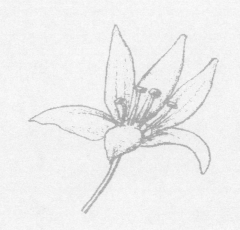

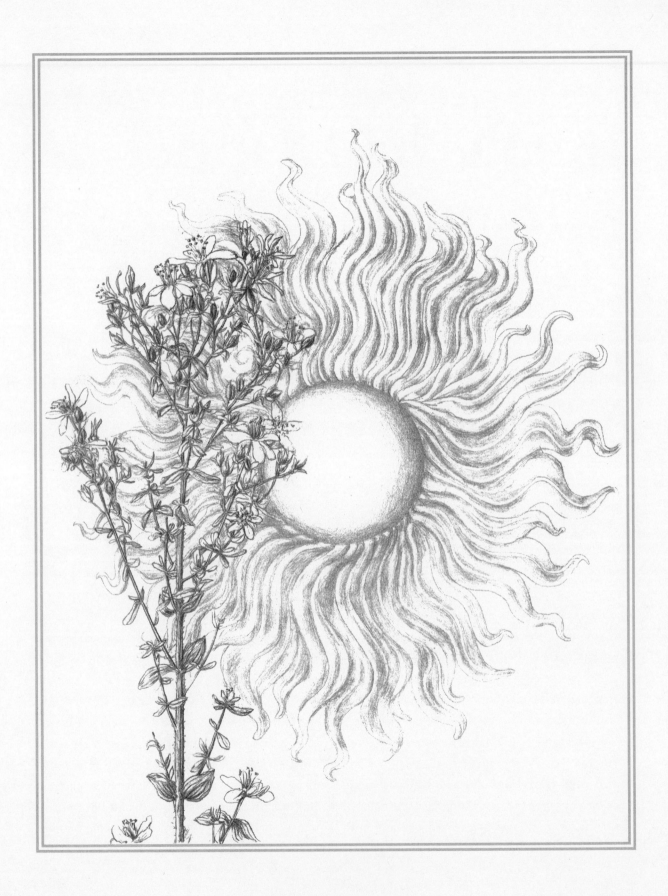

St. John's Wort

Hypericum perforatum

Perforate St. John's Wort, Amber, Goatweed, Johnswort, Klamathweed, Tiptonweed

St. John's Wort family — Hyperiaceae/Guttiferae

At the ancient celebration of summer solstice, St. John's Wort stands in full bloom. He is the most beautiful of the sun plants, filled with solar energy and thereby related to all benevolent spirits. People everywhere have recognized in this plant a salubrious, illuminated spirit with the power to chase away evil and darkness.

St. John's Wort, always associated with the summer solstice, carries within the secrets of this day. On June 21 the sun reaches its highest position to create the Earth's longest day and shortest night of the year, a union of light and darkness and of spirit and matter. Since the dawn of time, priests and priestesses symbolically consummated the cosmic event that common people celebrated with ritual and dance. Spiral dances, as noted in the chapter on Male Fern, symbolized the course of the sun, and all who joined in the dance became children of the light. Solstice bonfires symbolized the sun's power on Earth and those who jumped over the fires were healed of darkness and disease. Dancers wore head wreaths woven from plants that symbolized the unity of all things in the cycle of life and death—the union between our world and the other.

Sacred plants had a special connection to this feast. St. John's Wort, Male Fern, Mugwort, Arnica, and Calendula were all magical plants in which people saw the sun's power to banish darkness. By decorating their solstice altars with St. John's Wort and wearing wreaths from the flowering herb as they danced around the bonfire, they renewed their connection with the energies of light.

A feast day celebrated for so many millennia was unsuppressable—even following Christianization. Shifted three days, the pagan celebration became the Feast of St. John the Baptist. As we know, the summer solstice marks not only the sun at its highest position but also the turning point at which its strength begins to diminish, reaching its lowest point at the winter solstice. This process was represented since Paleolithic times by two counter-rotating spirals. Germanic mythology expressed it in the story of Baldur, the God of Light, whose head radiated fire like the sun itself. Fatally wounded by his blind brother

Hödur, who was the God of Time, Baldur later became St. John, since remembered for being beheaded on this day.

Such solstice stories seem imprinted in St. John's Wort, his golden five-petalled blooms radiating like small sun-wheels around a shower of bobbing stamens. Our forebearers saw in these flowers the captured power of the sun, each five-pointed star a sign of the benevolent powers. Ancient druids saw a resemblance to their sacred pentagram while Christians felt it symbolized the five stigmata of Christ.

When we rub the flowers between our fingers, the dark dots around the edges exude a juice or oil as red as the blood of Baldur or St. John. And when held up to the sun, the leaves appear perforated with needles. These "holes" are actually transparent oil glands (as are the flowers' dots with their red oil). For many people the perforated leaves came to symbolize the wounds of the martyrs. Others saw the plant's ability to take solar power and store it in these red droplets. Like the life's blood in our physical bodies, St. John's Wort oil was the sun's life blood, a ruby red oil that brought this life-giving energy to our bodies. It is said that St. John's Wort allows the powers of light to penetrate him completely so that he can pass them on to us. In this way he helps us open ourselves to lightness when our spirits are heavy and everything seems dark. This is how St. John's Wort illuminates the soul. And, truly, he is one of our best-known antidepressant medicinal herbs.

It is a miracle that what people recognized in a plant through deep understanding is now being confirmed on many levels. Even when we dissect this plant down to its smallest parts, again and again we encounter the theme of light. The red

on our fingers from rubbing the flowers is from hypericin, the primary constituent of St. John's Wort. It is a red pigment with skin-photosensitizing properties when taken internally. The connection between St. John's Wort and sensitivity to light was first observed in animals. Horses and cattle who ate too much of it developed white patches on their hides due to their increased photosensitivity, a condition called *Lichtkrankheit* ("light disease") in German.

Modern science confirms that the red pigment hypericin can stimulate cellular metabolism. By activating the cellular respiration that oxygenates our cells, it provides new energy to the smallest units of our biological organism. As the old ones said: *St. John's Wort stores the Sun's life energy in its leaves and flowers to give to us.*

Much of the traditional wisdom about this plant has merged with modern ideas. After all, something so deeply connected to people is not apt to be forgotten. Every story, ritual, and magical use is related to the sun's energy and the demon-banishing power of St. John's Wort, and many of these old customs have been passed down to us. For instance, it was common knowledge that the plant was strongest when gathered on St. John's Day and even more magical and healthful when picked in the early morning dew. This dew was thought to be the sacred water of fertility left from the wedding of Heaven and Earth on solstice night. And in Iceland on this day people would roll in it to become strong and vigorous.

From medieval days St. John's Wort was thought to banish demons. Peasants hung it in the stables to protect livestock from sorcery and placed a small tuft in their chamber windows to keep evil spirits from entering. The plant's power to undo spells resulted in names like "Chase the Devil," "Devil's Banisher," and "Flight of the Demons" (fuga daemonum). According to legend, the Devil himself perforated the leaves of St. John's Wort because he fretted about its healing power. However, rather than perish, the plant became a sure means of repelling evil spirits.

It was customary on St. John's Day until the last century to throw a wreath of the herb onto the roof of one's house as protection from lightning. Often it was sufficient to strew a bit of St. John's herb on the hearth to repel a thunderstorm. One story tells us that a miraculous voice from Heaven shared this secret when a terrible thunderstorm raged over the land:

Is there not an old wife who could pick some
 "Hard Hay" [St. John's Wort]
so that the thunder might be blocked?

Throughout the centuries bonfires illuminated the nights of the summer solstice and maidens wore wreaths (corona regis) of the flowering St. John's Wort herb for the dance around the fire. This pretty custom is still practiced in some regions—but few recognize it for its symbolic connection with the powers of light.

As familiar as I am with this plant, I have nearly forgotten to describe it. A few plants might be confused with it but only true Perforate St. John's Wort (*Hypericum perforatum*) is used for medicinal purposes. The healing powers of the other species are considerably weaker.

After all that has been said so far, the reader will not be surprised to learn that St. John's Wort prefers a sunny and warm habitat. He loves waysides, sparsely wooded areas, thickets, and open meadows. Modest in need, he easily grows—like a pioneer—on even the poorest of soils and is considered an indicator species for a particular meadow's lack of nutrients. The plant can reach three feet in height.

Let's look closely at the stem—or, even better, touch it—because the feel of it reveals an important feature. Erect and extremely woody, its inclusion in a mown field makes the hay hard—hence its name "Hard Hay." Running our fingers along the stem, we can feel two fine longitudinal lines. (Related species have four ridges). We cannot just pick St. John's Wort—the stem is too hard for that. We have to cut the plant with knife or shears in order not to pull up the roots. The stem's cut surface reveals a pithy, spongy tissue, which is another distinguishing characteristic. (As an aside, a plant stem with only two ridges is a rarity in botanical species native to my area of the world.)

The leaves have no stalks (sessile) and sit opposite each other, one above the other on the stem. Ovate to oblong and undivided in shape, the leaves when held to the light show many tiny dots, especially along the edge, leading to the name Perforate St. John's Wort. These dots make them look as if they were pierced with needles and are actually translucent oil glands. In medieval times this was seen as a clear signature of the plant's healing powers, and St. John's Wort was thereby recommended for the healing of wounds resulting from punctures or blows.

St. John's Wort's stem branches out bush-like at its terminal end, allowing the flowers to receive maximum sunlight. From June to September he pushes them forth—five lovely golden petals surrounding up to a hundred stamens arranged in three clusters. Indeed, the flowers produce so much pollen that pollinating insects revel in it. Covered with dark glands containing hypericin (up to 8%), the petals when rubbed secrete a red juice that stains the fingers and leaves a warm balmy scent. Face a St. John's Wort plant on a sunny day and you will surely feel its radiance and recognize a valuable healing plant.

Distinguished by its two-ridged pithy stem and numerous oil glands, Perforate St. John's Wort seems stronger and more vigorous than some of the other German native species that I list:

- Spotted St. John's Wort (*Hypericum punctatum, H. maculatum*) grows 6 to 16 inches high on a hollow stem with 4 raised longitudinal ridges. Leaves contain few oil glands.
- Mountain St. John's Wort (*H. montanum*) grows mostly in higher altitudes. It has an erect round stem, pale yellow flowers, and hairy leaves of which only the uppermost ones contain oil glands.
- Prostrate St. John's Wort (*H. humifusum*), aptly named, has a creeping nature and rarely grows higher than 6 inches. Its round stem has two ridges.
- Hairy St. John's Wort (*H. hirsutum*) is entirely covered with a soft woolly coat. The erect round stem can reach a height of 4 feet.
- Beautiful St. John's Wort (*Hypericum pulchrum*) is distinguishable from other species by its heart-shaped basal leaves. Its round stem can grow up to 20 inches high. The buds are conspicuously red on the outside due to glands in the ciliate calyx.

- Square-stalked St. John's Wort (*H. tetrapterum*), also native to Great Britain, has a roundish and squarish stem with 4 prominent "wings." It reaches a height of 2 feet. Leaves and flowers have few oil glands.

In the United States, Sunset magazine's *Western Garden Book* names over a dozen species found in North America—including Perforate St. John's Wort, Aaron's Beard or Creeping St. John's Wort (*H. calycinum*), Gold Flower (*H. moseranum*), and the Hypericums 'Rowallane,' 'Sungold,' and 'Hidcote.'

HEALING PROPERTIES

The most profound description of St. John's Wort is from 450 years ago. According to Paracelsus, the Swiss-born physician and alchemist, this plant was a God-given panacea to humanity. He wrote that God wanted physicians to recognize and choose the right remedy for their patients—and, to Paracelsus, God's will was especially visible in St. John's Wort:

Nothing chases away disease like strength . . . Therefore, we should seek medicines with the power and strength to overcome whatever illnesses they are used against. From this it follows that God has given to *Perforatam* [St. John's Wort] the strength to chase away the ghosts of nature, also worms, and to heal wounds and bone fractures, and all brokenheartedness . . . It is a truly a *universalis medicina* beyond mankind's creation.

Paracelsus prescribed St. John's Wort for depression, melancholy, and hysteria, calling these diseases without physical body and substance "phantasmas." He said that "alone in the spirit of contemplation a different spirit is born by which the human being is ruled."

Today's medical researchers are increasingly aware of the antidepressant effects of St. John's Wort, which has proved in clinical testing to have a central effect on the human brain. Naturopathic as well as folk medicine utilizes the herb as a nerve and wound remedy. We also know that it has a general tonic effect and recommend it for mental exhaustion, anemia, and recovery from severe illness.

Before describing its different applications, I would like to point out a peculiarity of St. John's Wort. Hypericin, the red pigment contained in this plant, heightens our skin's sensitivity to light. In fact, because too much sun or bright light can result in a skin rash, we should avoid exposure to bright sunlight or tanning during a course of treatment with the plant. This applies to all its preparations—tea, tincture, salve, and oil.

If you intend to use it for remedial purposes, gather the plant when it is in full bloom. This is because hypericin is found only in the flowers. To prepare a tea, use the whole plant minus the root because the flowers, stem, and leaves contain other important constituents such as tannins, essential oils, and flavons. Cut the flowering St. John's Wort above the ground, tie the plants in loose bundles that are not too large and hang them upside down to dry in a well-ventilated shaded area. Later cut the whole plant into small pieces to store. I like to hang a few bunches around my house to spread their pleasant balmy scent.

By the way, be sure that any St. John's Wort tea you purchase commercially does not contain

square stem parts. This would mean that inferior Hypericum species were used. (See the previous list of different species.)

Nearly everyone who discusses St. John's Wort indicates something about the preferred time to harvest it. My teachers did, reiterating that each plant has its favorable gathering time—usually when its chemical constituents are at their highest concentration. I gather St. John's Wort early in the morning between the summer solstice and St. John's Day (June 21 to 24). Let us again consult Paracelsus who gives us precise directions:

If one wants to use *Perforatam* against the phantasmas of which I earlier spoke, gather it according to the course of the celestial orbit. This is so that its influence can be also against those ghosts mostly in Mars, Jupiter, and Venus, and by no means according to the Moon, but contrary to it. Also not in the afternoon or at night but in the Sun's rising—

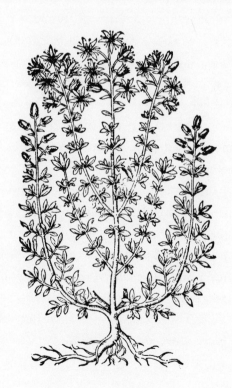

toward the Sun in aurora (that is, at sunrise) or in diluculo (that is, in the dawning). The best plants stand near other good plants or grow among them—and the longer the better, the more with flowers the better, and at the time when flowers are at their highest.

Homeopathy calls this herbal plant "Arnica for the nerves"—and it truly is one of our best nerve remedies. Made into a tea or tincture, it can lift our spirits. Especially beneficial for those who are easily excited or dejected, St. John's Wort strengthens the nerves and balances states of depression and nervous exhaustion. It is prescribed for headaches and concussions, insomnia due to nervous excitement and strain, and shock. For all of these conditions, you can either drink two to three cups of the tea daily or take 20 drops of the tincture three times daily as needed. In cases of severe shock (for instance, following an accident), I recommend sipping half a snifter of St. John's Wort tincture.

A simple home remedy is to add a little St. John's Wort to a favorite tea blend. Another is to fill a sleep pillow with its dried leaves and flowers. Both aid sleep, relieve mental excitability, and help restore a soul's disturbed balance. I list some other medicinal herbs that are commonly used for sleep disorders and to calm the nerves:

- Balm (*Melissa officinalis*) also affects emotional balance and is mostly prescribed for women. One of its components affects the heart, making it helpful for heart-related nervous disorders and as a daytime tranquilizer.
- Valerian (*Valeriana officinalis*) affects the body more than the mind for nervous

tension and rigidity. A tried-and-true sleeping aid, it is a useful daytime remedy for relieving stress.

- Hops (*Humulus lupulus*) is used as a tea or in a sleep pillow. Its calming, sleep-inducing effect makes it especially helpful for nervous stomach and difficulty falling asleep in the elderly. As an evening tranquilizer, it curbs sexual excitement.
- Sweetclover (*Melilotus officinalis*) is used as a tea or in a sleep pillow to aid sleeping and lift the spirits.
- Bitter (sour) Orange (*Citrus aurantium*) flowers are both a fragrant and calming addition to all teas for relaxation and for the nerves.
- Lavender (*Lavandula* spp.) flowers have a mild calming effect especially for nervous exhaustion. Its essential oil and sleep pillows are more powerful than the tea.
- Maypop Passionflower (*Passiflora incarnata*) is a Native American medicinal herb that affects the heart and circulatory system at the same time. It is a valuable addition to a nighttime tea for the elderly.
- Cowslip's (*Primula veris*) calming, balancing, and sleep-promoting effect, like St. John's Wort, is indicated in cases of melancholy and depression. One can sip the tea during the day because it does not make one tired.
- Sweet Woodruff (*Asperula odorata*) is especially prescribed for sleep disorders with heart conditions. Use it as a tea or in a sleep pillow.

St. John's Wort enjoys an equally fine reputation as a wound remedy. The red oil (which is the one primarily administered externally) should be present in all home pharmacies. An outstanding wound and burn oil, it has pain-soothing, anti-inflammatory, and healing properties and aids puncture wounds, contusions, abrasions, scar pain, neuralgias, trigeminal neuralgia, sciatica, gripes in infants and children, lumbago, and muscle strains. Where a large number of nerve endings are injured or where there is pulling or tearing pain, St. John's Wort is indicated. Furthermore, although I noted earlier that it can heighten sun sensitivity, St. John's Wort oil applied before sunbathing is also one of the best remedies for treating sunburn.

For treating wounds, saturate a piece of cloth with St. John's Wort oil and apply it externally. Use it as a liniment for rheumatism, lumbago, and the like.

Inflammation of the gastric or intestinal mucous membranes and nervous gastric pains also benefit from the oil. In such cases I recommend that the patient ingest about 10 drops on a sugar cube two or three times daily.

In pediatric medicine, the tea and tincture are prescribed for concentration problems, speech disorders, and bedwetting. For children I prescribe one to two cups of St. John's Wort tea daily along with the tincture twice daily. (The dosage is one drop of tincture for each year of age.)

St. John's Wort is available in herb stores as "Herba Hyperici." The homeopathic tincture "Hypericum" is prepared from the whole flowering plant.

Note: German herbal pharmacies no longer prepare St. John's Wort oil with olive oil. There-

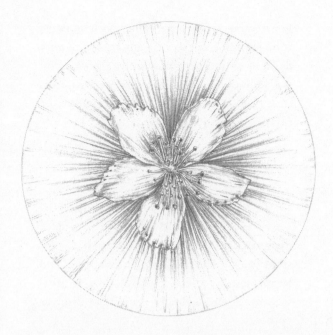

fore I recommend that readers ask at their local herb stores for herbal oil that is still prepared according to the traditional pharmacopeia.

❧ St. John's Wort Tea

Steep 1 teaspoon of the dried herb in 1 cup of cold water. Bring the mixture quickly to a boil, cover it, and let it steep for a little while. A daily dose is 1 to 3 cups.

For a course of treatment (for depression as an example), drink the tea for at least 6 weeks.

❧ St. John's Wort Oil

The best-known preparation is the ruby red St. John's wort oil. For this, gather the flowers and put them in a transparent jar. Cover them completely with cold-pressed olive oil or sunflower oil. Close the jar tightly and let it stand in the sun for 3 weeks. Strain the oil into dark bottles, carefully pouring off any cloudy or watery dregs that might have formed.

For treating sunburn and other burn wounds, combine some of this oil with a good quality flaxseed oil in a separate bottle. (Flaxseed oil has additional burn-soothing properties.) This special oil can also be worked into medicinal salves.

❧ St. John's Wort Tincture

Gather only the tops of the plant. Remove the leaves and flowers and put them in a dark glass jar. Cover them completely with a grain spirit or fruit liqueur. Close the jar tightly and let it stand for 3 or 4 weeks, shaking it occasionally. Strain the tincture into dark dropper bottles.

Veterinary Medicine

St. John's Wort oil is useful in treating wounds and sores in animals and humans alike. Again, as with people, too much St. John's Wort can induce skin damage from sun exposure. Therefore, do not allow livestock with light-colored hides to consume too much.

Cosmetics

It should be no surprise that St. John's Wort oil is a good skin-care product. The mild oil soothes the skin and heals inflamed, dry, and cracked skin. This is because St. John's Wort actually rejuvenates the skin and activates the skin's metabolism.

The tea applied as a compress or in a facial steam bath cleanses and invigorates the skin— especially if it is oily and blemished. A tea of Witchhazel and St. John's Wort in equal parts makes a facial wash that is especially suited for cleansing sensitive, inflamed skin.

To prepare St. John's Wort oil specifically for skin care and as a facial oil, steep the fresh flowers in wheat germ oil or sweet almond oil.

Cultivation

St. John's Wort is very ornamental in a garden. If you cannot yet distinguish the different wild species, first grow the true Perforate St. John's Wort in your garden and get to know it.

Various species are available as seeds or as starter plants. A hardy and modest plant harvestable for years, it likes dry calciferous soil and thrives best in sunny locations. Sow the seeds outdoors in June and July, later thinning seedlings to eight inches apart.

You can propagate St. John's Wort by dividing older rootstock. It also fits well into a rock garden. Two low-growing species, *Hypericum olympicum* and *H. polyphyllum*, make particularly fine ground covers. *H. olympicum* has large lemon-colored flowers and forms little patches of blue-green leaves. *H. polyphyllum* has yellow flowers and scaly leaves, growing about six inches tall. The smallest species is the four-inch *H. coris* with its pale yellow flower panicles. In partial shade Aaron's Beard (*H. calycinum*) is suitable; also called Creeping St. John's Wort, its leathery leaves make good foot-high ground foliage.

Other American species include *H. androsaemum*, a three-foot shrub with golden flowers;

H. beanii, a four-footer with willowy branches and bright flowers; and *H. frondosum,* a Georgia native. They all prefer mild coastal regions with moister conditions.

Note: Remember to only use Perforate St. John's Wort (*H. perforatum*) for medicinal purposes.

BOTANICAL CHARACTERISTICS

Name: *Hypericum perforatum* — St. John's Wort

Distribution: Temperate zones; Europe, North America, northwest Africa, northern Asia

Habitat: Dry sunny locations; forest fringes, slopes, waysides, moors

Description: Grows 30 to 40 inches tall on firm, two-ridged, pithy stems; branches bushlike at terminal end; sessile leaves, opposite growing on the stem; full leaves are ovate to elliptical, dotted with many oil glands; flowers are golden yellow and 5-pointed with numerous brownish stamens with dark glandular dots in their center. When crushed the plant gives off a purplish red juice that stains the fingers. Flowering time is June to September.

Confusion with similar plants: With other St. John's Wort species (see text)

Collecting season: From June to September, traditionally between the summer solstice and St. John's Day (June 21–June 24)

Active ingredients: Flowers contain hypericin (0.1 to 0.3%), tannins (up to 10%), and essential oil. Leaves contain essential oil, tannins, flavonoids, and hyperforin.

Astrological association: Sun

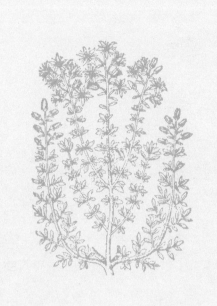

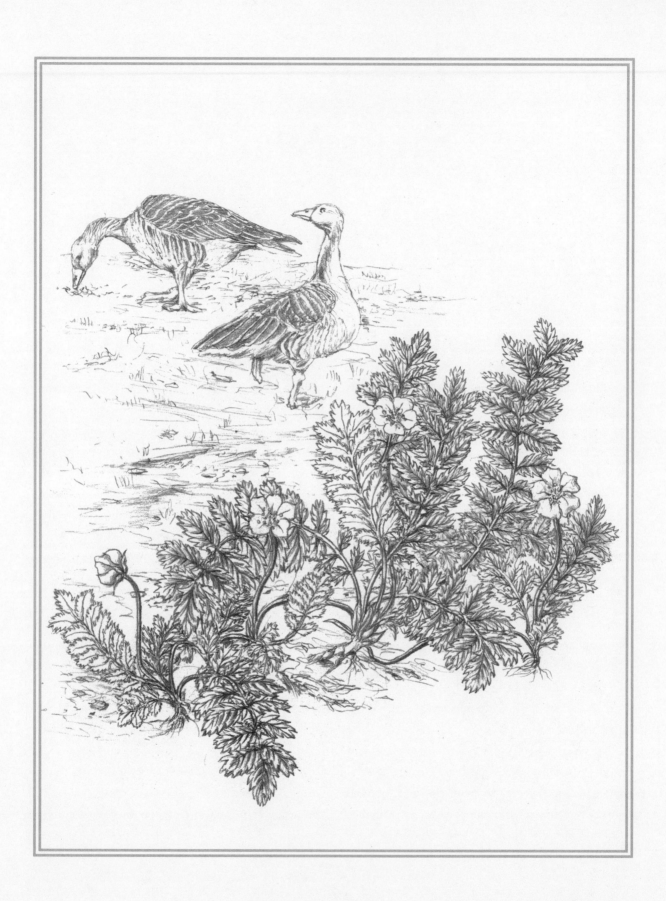

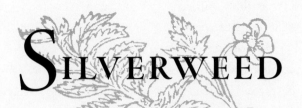

SILVERWEED

Potentilla anserina

Potentilla, Cinquefoil

Goose Grass, Five-Leaf Grass, Crampweed, Moor Grass, Silver Cinquefoil

Rose family—Rosaceae

ACCORDING TO LEGEND, on whose leaves do the fairies and plant spirits congregate in the moonlight to chat and to dance? Why, on the lovely silvery arms of Silverweed, of course! And it is only in the daytime that we larger folk can take a close look at this plant without fear of disturbing its merry nocturnal company.

Silverweed (or Potentilla as it is also called) is a cinquefoil that does not really merit the name of "five-leaf grass." Unlike Tormentil and most other species of this genus, its leaves are not fingered like hands. Instead, they are pinnate with one pair of leaflets arranged above another pair in a row along the stem. Silverweed's leaves look like small palm branches, their most beautiful feature being not their graceful, filigreed shape but rather the silvery white hairs underneath. After dark, the leaves shimmer dimly as if bathed in moonlight.

The basal rosette of a Silverweed plant can become a small carpet of plants. Clearly visible, runner-like stalks spread from the leaf axils to take root and form new plants as far as 16 inches from the mother plant. In fine weather we are able to admire Silverweed's golden yellow, radiating flowers that stand alone on long stalks grown just for them. When the weather turns foul, the flowers close halfway. And when it rains, the silver-green leaves crowd together to form a protective roof over the fragile yellow flowers, a protective gesture that has made Silverweed a symbol of Mother Mary. As far as the flower is concerned, with its five petals and five sepals Silverweed adheres dutifully to the rules of its noble Rose family. In fact, its flowers are similar to those of the Strawberry, a Rose family cousin.

We need not travel far to find Silverweed. It grows just about everywhere—in meadows, on rubbish piles, along roads and railway embankments, in town and the countryside alike. The most widespread and cosmopolitan of cinquefoil species, Silverweed has spread over most of the Northern Hemisphere and in many areas of the Southern Hemisphere. Believed to have originally flourished along salt marshes and dunes, Silverweed is now a companion to human settlements.

In contrast to Tormentil's preference for unworked grasslands, Silverweed likes nutrient-rich, dense earth—exactly the kind of soil that results from cultivation. For this reason, it has found its way to pastures, cattle runs, roadsides, and, historically, geese pastures. Hence, old German names for Silverweed are "Goose Grass" and "Goose Tansy." They like each other, the plant growing where the ground has been trampled by the tread of wide geese feet and fertilized by their droppings. Once it was commonly fed to goslings and, in truth, whenever I offer a variety of herbs to my geese, they choose their tasty namesake. This mutual fondness has led to

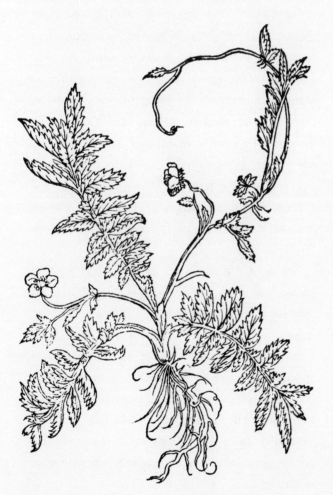

Silverweed's name of *anserina* from the Latin for "goose."

Silverweed belongs to folk medicine's repertory of regularly utilized plants. In the European countryside, many still recognize it as a remedy for animals and, in an emergency, for humans. In the alpine regions of the Allgäu and southern Bavaria, people use "Cramp Herb" or "Hedgehog Herb," as it is called, for wounds to prevent sepsis. Milk in which fresh Silverweed has been boiled is administered to the animal (or drunk by the human patient) while the steam-cooked herb is applied to the injury. This application with its long tradition in folk medicine is rarely mentioned in contemporary herbals. However, its explicit use in combination with milk suggests that Silverweed was part of the ancient German healing arts, whose practitioners recorded that the best method to ingest a plant's healing powers was a decoction in milk.

Administering herbs in milk is probably as old as humankind's botanical medicine. We know from ancient Babylonian and Assyrian medicine that a decoction of plants in milk was the most common type of preparation. Western folk medicine even ascribes magical powers to Silverweed —whoever digs up its root on St. John's Day (Midsummer Day) before sunrise can make an amulet from it that will help win the love of another.

HEALING PROPERTIES

"*Potentilla anserina* is a most valuable, antispasmodic remedy with which no unpleasant side effects need be feared." So writes the great herbalist Gerhard Madaus in his *Textbook of Biological Remedies*. And as far as healing is concerned, Silverweed has long been called Crampweed.

Herbalist Parson Kneipp has reawakened Silverweed, like many other forgotten herbs, from the long memory of folk medicine. Having used it on himself and patients, he praises its cramp-relieving nature. He points out its beneficial effect for abdominal cramps in infants and even describes a case in which he healed tetanus with a hot decoction of the herb in milk. Silverweed has an anti-spasmodic effect on smooth muscles and is particularly effective for stomach and intestinal cramps and pyloric spasms (especially in infants). It is effective for spasms of the uterus in cases of painful, cramping menstruation. Silverweed's astringent effect, while weaker than Tormentil's, is useful for cramping diarrhea.

For a general tonic, it is best to gather the flowering herb in May. However, if you plan to use the tea for cramping related to diarrhea, dig up the root in the fall, cut it into small pieces, dry it, and mix it with the leaves and flowers.

For muscle spasms, apply compresses of Silverweed that has been crushed or soaked in boiling water. Afterward, rub Mugwort tincture (*Artemisia vulgaris*) and/or Marjoram oil (*Origanum marjorana*) on the affected area. For the latter, mix six drops of essential oil of Marjoram with 50 milliliters of St. John's Wort oil (*Hypericum perforatum*) and shake it vigorously in a jar with a tight lid.

Silverweed is available in herb stores as "Herba Anserinae." "Potentilla anserina" is the homeopathic mother tincture.

❧ SILVERWEED MILK OR TEA

> 3 teaspoons fresh or dried silverweed
> 1 cup milk (or water)
> cinnamon and saffron (optional)

To prepare the milk drink (or tea), put the fresh or dried plant into the cold liquid, let it boil briefly, and drink it hot. A daily dose is 3 cups.

To treat painful menstruation, add a pinch of saffron and cinnamon, both cramp-relieving spices, to the hot silverweed milk. For a stronger effect, apply the boiled herb externally to the painful area. In addition, I prescribe hot mugwort foot baths and possibly a hot pack of hay flowers (flowering grasses) placed on the lower abdomen or the lumbar area.

VETERINARY MEDICINE

An old German name for Silverweed refers to animal diseases, indicating its use in veterinary medicines—"Scurfweed." Today when an animal is injured and especially when there is a risk of sepsis, farmers apply Silverweed simmered in milk to the wound and administer the milk to drink. Silverweed is also a well-known, proved remedy for colic. It was used when cattle ceased to ruminate, a sure sign of digestive problems. Yet another name—"Bullherb"—reminds us that once the herb was used for infertility in bulls.

CULINARY USE

We know from archeological excavations that Silverweed was gathered for food by people in

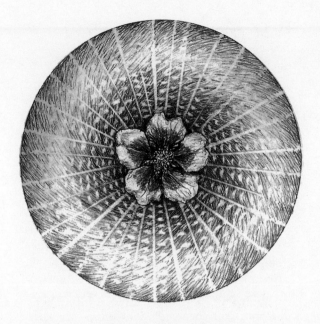

1 onion, chopped

soy sauce to taste

parsley to garnish

Roast the buckwheat in an oiled skillet; add the chopped onion. When the onion begins to turn translucent, stir in the silverweed roots and sauté them briefly, adding soy sauce and a little water until the roots are tender. Serve with fresh chopped parsley.

CULTIVATION

Silverweed is a very pretty groundcover, quickly propagating by its many runners to form a silver-green carpet. It likes sunny places and any type of soil. To cultivate plants for medicinal purposes, plant in dry places (where the leaves turn more silvery) and fertilize them only if necessary. Potentilla, as it is commonly known in nurseries, is especially pretty next to blue flowering plants in a rock garden. Evergreen perennials available in North American garden centers include *Potentilla cinerea* with its pale yellow flowers; *Potentilla nepalensis* "Miss Willmott" with salmon pink flowers; and *Potentilla tabernaemontanii* "Nana," whose dainty yellow flowers and creeping nature make an excellent lawn substitute in arid areas. Several decorative shrubs are commercially available under the name *Potentilla fruticosa.* Blooming from June through October, they range in cheery colors from gold to pale yellow, white, red, and bright yellow orange and can grow up to five feet tall.

prehistoric times. In England, the dried and ground roots have been used as a flour for baking bread. Similar in taste to parsnips or Jerusalem artichokes, they can be cut into slices and grilled or sautéed, and served with lemon juice, sour cream, or a sauce. They are also tasty in a raw vegetable salad.

The leaves of Silverweed are tender and can be mixed with other kinds of wild vegetables or used alone. These I cook in salted water until they are soft and dress them with soy sauce and roasted sesame seeds and sea salt or with sour cream or a bechamel sauce. I also prepare a Silverweed casserole by alternating layers of cooked buckwheat with finely chopped, cooked leaves, and grated cheese; my seasonings of choice are fennel seed, dill, and parsley.

℘ *Sautéed Silverweed Roots*

1 cup silverweed roots, finely chopped

1 tablespoon buckwheat,

whole and uncooked

BOTANICAL CHARACTERISTICS

Name: Potentilla anserina — Silverweed

Distribution: In temperate zones of the world

Habitat: Along waysides, pastures, rubbish dumps, railway embankments, and ditches

Description: Grows up to 1 foot 4 inches tall with long, thin runners (stolons) on whose nodes grow roots; leaves are green on top, silvery and hairy underneath, about 8 inches long, odd-pinnate with sharply incised, serrated leaflets; five-petaled flowers are bright yellow on single stems. Flowering time is May to September.

Confusion with similar plants: None

Collecting season: May, possibly until August

Active ingredients: Tannins, flavins, bitter resin bitter compounds

Astrological association: Moon / Jupiter

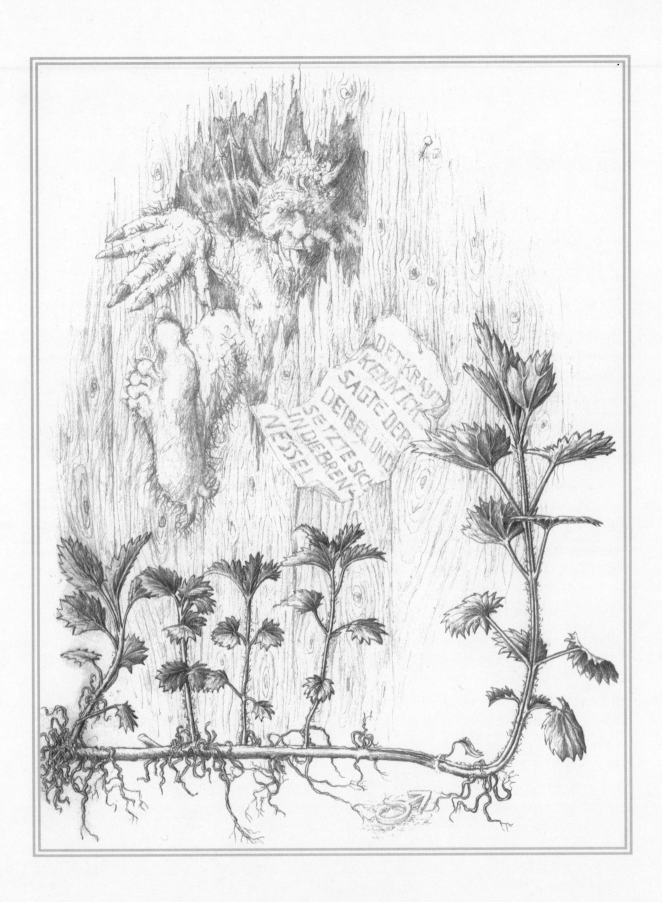

STINGING NETTLE

Urtica dioica – Big Sting Nettle, Common Nettle
Urtica urens – Small Nettle, Dog Nettle
Nettle family — Urticaceae

"I know this herb," said the Devil, and with pleasure sat down in a big thicket of Nettles right behind the house.

THIS EPIGRAM from the sixteenth century herbal of Dodonaeus fits right into our image of Stinging Nettle. Biting, stinging, dark, repulsing, often banding together in small plots of rough-legged warriors, they stand there as if daring us to come too close. Relegating her to the status of "weed," we leave her alone most of the time. Our great fortune is our failure to exterminate her.

Horace and Ovid lauded Stinging Nettle in antiquity. The Greek natural philosopher Phanias wrote an entire book in her honor, the Roman poet Catullus praised her, and Hieronymus Bock placed the plant at the beginning of his herbal. Indeed, all old and new medicinal herbalists give her special prominence as a potent healing plant. Even Albrecht Dürer, Germany's leading Renaissance artist, placed Stinging Nettle into the tender hands of an angel in one of his paintings to carry to the throne of God. And we moderns complain about it burning our fingers! We must be missing something.

The question is why of all plants should a Devil's weed be elevated to Heaven? And, truth is, we never have to go far to find these common plants. Next to our house or on any neglected piece of soil is where Stinging Nettle establishes herself. Although seemingly concerned with keeping us at a distance, she chooses to settle where we settle—in the city, in the countryside, near farms, and by the most deserted mountain cabin. Even where settlements overgrown with grass have long since been abandoned, Stinging Nettles still stand and indicate that humans once lived there. They turn up behind the house or garage where we put our trash, or beside the cesspool where the soil is saturated with dung or urine. Stinging Nettles seem capable of handling an excess of urea. Where we leave off tending the soil or make a mess—on dumps, abandoned lots, in trash piles, between the rusty watering can and old boards, the Nettles spread. They grow rampant and try to bring into balance what we destroy.

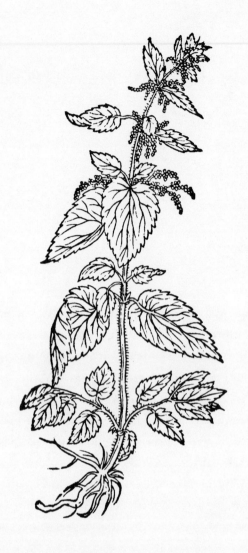

From the beginning, Stinging Nettle must have known that people would be destructive. It is as if she obtained a secret directive: "Stay with people, follow them at every turn, maintain order and heal. But guard yourself from them for once they recognize your greatness, they will eradicate you in their greed."

And so, our helpful plant spirit follows us in the disguise of a biting, burning, and unsightly weed. Had Stinging Nettle not defended herself so staunchly, she most definitely would be threatened with extinction by now. Her usefulness is beyond compare. In the spring she offers herself as a nourishing and tasty food source. With her roots and leaves, we dye wool and other fabrics. We even process her stem's tough fibers for weaving into cloth. In the Middle Ages, Nettle was used to make muslin, a fabric that is now produced from cotton. Today Nettle is largely valued for the chlorophyll that she contains in especially large quantities.

Followers of the old lore valued her as a great medicinal plant. Almost all of us get acquainted with Stinging Nettle through the itchy, burning rashes or single blisters that arise when we come too close to her. But what makes Stinging Nettle hurt so much? Pliny wrote in the first century A.D.: "Strange it is that without any thorn the wool of Nettle itself brings damage, and that from an ever so slight touch results itching and soon after blisters similar to burn marks." Through a microscope, however, we can see that the many hairs covering Stinging Nettle have a small head attached to a glassy, hollow body. This head breaks off at the slightest movement, the tip of the hair penetrates the skin, and a caustic juice flows into the wound causing itching

Here we are already on track of this herb's first virtue. Stinging Nettles have a healing influence on the workings of the Earth's soil. With their long, widely ramified roots they break up the dirt for the formation of humus. The withered plants enrich the soil with their high mineral content and transform excess nitrogen in the soil. These are the properties of Stinging Nettle that we can put to good use in our gardens. Planted beneath fruit trees, Nettles will increase the harvest. Planted near aromatic herbs, they heighten their scent.

and burning. "This plant contains much Fire," the old practitioners said. "The quality is warm and dry to the third degree."

With practice it is possible to dig out a Stinging Nettle plant without sustaining injury by striking at the widespread web of thin roots from which the mother plant sends up new shoots. These shoots, purple at first, turn green when they are a few inches above the ground—however, even the smallest bears the aggravating hairs! If digging reveals a single taproot, we have found Small Nettle or Dog Nettle (*Urtica urens*), a smaller and annual plant with shiny, roundish leaves. Common Nettle (*Urtica dioica*), also called Big Sting Nettle, is a perennial with larger, dull green leaves. However, size holds no promise—the smaller plant is more spiteful being completely covered with stinging hairs while Common Nettle has some that are harmless.

The leaves of both are aligned along the stem in an orderly fashion, each pair at right angles to those above or below it. This is easily discerned when you stand over the plant and look down at her. Stinging Nettle does not set a high value on flowers, her inconspicuous blooms are the purple hue of the early shoots. Common Nettle is a dioecious plant (her botanical name *dioica* means "two houses") and we find plants with only female flowers and others with only male ones. The small female flowers sport a purple tuft of hair. The male flowers are shaped like small, four-pointed stars. Each point rolls inward before pollination, opening abruptly when stimulated by warmth to spread a cloud of pollen in the air. The fruit of Stinging Nettle easily catches the eye because they hang on the stem for a long time—even after the stems drop their leaves in

the fall. And while her flowers may be plain, Stinging Nettle maintains a vital and colorful relationship with three very special butterflies. Peacocks, Small Tortoiseshells, and Red Admirals buzz busily around her, preferring her to those with more colorful flowers. They lay their eggs on Stinging Nettle, on whose leaves the hatched caterpillars feed exclusively.

Stinging Nettle clearly belongs to the legions of Mars. Tough, robust, and vital, her leaves are sharply serrated and prickly, often containing caustic juices. To the planet of the War God, the ancient Greeks and Romans assigned iron, the metal of war, along with its blood red color. Mars was later identified with the Devil, explaining Stinging Nettle's "devilish connection" described in rhymes and epigrams.

As a plant of Mars, Stinging Nettle can incite warmth in our bodies. In addition, she adeptly handles urea and waste products (remember her habitat near cesspools and outhouses . . .), making her ideal for treating rheumatism and gout. She aids the body in ridding itself of accumulated toxins in joints, muscles, and blood. The best course of treatment for rheumatism is to rub the joints with the fresh plant—truly a Martian therapy not for cowards!

Not surprisingly, iron is found in high concentration. This means that in the human body Stinging Nettle can stimulate the iron-producing organs as well as supplement iron. Mar's blood red color has its corresponding aspect in the healing power of Stinging Nettle. She is one of our greatest botanical blood-cleansers. In the month of March (Mars' namesake), when our sluggish bodies are full of mucus from the winter, a cleansing course of treatment with Stinging

Nettle is invaluable. Spring is when Stinging Nettle has an especially high content of iron to restore healthy pink complexions to pale iron-deficient people!

HEALING PROPERTIES

I personally swear by a spring course of treatment with Stinging Nettle to give my body a kick after the winter and chase away fatigue. In fact, the treatment makes me feel like I could uproot a tree! This cure cleanses the blood, stimulates the bladder and kidneys, promotes the function of stomach and intestines, and stimulates the pancreas. It furnishes important minerals and vitamins to the body—Stinging Nettle contains iron, xanthophyll, vitamins A and C, tannins, hormones, enzymes, calcium, sodium, silicic acid, sulfur, phosphorus, and a strong dose of Mars' warming energy. In addition, this medicinal plant is distinguished for its high concentration of chlorophyll and its positive effect when ingested as freshly pressed Nettle juice. The fresh juice holds the plant's full power and vitality. If you cannot gather Stinging Nettles to juice, ready-made juice may be available at your health food store.

Heinrich Pumpe, a proponent of the Kneipp method of hydrotherapy, experimented with Nettle juice. Here is his regimen:

Begin with a daily dose of 3 tablespoons of fresh Nettle juice. Every third day, increase the dose by 1 tablespoon until you are taking 10 tablespoons. This is the end of the treatment. Dilute the juice with water, buttermilk, or milk in a ratio of 1 part Nettle juice to 5 to 8 parts other liquid.

For years I have undergone a Nettle juice treatment every spring and my acquaintances, patients, and friends who try it are equally enthusiastic about its effect. The following regimen is a modified version of Pumpe's treatment that I developed for myself:

Start with 1 tablespoon of fresh juice, increase the dose daily by 1 tablespoon until you are taking 14 spoons of juice. Then proceed to decrease your daily dose by a tablespoon until you are taking only 1 tablespoon. This ends the treatment.

The juice is most effective when pressed from fresh Nettles. If you do not have the opportunity to gather them daily, you can preserve a stock of fresh plants for two or three days in the refrigerator rolled in a wet towel. Before pressing out the juice, be sure to wash the plants well. And do not let the juice sit for long because it deteriorates easily. By the way, it tastes a lot like fresh-pressed railroad tracks. Always mix it with buttermilk—at the beginning with five times the amount of juice. Later, when you are taking eight tablespoons or more of Nettle juice, mix it with three times as much milk. *Note: Do not overdose on the juice because it can lead to diarrhea or vomiting.*

Weaker in potency, dried Nettles make a good tea for diseases of the urinary tract, for blood-cleansing in cases of skin impurities, and for flushing out rheumatism and gout. (And I was not joking earlier when I said that courageous people can drastically increase the effects of the latter by beating the affected body parts with Stinging Nettles.)

Stinging Nettle is an old remedy for hair

growth. Clergyman Kneipp praised it for this, and I include his recipe:

> Boil 200 grams of fresh chopped Stinging Nettles in 1 liter of water for 30 minutes and strain the decoction. Rinse your head with this liquid before going to bed.

Of course, it will not return hair to a bald head. But hair lotions and hair oils that contain Stinging Nettle, Burdock root (*Arctium lappa*), and Birch leaves (*Betula pendula*) can strengthen the scalp, increase blood circulation, fortify the hair, and prevent premature hair loss.

Nettle seeds contain phytohormones and other substances that vitalize the body. Crafty horse traders have long used it to transform old or debilitated animals into resaleable specimens. And Roman poet Ovid describes Nettle seed's effect in a 2,000-year-old passage from his *Ars Amatoria* ("The Art of Love"). To intensify sexual pleasures, he says, "pepper the mix with the seed of Nettle." However, he prefers a mixture of honey, onions, eggs, and pine nuts . . .

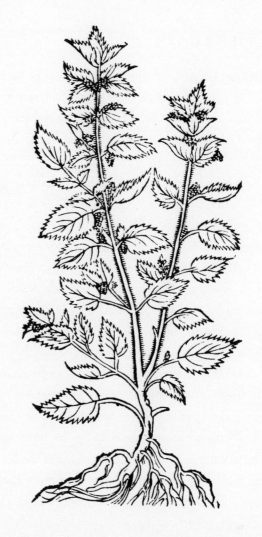

Modern-day naturopathic medicine recommends Nettle seeds for less tantalizing applications: as a tonic to stimulate bodily functions in conditions of exhaustion, in times of stress, and during recovery from illness. The seeds are recommended especially for elderly people.

Gather the mature seeds, dry them on a piece of cloth, and preserve them in a cardboard box or cotton pouch protected from moisture. Grind them as needed in a coffee grinder or with a mortar and pestle. Take one or two tablespoons daily. Add the seeds to baked goods or sprinkle them on buttered bread.

Recently, an extract from Nettle root has been administered successfully for diseases of the prostate. It is used in the manufacture of Bazoton, a prepared medicine commercially available in Germany. However, you can prepare a strong tincture from the root at home. For this purpose: clean the fresh roots, chop them finely, and put them in a mason jar. Cover them with 45% alcohol or grain spirit and let the jar sit for two to three weeks, shaking it occasionally. Transfer the strained tincture to dark dropper bottles. A dose is 20 drops taken three times daily.

Stinging Nettle tea is available in herb and natural food stores as "Herba Urticae." The homeopathic mother tincture is "Urtica dioica."

Cultivation

Welcome or not, Stinging Nettles are close at hand in nearly every garden. Instead of trying to eradicate them, we should make a small plot for them. They make a delicious vegetable dish—so why not eat them instead?

Stinging Nettles are a boon to gardening. They enrich the ground with minerals and, when left underneath fruit trees and shrubs, they improve the harvest. Planted next to aromatic herbs, they increase the content of their essential oils. A liquid fertilizer made of Stinging Nettle is excellent for garden plants as fertilizer, for pest control, and to support the formation of chlorophyll.

To prepare: Fill a large, nonmetal container with fresh Nettle plants. Pour rainwater over them and let everything ferment for two or three weeks. (Warm weather speeds up the fermentation.) As needed, strain the liquid and dilute it with water in a ratio of 1 to 10. With this diluted liquid you can water garden vegetables as well as container plants. It makes a good fertilizer for heavy feeders like tomatoes. Finally, when poured over compost, it stimulates decomposition. Here is a list of other herbal liquid fertilizers that can be prepared the same way.

- Common Comfrey (*Symphytum officinale*) or Canadian Comfrey (*Symphytum peregrinum*) fertilizer is especially good for fertilizing lettuce heads, potatoes, and tomatoes. It contains high quantities of calcium, potassium, phosphorus, and magnesium.
- Horsetail (*Equisetum arvense*) fertilizer prevents fungal infections and powdery mildew.
- Wormwood (*Artemisia absinthium*) fertilizer protects from pests.
- Male Fern (*Dryopteris filix-mas*) fertilizer drives away ants.

Since Stinging Nettle handles nitrogen so well, animal manure is prepared with this herb as well. First, you must ferment fresh dung from the stables according to biological principles before applying it to the field or the garden. Unfermented, it loses its nutrients before the soil can absorb them causing overly rapid growth and making plants susceptible to pests. Fermenting is initiated by adding a lot of fresh Nettle herb as well as biodynamic herbal additives to the dung. Inquire at your local library or bookstore for detailed information on biological gardening.

Veterinary Medicine

Stinging Nettle is a useful tonic and medicinal herb for many kinds of animals. It is wise to keep a stock of dried Nettle herb and seed on hand to feed them during the winter.

℘ Chickens

Stinging Nettle seeds strongly stimulate the laying capacity of hens. During the winter, mix them with the grain feed once in a while. This past winter, I withheld the seeds for comparison purposes—and the difference was enormous! With grain feed and Nettle seeds, we can avoid ready-made feed that contains fish meal, dyes, and toxic chemicals such as hydrochloric acid, DDT, and lindane.

❧ Dogs

A powder made from dried Nettle herb can occasionally be mixed into your dog's food. It will give your pet a shiny coat and help prevent rheumatic conditions.

❧ Geese and Ducks

Fresh, finely chopped Nettles make excellent fodder for rearing young geese and ducks.

Ducks: From the time of hatching until the tenth week, feed them barley meal, wheat bran, chopped Nettles, and rolled oats. Mix these ingredients in equal parts with enough sour cream to make a thick mash.

Geese: From the time of hatching until the second week, feed them hard-cooked eggs and Nettles, both finely chopped, mixed in equal parts, and unmoistened. From the third week on, feed them barley groats, wheat bran, and finely chopped Nettles. Again, mix them in equal parts without moistening them. Use this feed until the young geese are halfway fledged.

❧ Horses

Conventional wisdom says that Nettle seeds make horses strong and their coats shiny and silken. From the 1874 herbal of Ferdinand Müller: "Fed a moderate quantity of Nettle seeds for only eight days, horses become fat and beautiful." Not commonly known, this was a secret of cunning horse dealers. This remedy truly revitalizes the animals.

In fact, Nettles are a strong medicine and should not be fed in excess to a horse. A little of the seed scattered occasionally into the fodder is sufficient to keep the animal healthy.

❧ Dairy Cows and Sheep

Stinging Nettles stimulate milk production. During winter give a bunch of dried Nettles every day to cows and sheep.

Culinary Use

It may surprise the reader to know that Stinging Nettles are not just a cheap spinach substitute in times of hardship—they are a gourmet culinary secret! As a flavorful and aromatic spring vegetable, leaves of the young Nettle plants are favored. But we can use Nettles far into summer by snipping off only the uppermost sprouting tips. Like spinach, Nettles shrink considerably when cooked, so gather a basketful and remember to wear gloves or you may develop what our grandmothers called nettlerash! Carefully pluck the leaves from the stems and wash them. But have no fear: Stinging Nettles lose their "burning" properties in the cooking process.

The milder tasting leaves of Dead Nettle also make a good vegetable. (See the chapter on Dead Nettle.)

❧ Nettle Salad

Scald young stinging nettle leaves with boiling water; strain them. Chop them roughly and let them cool. Serve with your favorite salad dressing.

❧ Cream of Nettle Soup

4 handfuls stinging nettle leaves

½ garlic clove

2 teaspoons flour

1 tablespoon butter

2 cups milk

nutmeg

sea salt

fresh lemon

parmesan cheese

Steam-cook the nettle leaves with the garlic clove; pureé them in a food grinder or blender, and set them aside. In a small soup pot, whisk the flour into the melted butter, stirring for a few minutes. Slowly add the milk and, still whisking, simmer it until it thickens. Do not boil. Add the nettle pureé and season to taste with freshly ground nutmeg, sea salt, and a squeeze of fresh lemon. Garnish with grated parmesan cheese and serve with toasted garlic bread.

Stinging Nettle Soufflé

4 handfuls of nettle leaves

2 dinner rolls

2 cups milk

2 tablespoons butter

1 onion, finely chopped

1 egg, beaten

grated cheese

marjoram, lovage, oregano, or sage

sea salt

grated cheese

Steam-cook the fresh nettle leaves until they are limp; pureé and set aside. Cut the dinner rolls into small pieces, soak them in milk, and steam them until soft. Sauté the onions in the butter and combine them with the bread mixture; add the egg and pureéd nettles. Season to taste with sea salt and herbs of choice. Pour this mixture into a greased soufflé dish, sprinkle with grated cheese, and bake in a preheated 350° oven for 30 minutes.

Sautéed Stinging Nettles

Boil stinging nettle leaves in salted water until they are soft. Chop them and sauté with butter and diced onions. Season with sea salt and spices to taste and serve with crème frâiche.

Vegetarian "Meatballs" with Goatweed and Stinging Nettle

2 cups rolled oats (or cooked groats, millet, buckwheat, or rice)

milk

2 handfuls of stinging nettle leaves (*Urtica dioica*)

2 handfuls of goatweed leaves (*Aegopodium podograria*)

1 onion, chopped

flour

1 egg, beaten

nutmeg, oregano, and marjoram

sea salt

Soak the rolled oats in milk to cover; reserve. Steam-cook the nettle leaves until soft, adding the goatweed at the end because they cook faster; chop and set aside. Brown the onion in a well-oiled pan. Combine all ingredients in a bowl and mix them well, adding flour as needed to make a sticky mass. Shape into balls or patties, roll them lightly in flour, place them on an oiled baking sheet, and bake in a preheated 350° oven until browned and cooked through.

BOTANICAL CHARACTERISTICS

Name: Urtica dioica — Stinging Nettle

Distribution: Everywhere except in the Arctic, India, and South Africa

Habitat: Waysides, dumps, near stables, populated areas

Description: Grows from 1½ inches to 5 feet tall; square stem with elongated, coarsely serrated dark-green leaves, crosswise opposite; stem and leaves covered with hairs, small inconspicuous flowers in long, hanging panicles. Flowering time is May to October.

Confusion with similar plants: With Small Nettle (Dog Nettle, *Urtica urens*); 6 to 18 inches tall; juicy, green leaves. With Dead Nettle (*Lamium album*); white flowers, does not sting.

Collecting season:

    Fresh plants – March to June
    For tea – March to September
    Seeds – September to October
    Roots – Fall

Active ingredients: Nettle toxin, histamine, chlorophyll, vitamin C, formic acid

Astrological association: Mars

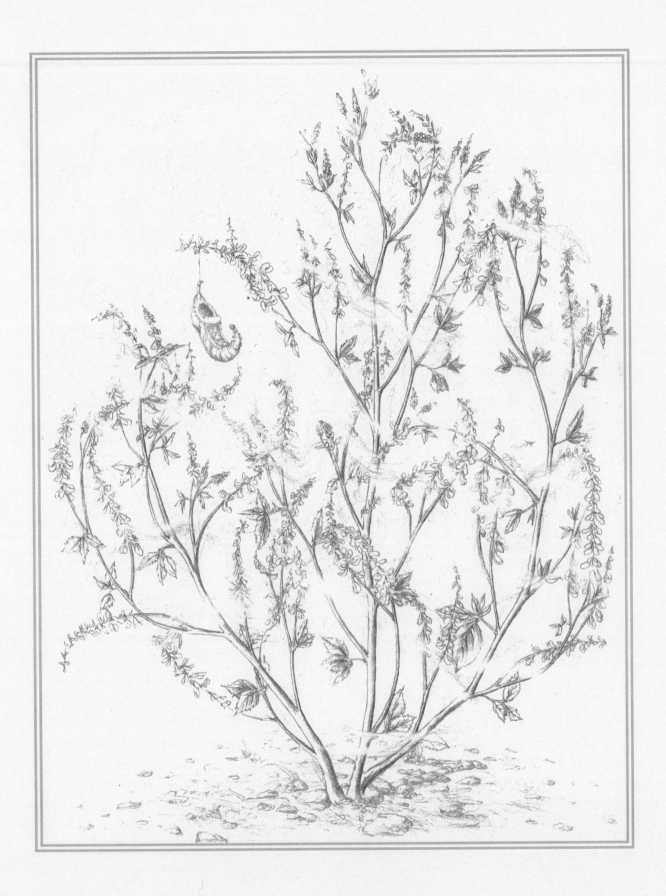

Sweet Clover

Melilotus officinalis – Yellow Sweet Clover
Melilotus albus – White Sweet Clover
Melilot, Common or Ribbed Melilot, King's Clover, Hay Flowers
Pea family — Fabaceae

EVERY TIME I ENTER MY ATTIC and walk past the bunches of Sweet Clover hung there to dry, a sweet scent surrounds me. It makes me put down my clothes basket, stick my nose into the herbs, and deeply inhale the fragrance. In fact, the one thing I regret about the German Alps is that the Jasmine of warmer climes cannot grow here. Sweet Clover, however, always consoles me because her perfume is nearly as sweet and lavish, smelling of honey, fresh hay, vanilla, and Sweet Woodruff. In winter I like to sleep on a Sweet Clover pillow and inhale the memories of summers past.

Her herbal scent has always been considered a good defense against the blues, and the old-fashioned herbal pillow is being rediscovered as a therapeutic method. Aromatherapy is a modality that treats patients with botanical fragrances. It is employed by many physicians and naturopaths (especially in France, Germany, and England) who recognize that certain smells can help a person regain mental and emotional balance. Certainly everyone can think of a particular scent that makes us feel happy or serene.

Whether it is the scent of a rose, of a wild flower meadow, or even of a pine forest, odors affect us predominantly through the psyche—which is why mental and psychological illnesses respond so well to aromatherapy. In the herbal workshops that are part of my naturopathic medical practice, I demonstrate how a particular plant's effect and essence is easily detected by its fragrance. [My book on the subject is available in English as the *Complete Aromatherapy Handbook: Essential Oils for Radiant Health* (Sterling Publishing, 1990).]

Let's climb back up to my attic and sit beneath the hanging Sweet Clover. When first picked, the scent was faint. Only as the herb withered and dried out did it develop a cloud of fragrance. This is explained by the presence of coumarin, an aromatic substance given off as the plant dies back, and is why plants like Sweet Clover and Sweet Woodruff containing coumarin have little fragrance growing out in the open. Sometimes I even imagine that Sweet Clover smells stronger at different times, making me think there is truth in her old name "Seventide" and in the belief that seven times throughout the day her odor increases—and especially prior to a change in the weather. Tabernaemontanus describes this in his 1731 herbal:

> The whole herb without the root has a scent like a pleasant-smelling pitch. But while standing in gardens, it has its scent seven times during the day and also loses it again as many times. Therefore it is called Seventide. After being picked and dried, however, it retains its fragrance, and when cloudy weather approaches the herb's scent is so powerful that everybody in the house where it hangs notices. Therefore we might also call it Weather-herb.

Stepping outside to look at Sweet Clover growing, we will find that the old German name "Stone Clover" reveals her preferred habitat. She is a plant of stone quarries and railway embankments, of roadsides and even waste dumps. The tallest Sweet Clover plants I ever saw, in fact,

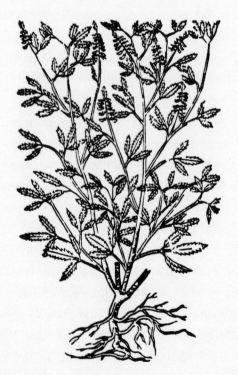

were over six feet tall and thriving in a gravel pit. Like her scent, the overall plant has a countenance that is light and full of grace—never heavy and earthy. She is so delicately proportioned that one could almost overlook her, or rather look through her. She would almost seem to take off and float if her deep-growing taproot did not anchor her securely on Earth.

There are two different species of this graceful plant; one flowers yellow and the other white. Yellow Sweet Clover is considered the true one; that is, the one gathered for medicinal use. However, both emanate the same sweet smell. The flowers, arranged in long racemes, are filled with a fine nectar. Accordingly, her Latin genus name is *Melilotus*, derived from the word for honey (*mel*). Her flowers are a favorite abode for visiting bees. Contemplating this herbal figure of gentility, we can easily sense that her smell chases away heavy thoughts and lightens the spirit.

Mother Earth holds some plants to be gentle or aggressive, light or heavy, male or female. Sweet Clover of old was considered a gentle plant of feminine beauty and purity. In ancient Greece she was dedicated to the nine beautiful daughters of Jupiter and Mnemosyne, the graceful muses and goddesses of song and poetry and the arts and sciences.

We know the ancient Germans assigned her to Ostara (or Eostre), the goddess of light, fertility, and spring. They celebrated her feast day in April, lighting Easter bonfires to symbolize the "rising up of the light" following winter's darkness. The women braided wreaths from flowering Yellow Sweet Clover to throw on the flames. Even the "eastern" direction of the sunrise was named after this ancient goddess of light. Today the name of our modern Easter holy day is but one element held over from those pre-Christian celebrations. Of course, the Blessed Mary eventually supplanted the old icon, and today in some regions Sweet Clover bears melodious names like "Our Dear Lady's Slipper."

The earliest recorded history tells us that many medicinal plants were dedicated to goddesses, a custom preserved in the Christian era by the offering of healing herbs to Mary. There were always more women's plants than men's plants—and very few gods were assigned an entire herb garden as was customary for goddesses. In most cultures women and priestesses gathered medicinal plants to heal family and tribe. Wisdom of the healing power of plants was gleaned from their experience and symbolized in fairy tales, legends, and folklore. Many women knowledgeable of herbal medicine stood accused of practicing witchcraft and suffered the cruelest consequences, taking to the stake their wisdom and experience. The so-called modern scientific method further reduced healing herbs to chemical formulas and material benefit.

Today, while few people still recognize the old connection between human, animal, and plant kingdoms, a growing number understand the values that moved women herbalists of the past. We find healing remedies for our illnesses outside in nature and feel gratitude and responsibility to place medicinal plants once again under the benevolent protection of Earth and her goddesses.

Healing Properties

Yellow Sweet Clover (*Melilotus officinalis*) with its greater flavon content is the species used for medicinal purposes. However, both Yellow and White Sweet Clover (*M. albus*) have the same amount of coumarins.

An ancient medicinal herb, Sweet Clover was considered by Hippocrates, Dioscurides, and Pliny a special remedy for sores. Known as Melilotus, it was much used in the past—every pharmacy sold Melilot plasters and every household kept small sachets of Sweet Clover in reserve.

Modern natural medicine administers Sweet Clover internally as well as externally. It is used externally as an anti-inflammatory whose softening and antispasmodic properties soothe pains and promote the formation of pus. Used in plasters, salves, herbal pillows, or compresses, it aids the healing of ulcers and sores, hardened lymph nodes, suppurating and firm milk glands, thick and swollen tonsils, and strongly purulent wounds, contusions, sprains, and bruises.

The quickest way to soften swollen glands, speed the formation of pus, and cleanse wounds, ulcers, and boils is to repeatedly apply a hot Sweet Clover sachet or pillow. You can easily make one from a piece of cotton, linen, or a cloth diaper and stuff it with Sweet Clover. Place the sachet in a large container and pour boiling water over it; let it steep for a few minutes. Carefully press out the hot water and apply the herbal compress to the area being treated, keeping it as hot as is tolerable. Wrap the affected area with a towel or a woolen shawl or blanket, leaving the sachet in place until it cools down. If you do not have a sachet or pillow handy, you can instead prepare a hot compress with Sweet Clover tea.

To treat hardening of the breast glands and for treatments following breast surgery, massage the area daily with a lymph salve. Rub it into the shoulder and upper arm area of the respective side. As an adjunct internal treatment, the patient can sip a tea made from Sweet Clover, Calendula, and Figwort.

A large pillow filled with Sweet Clover makes a wonderful sleeping pillow for a person suffering from nervousness and insomnia. If the smell is too strong, you can mix dried moss with the Sweet Clover. The following herbs also calm and promote sleep. They can be added to a Sweet Clover pillow according to personal taste, or rather, smell: Lavender (*Lavandula* spp.), Hops (*Humulus lupulus*), Valerian flowers (*Valeriana officinalis*), Sweet Woodruff (*Asperula odorata*), and Mugwort (*Artemisia vulgaris*).

As a special gift for someone, I sometimes make a scented sleep pillow filled with two parts each Sweet Clover and Rose Pelargonium leaves (*Pelargonium graveolens*) and one part Rose leaves (*Rosa* spp.). You can easily propagate Rose Pelargoniums in pots by sticking small cuttings into the soil. They root quickly and grow into large, handsome plants. Mine stand on the terrace throughout the summer. When I cut the leaves back to dry for pillows, new shoots reappear within a short time.

Pillows of Sweet Clover alone or combined with Sweet Woodruff (*Asperula odorata*) are good for repelling moths. Placed in closets and dressers, they also give a pleasant scent to laundry.

Sleep pillows keep their fragrance longer when Orris root powder is added to the herbal mixture. This natural and nontoxic fixative (which is the root of the Florentine iris) binds the scent and assures an herbal pillow's longevity. It smells pleasantly of Violets and is available in many herb stores. I make my own—when I decide to sacrifice my Garden Iris (*Iris germanica*) —by first digging up the fragrant rootstock in spring or fall, drying it thoroughly, and then grinding it into a fine powder.

My herbal first-aid kit always contains the remedies I include here for earaches and eye infections. In the case of the ear, after the steam bath I place a drop of St. John's Wort oil or Mullein oil in the affected orifice. For eye infections I administer pure Sweet Clover tea or, preferably, the herbal mixture described later.

Taken internally, Sweet Clover is calming and enhances sleep. Its coumarin content thins the blood and has a healing effect on the lymph system. Besides using an herbal sleep pillow to treat sleep disorders, I recommend enjoying an evening cup of hot Sweet Clover tea by itself or mixed with some Cowslip (*Primula veris*).

For varicose veins, to prevent the risk of thrombosis, for a heavy sensation in the legs, and for calf spasms at night, I suggest sipping a cup of Sweet Clover tea twice a day. In addition, I prescribe chewing two teaspoons of Milkthistle seeds (*Silybum marianum*) daily to support the liver. Compresses made with the herbal tea or fresh Sweet Clover plant alternated with Coltsfoot leaves (*Tussilago farfara*) are part of the treatment for varicose veins.

All diseases of the lymphatic glands are aided by a course of treatment with Sweet Clover. You can also mix it with Calendula (*Calendula officinalis*) and Figwort (*Scrophularia nodosa*). The dosage is a cup of tea taken twice a day. As with all herbal remedies, do not overdose. In the case of Sweet Clover, too much can lead to nausea.

Note: People who take blood thinners after suffering a heart attack or stroke should not take Sweet Clover at the same time. This is because its coumarin content also has blood-thinning properties.

Sweet Clover is available in herb stores as "Herba Meliloti." The homeopathic tincture "Melilotus officinalis" is prepared from the fresh leaves and flowers.

✄ Lymph Salve

250 grams lanolin

1 cup calendula oil (*Calendula officinalis*)

1 cup sweet clover leaves and flowers, dried slightly (*Melilotus officinalis*)

½ cup minced fresh figwort root (*Scrophularia nodosa*)

¼ cup minced belladonna leaves (*Atropa belladonna*)

1 tablespoon finely grated beeswax

10 milliliters conium 4x (*Conium maculatum*)

Melt the lanolin and slowly add the oil. Mix in the herbs and heat for 20 minutes, stirring constantly. (Do not boil.) Strain the mixture through a cheese cloth into a clean bowl. Stir in the melted beeswax, add 20 drops conium, and pour the mixture into salve containers. If the salve is too liquidy, add more melted beeswax; if it is too firm, add a little more oil.

Belladonna is not available commercially and can be omitted from this recipe. However, if you choose to grow your own be sure to treat the leaves with care. Never put them in your mouth because they are highly poisonous. Conium 4x is homeopathically prepared hemlock, a proven remedy for tumors.

Use this salve as an embrocation for hardened glands, sores, ulcers, and boils.

✄ Steam Bath for Earaches

2 parts sweet clover (*Melilotus officinalis*)

1 part high mallow (*Malva sylvestris*)

1 part german chamomille (*Matricaria chamomilla*)

1 part mullein flowers (*Verbascum thapsiforme*)

A steam bath to relieve the pain of a middle ear infection or a simple earache:

Add the herbs to a pot with enough boiling water to cover them completely. Remove the pot from the burner and, using a piece of paper or cardboard shaped into a funnel, guide the steam into and around the ear. (Be careful not to burn the patient.) You can reheat the herbs in the pot several times. *Note: Do not put the tea itself into the ear.*

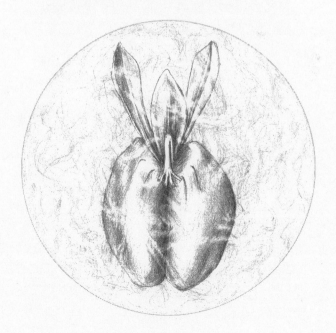

❧ Herbal Blend for Eye Infections

2 parts sweet clover (*Melilotus officinalis*)
1 part blue mallow
   (*Malva sylvestris mauritanica*)
1 part eyebright (*Euphrasia officinalis*)
rose water

Pour 1 cup boiling water over 2 teaspoons of the herbal mixture; let it steep until cool. To each cup of tea, add 2 tablespoons of rose water. Using an eye cup, wash the eyes with the tepid tea or administer it as a compress. (Never apply hot tea to the eyes.)

❧ Herbal Sachet

sweet clover (*Melilotus officinalis*)
German chamomile
   (*Matricaria chamomilla*)
flaxseed (*Linum* spp.)
mallow flowers (*Malva* spp.)

Mix the herbs in equal parts and stuff them into a small linen sachet. Place the bag in hot water for 10 minutes, squeeze out the excess liquid, and apply it to the affected area. This sachet softens and dissolves bruises, swollen lymph glands, boils, and sores.

CULINARY USE

Once Sweet Clover was used in Germany to make lemonade more aromatic. An extract of the plant was even added to tobacco to give it a pleasant taste. In recent years, however, synthetic coumarin has been substituted because natural coumarin in large doses is poisonous and its use is prohibited as a food additive.

Dr. Gerhard Madaus reports in his *Lehrbuch der biologischen Heilmittel* (*Textbook of Biological Remedies*, 1938) that people in the Swiss canton of Thurgau prepared Sweet Clover as a salad with vinegar and salt. I have tried it and found it palatable. However, I prefer using the dried flowers and leaves to flavor meat and fish dishes as well as desserts. For instance, I make a vanilla pudding by boiling some Sweet Clover with the milk and then straining it.

In one German region where it was once used to flavor cheese, Sweet Clover is still called "Cheese Herb." You can try adding some of the finely ground dried herb to yogurt, cottage cheese, and cream cheese.

Lastly, while the herb once enjoyed some fame in the production of liqueurs and brandy, today it is all but forgotten. Nonetheless, I include a traditional recipe here for your enjoyment—armchair or otherwise.

❧ Sweet Clover Liqueur

½ cup dried sweet clover, leaves and
   flowers (*Melilotus officinalis*)
½ cup linden flowers, fresh or dried
   (*Tilia cordata*)
½ cup dried rose leaves (*Rosa* spp.)
1 vanilla bean, split open
4 tablespoons honey
½ liter fruit liqueur ("Obstler")

Put the herbs and the vanilla bean into a mason jar. Dissolve the honey in a little bit of fruit liqueur and pour it over the herbs. Fill the jar with the remaining fruit liqueur and close it tightly. Let the mixture steep for 3 weeks in the cellar or a cool, dark place; shake the jar occasionally. Strain the liqueur into a clean bottle and let it stand for another 2 months in the cellar before serving.

CULTIVATION

There are several species of Sweet Clover. For medicinal purposes, we use Yellow Sweet Clover (*Melilotus officinalis*) and *M. altissima*, a high-growing species. White Sweet Clover (*M. alba*) is not used. Yellow Sweet Clover can grow from one to three feet high and prefers dry, rocky calcareous soil. *Melilotus altissima* also has yellow flowers but prefers a wetter habitat.

White Sweet Clover grows in the open in dry wastelands or hay fields. When large amounts of this species turns up in wet, moldy hay used as fodder, it can increase susceptibility to bleeding. In Germany this is called "Sweet Clover disease," and animals suffering from it can bleed to death if they have to undergo surgery.

Sweet Clover is a biennial plant. Seeds for all species are available commercially. Sow the seeds in fall or spring and later thin the seedlings 16 inches apart. In old peasant gardens, Sweet Clover was used as a border plant around beds to keep mice away.

COSMETICS

Sweet Clover is helpful for dilated or broken capillaries in the face. It removes stagnation from red blood vessels, firming the tissue and the walls. Use a strong herbal tea made from Sweet Clover twice weekly as a cold and wet compress or daily as a face lotion. (Also see the chapter on Hemp Agrimony.)

BOTANICAL CHARACTERISTICS

Name: *Melilotus officinalis* — Sweet Clover

Distribution: Temperate zones in Europe and Asia

Habitat: Waysides, dumps, and gravel pits

Description: Grows to 3 feet on a round, erect stem; leaves opposite, trifoliate ("ternate") with serrated margins; yellow flowers arranged in long racemes; a sweet scent develops when the plant withers. Flowering time is June to September.

Confusion with similar plants: With *Melilotus altissima* that is used like *M. officinalis*

Collecting season: Flowering plants – June to September

Active ingredients: Coumarin, flavones, tannins, mucilage, and choline

Astrological association: Venus / Jupiter

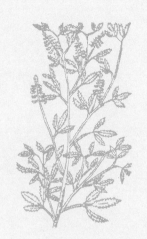

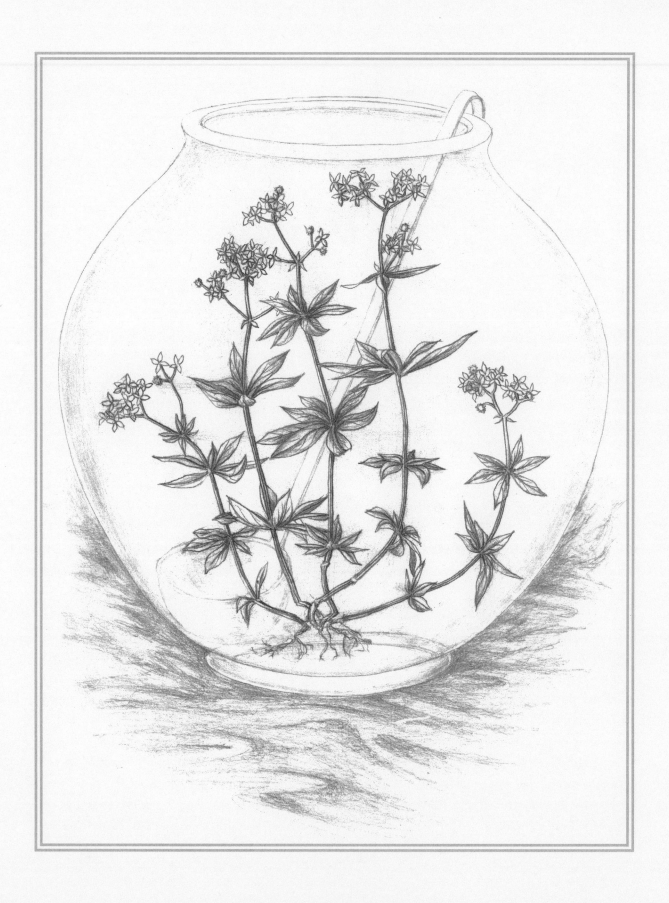

Sweet Woodruff

Galium odoratum (*Asperula odorata*)
Woodruff, Woodward, Master of the Woods
Bedstraw family—Rubiaceae

This herbal master was never honored with the hallmark "*officinalis*." It seems that only medicinal plants sold in the pharmacies of old were granted this sobriquet. Nonetheless, he was a favorite of folk medicine whose beneficiaries gave to him lovely, descriptive names like "Heart's Delight," "Mayflower," "Star Liver Herb," and "Woods Mother Herb."

Knowledge of Sweet Woodruff's healing power is all but lost. If not for the famous "Woodruff punch," it might possibly be forgotten entirely. This traditional May punch—Nicholas Culpeper's "May cups"—is mentioned as early as 854 A.D. when, according to the Benedictine monk Wandalbertus, one simply "pours sparkling wine over Woodruff fine."

Those tempted to start on the punch right away may leaf through to the recipes. The rest of us, however, will spend some time with the herb's vernacular names. Old herbals called it *Herba matrisylvae* or "Woods Mother Herb." At some point, however, the gender changed to "Master of the Woods." *Waldmeister* is still our German name for him as well as one of his vernacular English names. Rummaging further, we find that many Sweet Woodruff recipes were intended to address women's conditions.

Sweet Woodruff was among the group of plants known as "Mary's Bedstraw" or "Lady's Bedstraw" (which remains the common name of his cousin from the same genus, *Galium verum*). This name dates back to an ancient pagan custom of stuffing the pillows and mattresses of women in childbirth or childbed with certain herbs called "Lady's Bedstraw" that were supposed to ease labor and birth, strengthen mother and child, and protect against evil influences. Our Sweet Woodruff was tied around the calves of the bedded woman and stuffed into her pillow to bring restful sleep and strengthen her nerves. And because we know that infants' better developed sense of smell lets them perceive their environment through odors, the herb likewise treated the newborn. The scent so strengthened the hearts of mother and child that Sweet Woodruff bore the name "Heart's Delight."

Woodruff keeps not only heavy thoughts but also moths at bay. It seems that these creatures cannot stand the sweet smell, a fact that people have long taken advantage of by hanging sachets filled with dried Sweet Woodruff in trunks and wardrobes. It is truly pleasant to open one's closet in the morning and smell the herbal fragrance. For my scented sachets, I combine Sweet Woodruff with Sweetclover (*Melilotus officinalis*) because both plants contain coumarin glycoside, a compound that constitutes their unique smell. Interestingly, only withering plants give off the sweet odor, and both plants have a stronger scent when picked in the morning.

If you like the smell of Sweet Woodruff and

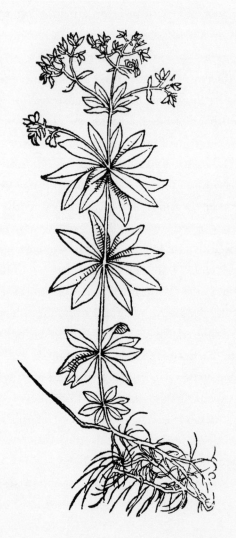

Sweetclover, you probably like the smell of fresh mown hay. I do—and so appreciate the nearby alpine fields of Sweet Vernalgrass (*Anthoxanthum odoratum*), a meadow grass with yellow heads and lanceolate leaves that, as it dies back, develops a characteristic fresh scent reminiscent of Woodruff.

The common name "May Herb" refers to the month in which it flowers and when Sweet Woodruff is gathered for the sweet punchbowl. (For medicinal purposes, however, it should be gathered after it flowers.) This is also the most enchanting time in the beech woods—Woodruff's favorite habitat. When beeches form their light green sun-dappled canopy, when bright spring flowers weave themselves into the forest carpet of light and shade, then from the dense bolster of Woodruff tender white star-shaped flowers beam as if saying: "Come, pick us, and we will delight your heart!"

At their side, Solomon's Seal bends gracefully toward Earth, dangling his white flowers like perfumed pearls. Further back, Ramsons emanates an entirely different smell. While in between, the green-flowering French Mercury pushes upward. Each of these plants love the humus-rich soil beneath the beech trees and hurriedly nurture their flowers. This is because soon the leafy overhead canopy will close off the sunlight.

The white Woodruff flower carpets fade beneath the trees in July. The flowers become tiny fruit-pellets with bristly hairs that, when mature, separate into two single-seeded small nuts. The thick hooked bristles easily attach to the fur or clothing of passersby who unwittingly carry off and disperse the seeds. Soon the weight of falling leaves bends our "Master of the Woods" to the ground to lie until spring's warmth penetrates the bare beech branches. Heeding Nature's call, Sweet Woodruff roots again and sends forth fresh new plants.

HEALING PROPERTIES

Sweet Woodruff has calming and antispasmodic qualities. It strengthens the heart and is a remedy for both the liver and the gallbladder. Its calming effect is especially helpful for migraines, nervous anxiety, and heart palpitations. It is a suitable addition to tea blends for promoting sleep and steadying the nerves. Headache sufferers can sometimes alleviate their pain by applying the fresh, mashed herb to their foreheads.

It also soothes cramps. German herbalist-cleric Pfarrer Kneipp, the father of hydrotherapy, administered the plant to patients suffering from gripping abdominal pains—and praised its effect. However, its antispasmodic properties are weaker than those of Silverweed (*Potentilla anserina*), although we can still add Sweet Woodruff to tea blends that treat stomachache, colic, and painful menses. It supports the effect of the other herbs and adds a pleasant taste and fragrance to the tea.

Also remember that Sweet Woodruff was once called "Star Liver Herb." Woodruff tea is a good adjunct when treating liver and gallbladder conditions. Because it stimulates the bladder and the kidneys at the same time, it is especially recommended for liver diseases accompanied by water retention.

With its coumarin content, it also belongs with the mild remedies that treat the veins. As a tonic, Sweet Woodruff has a mild stimulating and balancing effect in all areas. It is not a drastic remedy. Therefore it is a welcome addition to your "house" tea blend.

If you intend to use it in a remedial tea, gather Sweet Woodruff when it flowers. Spread it out in thin layers, drying the entire herb without the roots. Pure Woodruff tea is prepared as a cold infusion by steeping one teaspoon of the dried herb in a cup of cold water overnight. Strain off the liquid and, for a daily dose, drink two cups—and no more than two cups.

For a while Sweet Woodruff fell into disfavor and was considered carcinogenic. However, recent studies refute this. While it is true that Woodruff's ingestion in large amounts can lead to headaches and nausea (due to the coumarin content), each and every medicinal plant has a "reverse" effect. This simply means that going beyond any given plant's therapeutic dose can cause the disease that it supposedly cures (and is why Woodruff can heal headaches as well as induce them). *As a final caution: Do not ingest Sweet Woodruff or Sweetclover concurrently with blood-thinning medications.*

Scientific experiments of our time have isolated single constituents from individual medicinal herbs, administering them in mega doses to laboratory animals. It takes no leap of imagination to realize that isolating chemicals from the well-balanced entirety of a plant's active ingredients will cause side effects—maybe even carcinogenic ones. The unfortunate result of such lopsided experimentation is that several valuable medicinal plants have been removed from our herbal shelves. In Germany, for example, we can no longer purchase Birthwort (*Aristolochia clematitis*), a once reliable medicinal plant, and Comfrey

(*Symphytum officinale*) is currently under discussion and being sold commercially minus one of its chemical constituents. I believe there have been similar repercussions in the United States.

Sweet Woodruff is available in herb stores as "Herba Asperulae." The homeopathic mother tincture "Asperula" is prepared from the fresh herb.

℀ A Tea for Migraine Headaches

2 parts sweet woodruff
  (*Galium odoratum*)
1 part lavender flowers (*Lavandula* spp.)
1 part thyme (*Thymus vulgaris*)
2 parts cowslip flowers (*Primula veris*)

Pour 1 cup of boiling water over 2 teaspoons of the herbal blend. Let the mixture steep covered for 5 minutes, strain, and sip sweetened with honey.

℀ "Heart's Delight" Tea

the traditional recipe:

25 grams *Herba Asperulae*
20 grams *Flores Crataegi*
20 grams *Flores Aurantii*
15 grams *Flores Paeoniae*
25 grams *Flores Malvae*
20 grams *Folia Melissae*

modern equivalents:

25 grams sweet woodruff
  (*Galium odoratum*)
20 grams hawthorne flowers
  (*Crataegus monogyna*)

20 grams bitter orange flowers
  (*Citrus aurantium*)
15 grams peony flowers
  (*Paeonia officinalis*)
25 grams blue mallow flowers
  (*Malva sylvestris mauritanica*)
20 grams balm leaves (*Melissa officinalis*)

Stir 1 teaspoon of the herbal blend into cold water, cover it, and bring the mixture to a boil. Remove the pan from the heat and steep the tea for 5 minutes. To calm and strengthen the heart, drink 3 cups daily.

This tea's effect is enhanced by having the patient rest at night on a sweet woodruff sleep pillow (see the following recipe).

℀ A Sweet Woodruff Sleep Pillow

1 part sweet woodruff (*Galium odoratum*)
2 parts hops (*Humulus lupulus*)
4 parts forest moss (Musci family)

Stuff the mixed dried herbs into a pillow. For my sleep (or dream) pillows, I prefer to use untreated, naturally dyed fabric that is pleasing to the eye as well as to the touch.

℀ A Scented Pillow for Men

2 parts sweet woodruff
  (*Galium odoratum*)
1 part sage (*Salvia officinalis*)
5 parts forest moss (Musci family)
2 tablespoons finely crushed juniper
  berries (*Juniperus* spp.)

Sweet Woodruff is especially suited for scented pillows and this herbal blend has been particularly chosen for men.

❧ A "House" Herbal Tea Blend

> sweet woodruff (*Galium odoratum*)
> thyme (*Thymus vulgaris*)
> wild strawberry leaves
>   (*Fragaria vesca*)
> blackberry leaves (*Rubus fruticosus*)
> calendula flowers
>   (*Calendula officinalis*)
> sloe flowers (*Prunus spinosa*)
> apple and pear peels
>   (*Malus* spp. / *Pyrus* spp.)
> cocoa shells

This particular tea blend can be adjusted to suit your personal taste. Experiment to find a combination that suits you and your family.

To prepare: Steep 1 teaspoon of the herbal blend in 1 cup of cold water. Bring it to a quick boil, strain, and serve.

CULINARY USE

In May when the herb is still fresh and flowering, many people put it in wine and drink it, thinking that it is good for the liver and strengthens the same. They also say it strengthens and delights the heart!

This lively exhortation for the May feast with Sweet Woodruff wine comes from the year 1731.

The following recipes include a contemporary Sweet Woodruff wine punch that you can easily make at home—as well as a nonalcoholic version. Historically, other herbs were added to the Woodruff punch, as you will note in the directions for enlivening a cloister's punch bowl. And finally, see how your family and friends like my light and airy dessert creme.

❧ Sweet Woodruff Punch

> 1 bunch sweet woodruff
> 1 bottle white riesling wine
> 2 tablespoons sugar
> 1 bottle champagne

Gather the sweet woodruff before it flowers and let it wither slightly. Tie it together with twine and place it in a punch bowl, pouring the wine over it. Let the mixture steep for 2 hours in a cool place. Dissolve the sugar in a little hot mineral water and stir it into the punch. Add the champagne and serve immediately.

❧ "Virgin" Woodruff Punch

Let a slightly withered bunch of sweet woodruff steep in apple juice for several hours. Add mineral water to taste and garnish with a dash of freshly ground cinnamon.

❧ An Olde Cloister Punch

> 1 bunch sweet woodruff
>   (*Galium odoratum*)
> 1 handful wild strawberry leaves
>   (*Fragaria vesca*)
> 1 handful of black currant leaves
>   (*Ribes nigrum*) mixed with
>   ground ivy (*Glecoma hederacea*)
> 150 grams powdered sugar
>   (about 5½ ounces)
> 3 liters white wine

Place the herbs in a punch bowl, sprinkle the powdered sugar over them, and let them steep for 2 or 3 hours in a warm place. Add the wine and let the mixture steep for another 3 hours. Remove the herbs and serve the punch chilled.

This refreshing May bowl is said to strengthen the heart and stimulate digestion.

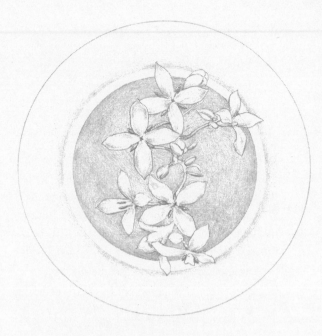

❦ SWEET WOODRUFF "WINE FOAM CREAM"

1 bunch sweet woodruff

½ liter white wine

1 snifter cognac

80 grams sugar (about 3 ounces)

4 eggs

the juice of half a lemon

a little grated lemon peel

1 packet plain gelatin

Place the sweet woodruff in a large pot and pour the wine over it. Let it steep for 3 hours; remove the herb. Add the cognac, sugar, 1 whole egg plus 3 egg yolks, lemon juice, and lemon peel to the wine. Heat the mixture very slowly, whisking constantly until the liquid becomes foam. Separately beat the remaining 3 egg whites until they are frothy, fold them into the wine foam with the dissolved gelatin. Serve it still warm with a plate of macaroons or sweet biscuits.

CULTIVATION

Sweet Woodruff makes a good ground cover under trees or other shady spots. Once it takes root, it spreads quickly to form a scented carpet. It is available commercially as seeds or starter plants. Sow the seeds outside in August (they are sometimes slow to germinate). In the fall, thin them to 8 inches apart. In the spring, you can propagate them by dividing the rootstock. Woodruff has a particular way of spreading—its burr-like seeds stick to the feathers of birds or the fur of animals who then carry them to other places. Because they are such good company, I plant Solomon's Seal (*Polygonatum odoratum*) among the Sweet Woodruff under my trees.

Sweet Woodruff also does well under fruit trees. For a first planting, mix loamy soil with beech leaves. It is not just a folk tale that it grows best under beeches.

BOTANICAL CHARACTERISTICS

Name: *Galium odoratum / Asperula odorata* — Sweet Woodruff

Distribution: Central Europe, Asia, North America

Habitat: Beech forests and mixed woodlands; loves nutrient-rich leaf mold and shady spots

Description: Grows 4 to 12 inches tall around an erect triangular stem; dark green lanceolate leaves are arranged in a star shape; small four-pointed star-shaped white flowers later turn into 2 tiny fruit-pellets; a thin, creeping root; a characteristic Woodruff fragrance; usually grows in clusters.

Confusion with similar plants: With Catchweed (*Galium aparine*) that has similar leaves but hairy hooks; also with Wood Bedstraw (*G. sylvaticum*). Neither plant is poisonous nor has the characteristic Woodruff scent.

Collecting season: May to June; for culinary purposes, before flowering; for medicinal purposes, after flowering

Active ingredients: Coumarin glycoside, tannin, and bitter compounds

Astrological association: Venus / Moon

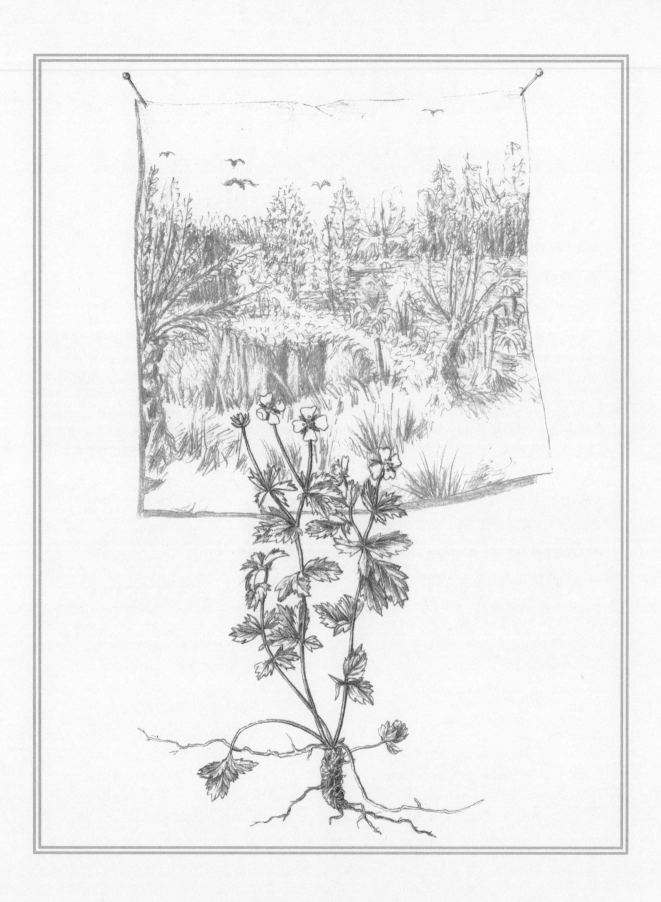

TORMENTIL

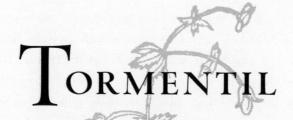

Potentilla erecta (*Potentilla tormentilla*)
Tormentilla Cinquefoil
Tormentilla, Shepherd's Knot, Upright Septfoil
Rose family — Rosaceae

A FIRST GLANCE at this inconspicuous little plant with her friendly, golden yellow flowers makes us question why the ancient ones called her Potentilla after the Latin word for power (*potentia*). The explanation hides underground with the plant's root, the holder of healing powers so wondrous that its bearer was granted the honorable title of "Powerful One."

The short, stocky root lies obliquely in the ground, irregular and knobby. Slicing into it, however, we observe a strange thing. The yellowish-white cut turns blood red as if we had cut our finger. "Blood Root" (*Blutwurz*) is still this plant's German name, the blood-stained root a clear sign that it was to be used for all kinds of bleeding. In his 1532 herbal, Otho Brunfels described Tormentil as "the most exquisite blood-stiller."

A good hemostatic remedy must have astringent properties, and our forebears recognized this in the plant's appearance. The sturdy rootstock, as if contracted into itself, grows thick and knobby—not wide. Likewise, it does not absorb much water even though it frequently grows in marshy soils. And if we chew a bit of the fresh root, its tart astringency is strong enough to numb our mouths. Even the upper part of the plant seems to grow in a gesture of contraction. The individual leaf sections, usually numbering three or five, all point toward the center. It was obvious to our ancestors that a plant with such contracting energy must also be able to bind broken blood vessels in our bodies.

Modern scientists have run Tormentil through numerous laboratory tests, dissecting it, analyzing it, and thereby confirming the old healing hallmark of the plant. Tormentil contains an extremely high percentage of tannin—up to 20% in some plants. It surpasses even Ratanyroot (*Krameria triandra*), a plant from the Andes long considered to be the remedy with the highest tannin content. Tannin gives Tormentil its strong astringent quality, while its antiseptic properties are most likely due to the red Tormentil dye.

Old German names like "Bloodwort," "Dysentery Herb," and "Dysentery Root" reveal another area of application. In earlier times Tormentil was used to treat dysentery, enteric fever, and infectious conditions of the intestines, especially when the patient's bowel movements were black and tarry with blood. It was also said to aid intestinal diseases combined with colic, indicated in its name "Tormentilla," again from Latin but this time the word for colic (*tormentum*).

Naturopathic physicians still use Tormentil to treat the aforementioned conditions, the healing benefits derived from the herb's combination of active ingredients. In short, Tormentil disinfects, repairs broken blood vessels in mucous membranes, soothes inflammation, and strengthens mucous membranes of the stomach and the intestines. We also know that Tormentil's high tannin content combined with its network of other constituents makes this plant's effectiveness superior to chemically pure tannin medicines. This natural tannin is more easily digestible because it binds to proteins and ensures a slow secretion over a longer period, a kind of stored time-release effect. As a result, Tormentil is a sovereign remedy for treating inflammatory and infectious processes of both large and small intestines.

Although a member of the Rose family, Tormentil has an inconspicuous appearance that hardly resembles a rose. I can clearly remember, however, when I first associated Tormentil with roses. It was the moment that I first grated the fresh root to prepare a tincture—and noticed a sweet rose-like scent. Later on, in a book listing the constituents of Tormentil, I saw that besides tannin, dye, and so on the root also contained a rose-like essential oil.

The palmate leaves, parted like fingers on a hand, classify Tormentil as part of the Cinquefoil (meaning "five leaves") genus that comprises

some 300 different species. Native European species are often confused with one another although they can be easily distinguished with a close examination. At flowering time Tormentil has a single unmistakable characteristic—her golden yellow flowers have only four petals while other Rose family members have five petals. In truth, flowers sporting four petals are a rarity in native European flora.

We must gather Tormentil's root in early spring or late fall when the plant is not flowering. And without the four-petaled flower as our signpost, we are forced to rely on other characteristics for its identification. We can look for her in dry or wet grasslands, along damp and boggy forest fringes, as well as high in the mountains where she will climb up to 8,000 feet. In the bog she is smaller and presses close to the ground. The drier the habitat the more expansive she becomes, growing to a height of one to two feet. Depending on the environment, Tormentil's slender and branching stems seem to hug the ground before eventually rising skyward. The coarsely toothed sessile leaves attach directly to the main stem. Dark green and almost shiny, they have five parts lower on the stem and three parts higher up. The golden yellow flowers perch above the stems as if atop a throne of four-leafed sepals.

In alpine meadows of higher altitudes grows a little sister of Tormentil—the Golden Cinquefoil (*Potentilla aurea*) growing only eight inches tall. Her leaves are smooth on top and shiny below, the lower-growing ones woolly and gleaming like silk. The root is also used for medicinal purposes. Once discovered, Golden Cinquefoil will catch your eye again and again, her friendly yellow five-petaled flowers beckoning from afar.

Another medicinal species of Cinquefoil hides behind the mysterious name "Pentephyllon" of Dioscurides. We know her as Creeping Cinquefoil (*Potentilla reptans*). Once a famous medicinal herb sold in pharmacies under the name "Herba Pentephylli," she was touted as a hemostatic and binding remedy—like Tormentil. Today she has disappeared completely from our medicinal treasure chest.

Once upon a time, this herb was believed to be magical. Occasionally I find her mentioned in old German books by names indicating such a use: "Hand of Mars," "Finger of Hermes," or "Smoke Herb." Legend says that when gathered an hour before noon and nailed to the stable door, Creeping Cinquefoil offered protection from sorcery. The plant was a common ingredient of the powdered incenses burnt to chase away evil spirits. In the Catholic areas of southern Germany, the church adapted this ancient custom to its own purposes. Wreaths were woven from the herb, brought to the church, and left to hang for the eight days preceding the Feast of Corpus Christi. These "smoke wreaths" were then carried in the ensuing religious procession. According to Robert Ranke-Graves's 1981 book *Die Weiße Göttin* ("The White Goddess"), Cinquefoil had widespread ritual use and was an important ingredient in the "flying ointments" used by witches in medieval times.

Frequently confused with Tormentil, Creeping Cinquefoil has leaves with long petioles that are parted into five fingers. Their edges are strikingly serrated and scalloped (crenate). Reminiscent of strawberry plants, her creeping stems, up to three feet long, repeatedly root at the nodes. She flowers from May to August with sunny yellow

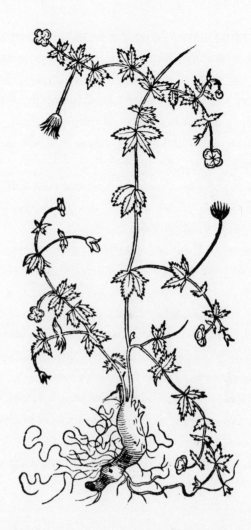

flowers of five petals sitting individually on long slender stalks.

HEALING PROPERTIES

A vial of Tormentil tincture or root powder should be present in any home pharmacy as a reliable and safe remedy. Both are made easily at home—with a few precautions. Due to its high tannin content, Tormentil reacts incompatibly with iron, copper, iodine, and bismuth—and also with Roman Chamomile (*Anthemis nobilis*).

Therefore when making the herbal preparations, it is important not to bring Tormentil root in contact with rusty iron or the aforementioned metals. And never mix it with Chamomile. Also, because the concentration of tannin in the dried root decreases significantly over time, it advisable to prepare tea, powder, and tincture anew every year. When you follow these simple instructions, nothing can go wrong with the preparation of your Tormentil remedies.

Tormentil is used internally and externally. The first area of application is acute and chronic inflammation of the small and large intestines, any type of diarrhea (as in a summer intestinal flu), intestinal infections, and even enteric (paratyphoid) fever, intestinal bleeding, and gastroenteritis. If you travel to countries where exposure to intestinal infections (such as cholera) is likely, be sure to carry a vial of equal parts Tormentil tincture and Herb Robert tincture. For gastric or intestinal bleeding, Tormentil is a good

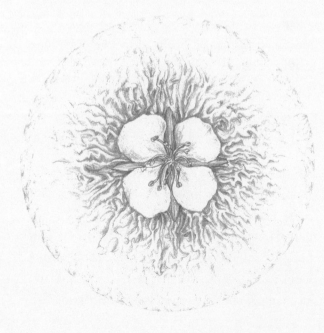

adjunct treatment. It also stanches excessive menstrual bleeding when administered alternately with a tea or tincture of Shepherd's Purse (*Capsella bursa-pastoris*).

A course of treatment for these illnesses is 40 drops of the tincture taken three times a day. In especially acute cases, you can administer a higher dose of the tincture or use the powder (one pinch three times a day). Finally, Tormentil powder and tincture have both proved to be more effective than the tea.

Applied externally, Tormentil is one of Nature's best hemostats. It is especially useful for heavily bleeding wounds and cuts. To use: First disinfect the wound with Arnica tincture and then sprinkle it with the finely ground root powder of Tormentil. The wound will soon stop bleeding. You can also soak a compress with Tormentil tincture.

I highly recommend using Tormentil tincture or the herbal toothpowder included in the recipe section for inflamed, bleeding, or receding gums, periodontal disease, gingivitis and canker sores, and all inflammations of the oral and pharyngeal cavities. Likewise red Tormentil salve aids diaper and other rashes, impure skin (especially oozing eczema), rough and chapped skin, and cracked skin and lips.

As for Tormentil wine or "Vinum Tormentillae," Tabernaemontanus wrote in 1731:

> From Tormentil one can make as useful a wine as from Cinquefoil. It serves to dry up and consume the primary discharges from eyes, nose, and ears and similarly to prevent tuberculosis, to strengthen the offspring in a woman's womb and fend off miscarriage, and to protect people from poisonous pestilent air. In sum, this wine can be used curatively

against all the illnesses I mentioned under the internal use of Tormentil.

Truly, Tormentil can help us with so many ailments that we should gather it with gratitude!

When we use Tormentil's root for remedial preparations, there is no need to discard the rest of the plant. Instead, we can dry it carefully and break or crumble it into small pieces to add to other herbal tea blends for the stomach. Although weaker than the root, it still retains a strengthening, invigorating effect.

Tormentil root is available in natural food stores or herbal pharmacies as "Rhizoma Tormentillae" and the tincture as "Tinctura Tormentillae." If possible, have the attendant or pharmacist grind the root into powder when you purchase it. This is because, as mentioned earlier, older powders are less potent.

❧ Tormentil Tea

Gather the root in early spring or late fall, when the plant concentrates all its energies in the root. Dig it out carefully, wash it, and cut it into small pieces. Dry these thoroughly by spreading them on a cloth or a fine mesh screen. Slicing the root, you will note the obligatory number five of the rose family. A faint five-pointed star will appear on the cut surface of each slice of root, becoming more obvious as they dry.

To prepare the tea: Take 1 teaspoon of tormentil root, cover it with cold water, and simmer the mixture in a covered pot for 10 minutes. A daily dose is 3 cups.

❧ Tormentil Powder

Tormentil powder is prepared from the dried root. Using a clean coffee or spice grinder,

pulverize the pieces of dried root as finely as possible. Store the powder in a tightly lidded mason jar—never use a metal tin.

A dose is 1 pinch taken 3 times daily.

❧ Tormentil Tincture

The strongest tincture is prepared from the fresh root. For this purpose, crush the cleaned root in a stone mortar, fill a dark mason jar halfway with it, and top it off with a grain spirit (90% alcohol) or fruit liqueur. Let the mixture sit for 2 to 3 weeks, shaking the jar occasionally. Strain the tincture into dark dropper bottles.

A course of treatment is 30, 40, or 50 drops taken several times daily.

❧ Bloodroot Schnapps

This cordial is an old folk remedy for stomach and intestinal conditions:

In a jar, put 1 handful freshly cut tormentil root and 1 quart spirits (such as vodka or a fruit liqueur). Cover the jar tightly and allow the mixture to steep for 2 or 3 weeks. Strain the liquor into a glass decanter and sip a small amount as needed.

❧ Tormentil Wine

Red wine and tormentil are perfect companions because red wine also contains tannin.

To prepare: Pour a liter of good red wine over 2 handfuls of freshly cut tormentil root. Let the mixture steep, covered, for 3 weeks before straining into a glass decanter. Enjoy the wine by the snifter.

❧ HERBAL TOOTHPOWDER

> tormentil root (*Potentilla erecta*)
>
> sage leaves (*Salvia officinalis*)
>
> linden coal (*Carbo Tiliae*, coal from
>
>   linden wood *Tilia cordata*)

Combine the ingredients in equal parts, grind them finely in a clean coffee or spice grinder, and store the powder in a glass jar. This toothpowder is used to cleanse and strengthen the gums.

❧ TORMENTIL SALVE

> 2 ounces lanolin (60 grams)
>
> a handful of finely chopped fresh
>
>   tormentil roots
>
> ½ fluid ounce tormentil tincture
>
>   (15 milliliters)

I encourage the reader to review the more extensive directions on preparing salves found in my chapter on Comfrey.

Slowly melt the lanolin in a double boiler. Add the tormentil root pieces and stir constantly for about 20 minutes. (Do not let it boil.) Strain the mixture through a cheese cloth, reheat slowly, and stir the tormentil tincture into the mix. Stirring occasionally, set the pan aside to cool slightly before transferring the salve into salve pots.

VETERINARY MEDICINE

Tormentil can be used for diarrhea in all animals and administered as a root powder, tincture, or decoction. A daily dose of the decoction for diarrhea is a pint for dogs and a quart for horses and cattle. The salve makes an effective treatment for eczema, lichens, and skin rashes. For wounds and injuries, especially with heavy bleeding, you can apply the finely ground powder or tincture as a compress.

Historically, Tormentil was a common medicinal plant employed by shepherds. Hieronymus Bock refers to this in his 1577 herbal:

> One can hardly find a root that serves better against all abdominal flows red and white [diarrhea with mucus and blood]. From Tormentil one can prepare confections, tablets, powder, electuaries, potions, sachets, and whatever anyone considers good for its use. Shepherds have learned this and know how to help their diseased sheep with it.

CULTIVATION

Tormentil is a hardy plant that makes few demands on the soil. Its natural habitats are wet or dry meadows. If you indulge a desire to start a wildflower meadow, plant a few Tormentil seedlings or add some Tormentil seeds to your mixture. Tormentil also tolerates shade and can be planted as a ground cover beneath trees. Sow the seeds in the spring and later thin seedlings to about three inches apart. Tormentil will thrive in a peat bed. After the second year, the roots can be harvested. Seeds and starter plants are available commercially.

Botanical Characteristics

Name: Potentilla erecta — Tormentil

Distribution: Europe, northwest Africa, northern Asia, and North America

Habitat: Dry and moist grasslands, boggy forest fringes

Description: Grows 4 to 15 inches tall; stem initially prostrate then erect (decumbent), thin, branching, with leaves; basal leaves on petioles, mostly five-fold, stem leaves are ternate (three-fold); golden yellow flowers have four petals. Flowering time is May to August.

Confusion with similar plants: With Creeping Cinquefoil (*P. reptans*) who is mostly creeping and not erect; leaves are mostly five-fold and flowers have five petals.

Collecting season: Root – March to April, October to November

Active ingredients: Tannin, dye, resin, and some essential oil

Astrological association: Saturn / Mercury

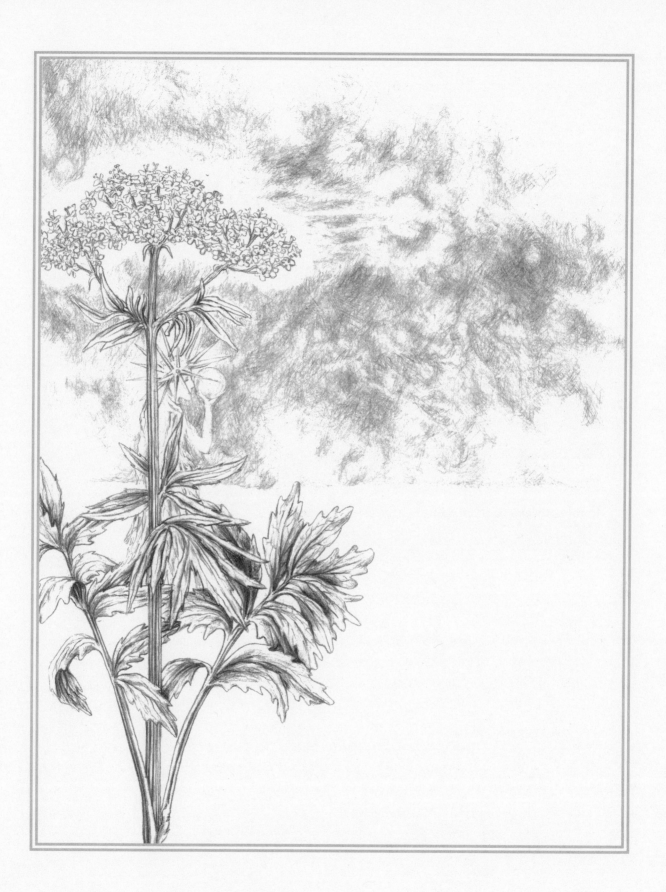

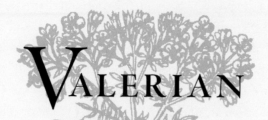

VALERIAN

Valeriana officinalis

Garden Heliotrope, True Wild Valerian, Fragrant Valerian,
All Heal, Vandal Root, Tobacco Root, Setwall
Valerian family — Valerianaceae

THERE IS NO NEED TO WORRY about Valerian's good name. He is already one of the most popular indigenous medicinal plants. In the course of centuries he has witnessed changes— being praised first for one healing property and then for another.

The ancient Greek and Roman physicians knew him by the mysterious name "Phu." Dioscurides valued the herb Phu as a remedy to warm and to promote menstruation and diuresis. Hippocrates, Paracelsus, and St. Hildegard von Bingen all considered Valerian to be a reliable cure. He was even grouped among the aphrodisiacs, as we conclude from a fifteenth century manuscript that reads: "To create good friendship among men and women, take Valerian, grind it into powder, and give it to drink in wine."

The Neapolitan scholar of jurisprudence, Fabio Colonna, even dedicated a book to Valerian two centuries later. Colonna suffered from epilepsy and in his search to cure his affliction he came across Valerian. He was healed with its help, studied botany, and wrote a book describing Valerian's healing properties. This was the first time Valerian was cited as a great remedy for the nerves, a reputation that stays with him today.

During the Middle Ages, Valerian was considered a panacea. His Latin name "Valeriana" derives from the Latin word *valere*, meaning "to be strong, well, and worthy." Even today, one of Valerian's English names is "All Heal." Valerian was known in medieval times to not only heal the nerves but offer protection from the plague and other epidemics. His old German name, "Theriak Herb," reminds us of this application. Theriaca herbal mixtures were especially potent and costly remedies whose ingredients were kept secret. Angelica was another "Theriak" herb.

Medieval people had a simple explanation for why Valerian was especially good for contagious diseases. The fairy mistresses of the woods supposedly revealed the secret during the time of the plague. Even the birds knew and chirped it to the people:

If you eat Valerian and Saxifrage
You will not grapple with the plague.

Had you drunk Valerian and Pimpinell*
You would not be dead, but well!

Long after the "black death" terrorized Europe, people still used Valerian as a remedy against contagion. They wore the herb around the neck as an amulet, chewed on it, and even burned the powdered root like incense.

It is especially noteworthy that old books on herbal medicine primarily praise Valerian as an eye remedy, an area not mentioned in modern literature. One old rural herbswoman (*Kräuterweiblein*) with knowledge of traditional herbal lore told me of this application. Valerian, she said, is good for the light—"light" meaning the eyes. This gives credence to the old German tale of the goldsmith from Würzburg, who so strengthened his eyes with Valerian that he was able to engrave a recognizable image of a lion on a broken sewing needle!

Contemporary considerations have reduced Valerian's healing properties to a single primary effect. For a long time he has been thought of as a remedy to calm the female nervous system. At the turn of the century, ladies even carried a vial of Valerian "just in case." Today's medical establishment has put Valerian through the rigors of so-called scientific laboratory examinations, earning for this herb of antiquity the seal "tested and considered medicinal." His antispasmodic effects on the central nervous system in humans and animals are considered proved, but nothing is mentioned of Valerian's other medicinal attributes.

After this brief excursion through Valerian's medicinal history, let us take a walk with him in Nature. Perhaps we will then grasp more of his true character and understand the meaning of some of his old names.

Valerian awaits us in the forest, in a small clearing, along the edge of a trail, in a wet, deciduous wood or mixed woodland, in a wooded marsh, or close by a river. He likes the wet element and wilts quickly when picked. The spirits of water and of the moon, water nymphs, and fairies are said to dance around him on moonlit nights. From them he acquires names like "Moonwort" and "Elfherb." Valerian has a graceful stature, fully an elfin plant. The high and slender, quickly shooting stem is adorned by fine, feathered (pinnate) leaves—not too many but enough to contrast nicely with the furrowed stem. An umbel-like flower head, a corymb, composed of white and pinkish flowers crowns the plant. One might think that such a flower head would make Valerian a member of the Carrot family (Umbelliferae) like Angelica and Chervil. He, however, has his own particular plant family—the Valerian family (Valerianaceae) with its 350 species.

There is nothing heavy or dark about Valerian. Like an airy pink cloud, the flower hovers over the graceful stem and foliage, straining toward the light. My ancestors called him Baldrian, perceiving in him the favor and radiant energies of Balder, their god of light, purity and kindness. *Balder* actually means "the most helpful" and the old Germanic people thought of Valerian as a plant offering succor for all ailments.

Valerian obtained a second seat of honor in Nordic mythology, this time in the gentle hands

---

* The Latin name for Great Burnet Saxifrage is Pimpinella Major.

of the goddess Hertha, who used him as a riding whip when racing through the forest on her Hops-bridled stag. The herb symbolized the appeasing powers that could tame a wild beast, a beautiful image for the calming properties of the good woodland spirit who could tame wild tempers and soothe agitated nerves.

However, there is one animal driven crazy when it smells Valerian. "Cat Herb," "Madcap," "Catwort" are old names that grew out of our domesticized beast's intense acquaintance with Valerian. In fact, I used to wonder why the tall stems of my lovely Valerian shrub often laid on the ground, bent and trampled. Finally I caught our cat jumping into it, stamping branches to the ground, and rolling around on them. She was quite literally mad from smelling the "Madcap" growing in my garden.

Valerian does have a strange scent. The root smells acrid, a bit like cat urine, especially when dried. Regarding the flowers, I hesitate to say whether their scent is pleasant or unpleasant. On sunny days a strong, enveloping odor that is sweet and warm surrounds the Valerian plant in my garden. But rain makes the flowery scent oddly "cat-like" again. Saved for more sensitive noses, some members of the Valerian family produce especially pleasant scents. To find them, however, we must climb the alpine mountains where other Valerian species thrive. Here we encounter Mountain Valerian (*Valeriana montana*), whose leaves are not as finely feathered as those of his valley brother and stand out opposite the stem. We also find "Rocky Valerian" (*V. saxatilis*), small and inconspicuous compared to the tall Common Valerian. A close relative is "True Speik" (*V. celtica*) and here again

we can use our noses. His rootstock emits an aromatic, strengthening smell that tells us why, since antiquity, this particular Valerian has been valued as incense. Unfortunately decimated in the wild, he currently enjoys protected status in Germany. The crowning jewel of all Valerian scents, however, comes from the East Indian Spikenard (*Nardostachys jatamansi*), a member of the Valerian family that thrives on the southern slopes of the Himalayas. From it was manufactured the best nard oil in old Tarsus. Sold in vials of alabaster and used for ritual anointment, it was considered the most precious of oils. We can find Valerian on many Christian images from medieval times.

On the rocky mountain slopes in the highlands of Mexico, at 6,000 to 9,000 feet grows Mexican Valerian (*V. mexicana*), a variety frequently used in today's commercially available Valerian remedies. The flowers are similar to those of my alpine Valerian. In contrast, the leaves are not pinnate but entirely simple leaves arising from the stem. The roots of this Valerian become quite large—as big as the healthiest horseradish roots. And the plant itself is enormous—growing up to six feet tall. Native Mexicans have long used this root as a tonic. In fact, the concentration of active ingredients in Mexican Valerian is six times greater than that of Common Valerian and proved to be a potent tranquillizer, especially for restlessness due to stress, insomnia, and physical imbalances. Mexican Valerian has only recently gained attention because its active constituents are lost in its conventional preparation as a tea. The constituents of this Valerian are found in several anti-stress remedies of plant origin.

Commonly called Garden Heliotrope in the United States, *Valeriana officinalis* was brought to North America by European settlers. It is now found nearly everywhere—particular east of the Mississippi River—having escaped, as it were, from cultivated gardens. Another Valerian, Centranthus ruber (*V. rubra*), is a showy, invasive, drought-resistant variety that is naturalized in many parts of the West. Arizona Valerian (*V. arizonica*) is yet another American native that grows from Colorado to Utah and south to Arizona and New Mexico. Other native Valerians abound.

HEALING PROPERTIES

"All forms of nervous conditions, convulsion, or pain call for Valerian!"

So writes Pfarrer Kneipp, the German herbalist-clergyman who originated modern-day hydrotherapy treatment. And, in truth, this herb really is one of our safest and most reliable nerve remedies, a veritable balsam for our nerves. Valerian enhances the ability to sleep through relaxation. It does not make one tired and therefore can be taken during the day for mental exhaustion and overwork. It is neither numbing nor addictive. With the dangers of strong soporifics and narcotics becoming increasingly obvious, more and more people are turning to Nature's drugstore for sleeping aids. Light sleeping difficulties can be remedied with Valerian, Hops, Balm, and St. John's Wort. This therapy is supported with herbal baths, with essential oils of the aforementioned herbs, and with what we call "sleep pillows" or "dream pillows." Valerian

and Hops relax the body and the mind; Balm and St. John's Wort calm and balance the effects of emotional strain. Valerian can relax headaches, nervous heart disorders, mild hyperthyroidism, biliary dysfunctions, and stomach and intestinal cramps.

When administering or taking a treatment that incorporates a medicinal plant, satisfactory results can be expected only when the remedy—Valerian in this instance—is administered properly and in the correct dosage. Again, in the case of Valerian, only the roots are used medicinally. They should be dug up in the fall, cleaned, and dried carefully and thoroughly in an airy place. To preserve their full aroma, I store them whole and cut them into pieces immediately before using them.

Valerian root is available in natural food stores and naturopathic pharmacies as "Radix Valerianae." The homeopathic mother tincture is "Tinctura Valerianae."

ℰ VALERIAN TEA

In a container place 2 teaspoons of finely chopped valerian root per cup of cold water. Let it steep during the day. In the evening, strain the tea and warm it to suit your taste. Drink 1 to 2 cups before retiring.

ℰ VALERIAN TINCTURE

For the tincture, fill a mason jar with freshly chopped valerian roots and grain alcohol or fruit liqueur. Close the jar tightly and let the mixture steep for 2 weeks before straining it into dark dropper bottles.

Take 1 or 2 teaspoons of the tincture before bedtime.

VALERIAN WINE

In a quart jar, place 1½ cups of freshly chopped valerian roots. Add 1 tablespoon of minced organic orange peel and fill the jar with a good white wine. Close tightly and let the wine steep for 2 weeks before straining it into a wine bottle or decanter.

Enjoy this wine by the liqueur glass before bedtime. And by the way, in the fairy tale, the eye-strengthening recipe of the goldsmith of Würzburg was to daily ingest a pinch of powdered valerian root in wine.

A TEA TO STRENGTHEN THE NERVES

This recipe is from C. W. Hufeland (1762–1836), court physician to Friedrich Wilhelm III and one of our greatest naturopathic physicians.

> valerian root
> wood avens root
> peppermint leaves
> bitter orange leaves

Combine equal parts of these herbs, dried and freshly chopped or crushed; store them in a lidded jar. Pour 1 cup boiling water over 1 teaspoon of the tea blend, letting it steep before drinking.

A daily dose is 2 to 3 cups.

Dr. Hufeland wrote a book originally called *The Art of Extending Human Life* that clearly described the principles of holistic treatment and lifestyle. Immensely popular, in its third printing it was renamed *Macrobiotics*, a term first coined by the author in 1805.

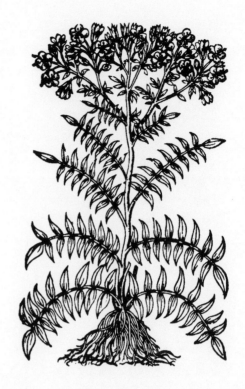

VALERIAN SLEEP PILLOW

This sleep pillow is most effective when used in conjunction with a course of treatment with valerian tea or tincture. To make, fill a small pillow form with dried valerian flowers, adding balm and hops if you desire. (I always use untreated fabric made from natural fibers.) Lay your head on the pillow when resting.

EYE-STRENGTHENING TEA

> 2 parts valerian flowers
> 1 part eyebright
> 1 part rue

Pour 1 cup boiling water over 1 teaspoon of the herbal mixture. Let it steep, covered, until the tea cools to body temperature. Strain off the liquid and use it in an eyecup to bathe the eyes. You may also soak a small compress in the tea to place over strained, reddened eyes.

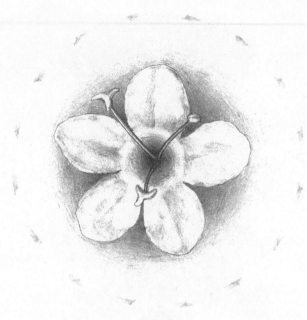

VETERINARY MEDICINE

Valerian has a calming and relaxing effect on animals as well as on people. It has proved its worth especially in cases of cramps and colics. You can administer either Valerian tea, tincture, or powder.

CULTIVATION

Valerian was never missing in the old rural gardens because people wanted this healing plant nearby. In today's vegetable gardens we can still find a variety of Valerian—a salad green known as mâche, lamb's lettuce, or corn salad (*Valerianella olitoria*).

Planted in a garden, Valerian enhances the growth of vegetables and helps them to flourish. The herb attracts earthworms, our small but irreplaceable garden helpers who aerate the soil and produce the best compost. In fact, mixing Valerian into the compost will increase the earthworms' transforming activity.

In the bio-dynamic gardening principles of Rudolf Steiner, a Valerian preparation sprayed on tomatoes in late fall and on flowering fruit trees in spring protects them from frost by utilizing the herb's warming effect. Remember the warm, sweet scent of Valerian in summertime? Well, gardeners can use these warming energies to protect their plants. When treated with a Valerian preparation, balcony and container plants grow longer and more abundantly while beans, peas, and strawberries develop more flowers. Briefly soaking tomato, leek, and wheat seeds in diluted Valerian extract strengthens the plants and makes them more resistant. (*Note*: Do not treat legume seeds this way.) To prepare this dilution according to bio-dynamic principles, add 50 drops of Valerian extract to five quarts of lukewarm water and stir for five minutes.

The extract can be purchased from sources that carry products for biological gardening. You can also make your own by processing fresh Valerian flowers in a juicer and mixing it with rainwater in a ratio of about 70% Valerian juice to 30% rainwater. The extract keeps well in bottles. For watering and spraying, mix this extract in a 1-to-10 ratio with rainwater and stir for about three minutes.

Valerian makes no great demands on soil—although it prefers a moist location, repaying deep soil with good root growth. It grows in partial shade as well as in bright sunlight. You can fertilize it with decayed manure. Seeds and starter plants are available commercially. The seeds take three to four weeks to germinate before showing the first sprouting leaves. I sow them in a glass-covered seed tray in early spring or outside after mid-May. Because Valerian needs light for germination, you should press the seeds lightly into the soil without covering them. Later you can transplant seedlings two or three feet apart. (The Valerian in my garden grows nearly five and a half feet tall!) And while they do take time to develop, by late summer you will have impressive plants. Valerian also grows in containers but it must be kept well watered.

When cultivating Valerian for the roots, cut off the flowers as soon as they open in order to stimulate root growth. The roots are ready to dig up by the second or third year once the foliage has died back completely. Valerian plants form runners that can be separated and transplanted in the spring.

BOTANICAL CHARACTERISTICS

Name: *Valeriana officinalis* — Valerian

Distribution: A European native now found throughout the world

Habitat: Wet meadows, clearings, deciduous forests, or mixed woodland

Description: Plants grow 2 to 5 feet tall; leaves are odd-pinnate and opposite; stem is hollow, furrowed, with short hairs at the base and smooth above. Flower is a cyme, white to pale violet in color. Root is brown, whitish inside, and strong smelling with many root fibrils. Flowering time is July to August.

Confusion with similar plants: Possibly with Hemp Agrimony although it lacks the typical Valerian smell.

Collecting season:
    Flowers – July to August
    Root – October

Active ingredients: Essential oil, isovaleric acid, valepotriates

Astrological association: Mercury / Sun

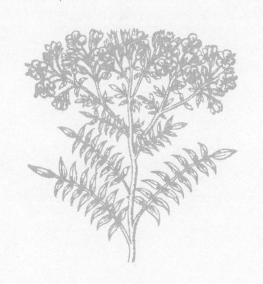

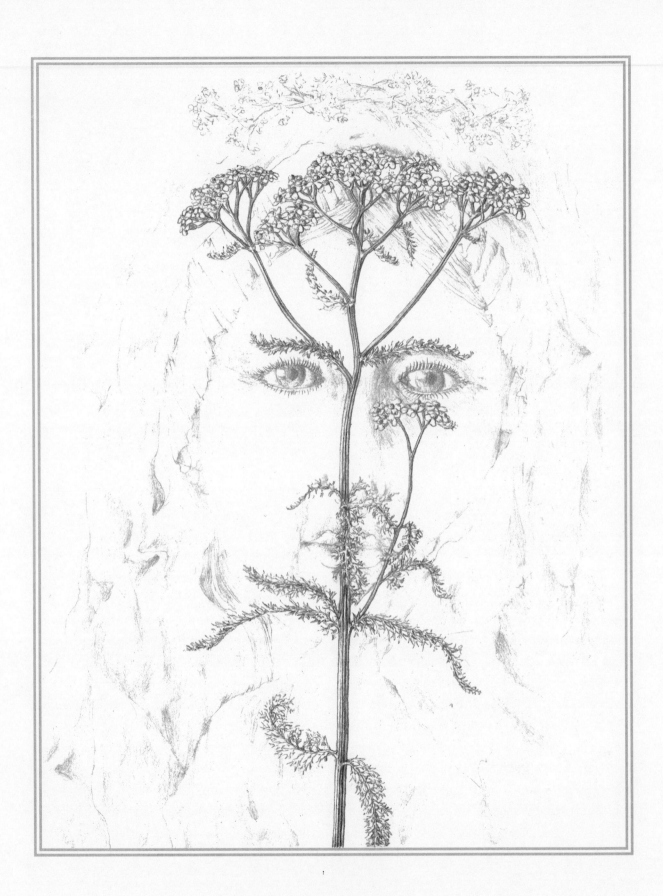

YARROW

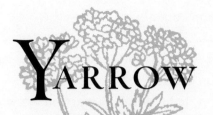

Achillea millefolium
Noble Yarrow, Milfoil, Thousandleaf, Sanguinary,
Nosebleed, Soldier's Woundwort
Daisy family—Compositae / Asteraceae

TO FIND YARROW'S MENTION in medieval manuscripts we would look for the provocative name *Supercilium Veneris*—or "the eyebrow of Venus." This tender plant with her filigree leaves was entrusted to the Goddess of Love, Beauty, and Grace.

Historically, plants named after goddesses have been healing remedies for women. Still called "Woman's Herb" or "Woman's Gratitude," Yarrow was included in the sacred bundle of herbs carried by women on the ancient pagan day of the Goddess that later became the feast of "Mary's Ascension." (I discuss this tradition in further detail in the chapter on Mullein.)

Not surprisingly, astrological-based herbology assigned Yarrow to the planet Venus and used her to treat diseases of the venous system such as varicose veins and enlarged veins (hemorrhoids). Today we know Yarrow can indeed strengthen the venous system of blood vessels by promoting the return of venous blood to the heart, thereby reducing strain on the heart and circulatory system. Modern naturopathic medicine uses Yarrow for menstrual problems, lower abdominal cramps,

and vaginal discharge. "Women would be saved much trouble if once in a while they would reach for some Yarrow," declared Pfarrer Kneipp and promoted it in his practice of aromatherapy. Likewise, the bladder and kidneys are Venus assignations, and modern science concurs that Yarrow's high potassium content stimulates and strengthens these organs without irritating them.

Yarrow's modern Latin name is *Achillea millefolium* and in it lies another story . . . When, in the Trojan war, Achilles was struck in the heel by an arrow, the Greek goddess Aphrodite (counterpart to the Roman Venus) entreated him to use Yarrow on his wound. Achilles may have been familiar with the plant because legend has it that the Centaur Chiron initiated him into herbal lore. People have since treated wounds with the help of Achilles' fabled herb, calling her "Stop Bleeding Herb," "Soldier's Herb," and "Wound Herb." For centuries she was used to treat injuries contracted through contact with iron. The French referred to it as "Carpenter's Herb" (*herbe des charpentiers*) because woodworkers frequently injured themselves with tools like axes, hammers, and saws.

Today herbalists primarily use Yarrow for internal bleeding. This area of application was noted in the first century A.D. by Abbot Wahlafrid Strabo, a plant lover from the island of Reichenau in Lake Constance on the border of Switzerland, Austria, and Germany. In his poem "Hortulus" written about herb gardens, he writes:

> Surely physicians use her as a medicine in their profession. She withdraws, when drunk as a remedy, as much blood from the body as she wholesomely returns juices to it.

Strange contradictions attract the attention of those who study Yarrow's applications closely and observe her effects on the human body. Yarrow heals both excessive and scanty menstrual bleeding. With the herb one can easily cause a nosebleed as well as quickly stop one by snuffing the fresh juice. While an overdose of Yarrow tea can lead to internal bleeding of the kidneys, it has likewise proved beneficial in cases of kidney bleeding. Regarding the skin, another Venus-related organ, Yarrow treats rashes, inflammations, and chapped conditions. However, she can cause allergic reactions of the skin (contact dermatitis) in sensitive people.

In other words, this healing plant seems to have a balancing effect that makes it applicable in many different kinds of complaints. With good reason she is sometimes called "All World's Heal." Hieronymus Bock in his 1577 herbal reveals his astonishment about her nature:

> This herb has such a contradictory nature that when one crushes it and places it on a bleeding wound, the blood will stand still. At the same time, when one puts a leaflet into the nose, in a short while the blood will follow.

Now I think it is time to learn from the plant herself. By the way, I rarely meet a person who does not know what Yarrow looks like. She is one of those plants usually associated with childhood memories of a Sunday walk or the smell of warm meadow grass. Preferring the dry warmth of sunny meadows, grassy knolls, waysides, and ridges, her shallow root thrusts firmly into the arid, rocky soil and sends out numerous pale brown root branches. Some stolons thicken and take on a purplish hue; from their ends, a new Yarrow plant or infertile leaf shoot grows. Her plant life begins with a kind of basal rosette that barely grazes the ground. In contrast to Broad-leaved Plantain's fierce grasp of the soil, Yarrow chooses a gentler connection.

However, do not mistake her gentle nature for weakness—she is quite sturdy! She winters over with a few leaves that by March and April are already light green and juicy. These leaves are a special characteristic of Yarrow—infinitely divided and shaped like filigree. Her Latin name *millefolium* ("thousand leaf") refers to this fine partition. Oddly, when we stroke our cheeks with her delicate leaf, it feels course. This is because each feathery leaflet has a tiny, white bristle at the tip. And it was these bristles that injured his mucous membranes and caused old Hieronymus's fabled nosebleed!

From the basal rosette slowly rises a sturdy stem that can reach 20 to 30 inches; the stalked leaves grow in stair steps, becoming darker as they go up. At its terminal end, the stem branches out into a single or sometimes several flower corymbs composed of many single, small flower heads. We usually encounter White Yarrow in the wild although some plants bloom a tender pink. Yarrow often keeps her flower until after first frost—as if she has soaked up enough warmth in her sunny spot to hold out against the approaching winter.

The entire plant emanates an aromatic, warm fragrance that is especially strong during its midsummer flowering. Rubbing a leaf or flower between our fingers and inhaling this odor, we can sense Yarrow's warming and cramp-soothing properties. Her herbal powers come from the essential oil that penetrates all of her parts. This particular plant oil contains an early stage of azulene, an azure blue oil that is only freed in the rising water vapor of steam distillation. Azulene has strong anti-inflammatory and antispasmodic properties, strengthens the immune system, and balances the nervous system. (German Chamomile contains more azulene than does Yarrow—but only in the flowers.) Because she is permeated with it, Yarrow can with subtlety direct the energy of this constituent and influence the illness on a more psycho-emotional level. She brings a gentle warmth into our bodies, simultaneously loosening and strengthening wherever there is tension.

The balancing element that works on us shows in her general botanical stature. Her delicate filigree leaves give her an airy quality. Her volatile essential oil seems ethereal. At the same time her stem is erect and unyielding. Were we to compare her with Comfrey or Burdock, we would call them earthy and heavy—more like elephants at work on another level in our bodies, preoccupied with the formation of matter. Or to compare her with Angelica, another stomachic plant who aids gastrointestinal conditions while calming and balancing the nervous system . . .

Well, Angelica conveys strength like a comforting pat on our shoulder. Yarrow, on the other hand, conveys the balance needed when tension, stress, and cold prevent us from feeling the warmth of our own souls.

Finally, I owe an explanation to my readers with a fondness for puzzling out plant names. The German name for Yarrow is *Schafgarbe* or "Sheep Healer." As in the case of Boldu and many other plants, people have learned from animals. Long ago, shepherds observed that sick sheep ate large amounts of Yarrow and healed themselves. The second part of the German name comes from the Old High German word *Garwe* ("healer"), which is probably the root of the Anglo-Saxon word *gearwe* from which the English common name "Yarrow" is derived. No damage comes to the plant when sheep and other animals graze upon her—she quickly grows back.

Even in the highest alpine pastures we find Yarrow. At 9,800 feet Musk Yarrow (*Achillea moschata*) grows between rocks and boulders, stretching her white flowers skyward. Only four to six inches tall, she is much more aromatic than her sister from the lowlands. In fact, the entire plant emanates a musk-like scent. The Swiss call her "Iva Herb" and value her as a remedy for both sheep and shepherd. There the famous Iva liqueur is distilled and administered for stomachaches and cramps. So when mountain hikers are injured or develop stomach problems, they—like sheep—can turn to Musk Yarrow.

In these reflections on Yarrow we have unwittingly encountered one of the oldest medicinal plants known to humankind. She has accompa-

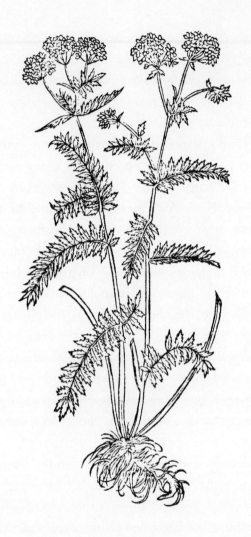

It is the variety of different active ingredients and medicinal constituents present in Yarrow that presents such a range of medical applications. Besides the essential oil with its azulene, Yarrow also contains the bitter compound achilleine, tannins, phosphorus, asparagin, inulin, resin, nitrates, propionic acid, proteins, acetic acid, malic acid, and probably others. Their effects on the body are anti-inflammatory, antispasmodic, antiseptic, blood-stanching, blood-forming, blood-cleansing, stimulating, and tonic. Whew!

Yarrow can be taken in the form of herbal tea, tincture, fresh juice, or medicinal wine. It can be used in a bath or on compresses. However, because the fresh juice can cause an allergic reaction (such as contact dermatitis) in sensitive people, especially when the skin is then exposed to the sun, people with these tendencies should first perform a patch test.

For the tea, gather the flowering plants on a sunny day. You can cut the plants a few inches above the ground and hang them up to dry in small bunches or spread them loosely over a frame covered with fabric or wire mesh. When the plants have dried thoroughly, cut them into small pieces and store them in a clean, dry container with a tight-fitting lid.

Yarrow tea is most effective when ingested in small sips throughout the day. It is best to prepare the daily amount in the morning and then sip it occasionally until evening. *Note: An overdose can quickly cause a reversal effect, making it important to pay attention to the quantity.* A course of treatment with Yarrow should not last over four weeks, during which the patient should avoid wine and coffee if possible. Fresh Yarrow juice has a stronger effect

nied us for millennia as a helpful and benevolent spirit from the plant kingdom. Estimated to be 60,000 years old, a grave excavated in Shanidar in modern Iran held the pollen-grains of eight medicinal plants. Yarrow was among the sacred herbs accompanying the dead on their journey.

HEALING PROPERTIES

Writing this, I stop in amazement as I consider the multitude of ailments for which Yarrow is valued. It is simply mind-boggling!

than the tea. This is because it still contains all the vital ingredients—especially chlorophyll, which is said to contain a substance similar to vitamin A.

It is the combination of essential oils, bitter compounds, and tannins that makes Yarrow such a good gastrointestinal remedy. Modern herbal medicine counts Yarrow among the bitter remedies. It is especially well-suited for stomach and intestinal disruptions that are accompanied by cramps. In inflammatory conditions of this region (as in gastritis), it lets the inflammation die down. It redresses a lack of appetite by stimulating the digestive glands. Finally, it expels gas and eases the uncomfortable cramping of flatulence. Yarrow also works well in tandem with other herbs geared to the specific malady.

For women, Yarrow brings welcome relief from all tensions of the pelvic area. This is especially true for menstrual cramps but also for spotting between periods and scanty or excessive menstruation. Yarrow helps to balance the changes a woman experiences during menopause. The application of warm compresses made with the tea or fresh juice supports the course of treatment very well. For this purpose, you can saturate a compress with hot Yarrow tea and apply it to the sacral area. Place a hot water bottle over it, a towel and blanket on top of that, and leave the lot in place until the compress cools. For acute cases, this can be a daily treatment. (When using Yarrow in the treatment of gynecological diseases, I prefer the pink-flowering plants.)

Yarrow is also proved to be an effective adjunct treatment for bladder infection, weak bladder function, and all kidney diseases. It warms and strengthens these organs and stimulates urination without irritation.

A special field of application for Yarrow is bleeding, especially of a light red color, from the rectum, from hemorrhoids, or from the uterus, bladder, and kidneys. To support the treatment of these conditions, Yarrow can be administered as fresh juice.

As I mentioned in the early part of this chapter, Yarrow is a tonic for blood vessels—in particular those of the venous system. It helps strengthen the blood vessels in hemorrhoids, varicose veins, and during pregnancy. It eases circulation in cases of high blood pressure and is a good adjunct treatment for angina pectoris when taken as a course of treatment with the fresh juice.

Yarrow strengthens a nervous heart and calms the nerves.

For rheumatism, lower abdominal problems, and kidney and bladder conditions, Yarrow baths are beneficial. For these conditions, we can make a strong tea and add it to the bath water.

To heal and disinfect wounds, freshly mashed Yarrow can be applied as a compress and the tea, juice, or tincture used to wash the wounds. It has blood-clotting properties and promotes scar formation. It even soothes the incessant itching of insect bites.

Note: People who are allergic to plants from the Daisy family—especially Yarrow—should abstain from applications of this plant.

Yarrow is available in herbal pharmacies and natural food stores as "Herba Millefolii" (flowers and leaves) and as "Flores Millefolii" (flowers only). The homeopathic tincture "Millefolia" is prepared from the fresh herb.

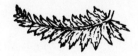

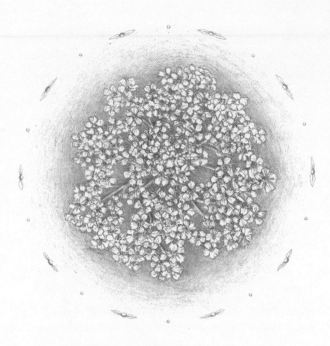

𝒴ᴀʀʀᴏᴡ Tᴇᴀ

In a small pan, combine 1 teaspoon of the dried herb, chopped or crumbled, with 1 cup cold water. Cover the pan and bring the mixture to a quick boil, letting it steep for a while before straining it.

A daily dose is 3 cups.

𝒴ᴀʀʀᴏᴡ Jᴜɪᴄᴇ

Gather the youngest leaves possible and process them in a juicer. Dilute this concentrated juice with equal parts of whey or water.

A daily dose is 3 tablespoons.

𝒴ᴀʀʀᴏᴡ Tɪɴᴄᴛᴜʀᴇ

Mix the fresh juice with an equal amount of wine spirits (70% alcohol). Let the mixture steep in a closed container for 3 weeks before straining it into clean dropper bottles.

A dose is 30 drops taken 3 times daily.

A Hᴇᴀʀᴛ Wɪɴᴇ ꜰᴏʀ Cᴀʟᴍɪɴɢ ᴀɴᴅ Sᴛʀᴇɴɢᴛʜᴇɴɪɴɢ

2 handfuls minced fresh yarrow herb
(*Achillea millefolium*)

2 handfuls minced fresh balm herb
(*Melissa officinalis*)

2 tablespoons minced fresh valerian root
(*Valeriana officinalis*)

1 teaspoon ground cinnamon

a liter of good red wine

Prepare the herbs and combine them with the cinnamon and red wine. Let the mixture steep, tightly covered, for 3 weeks in a cool, dark place. Strain the wine into dark bottles with a cork or lid.

Sip 2 liqueur glasses full daily.

Vᴇᴛᴇʀɪɴᴀʀʏ Mᴇᴅɪᴄɪɴᴇ

Yarrow aids sheep, goats, horses, and cattle suffering from gastrointestinal problems and flatulence. To treat them, add the herb to their fodder or administer it as tea or tincture. Interestingly, if we rub down the animals with enough fresh Yarrow juice to stick to their hides, pesky flies and other insects will be kept at bay.

Cᴏsᴍᴇᴛɪᴄs

Yarrow's germicidal and anti-inflammatory properties make it a good dressing for inflamed, irritated, oily, and blemished complexions. It strengthens, firms, and cleanses the skin. However, as I have noted several times, people who are sensitive and allergy-prone should not use Yarrow.

For a facial mask, mash some fresh leaves and place them on the face for 10 or 15 minutes. Likewise, applications of compresses saturated with Yarrow tea are well-suited for cosmetic treatments.

I find that facial steam baths are helpful in treating oily, blemished skin. For this purpose, I bring water to a boil in a pot, throw in a handful of fresh or dried Yarrow, and then transfer the pot from the stove to a counter or table where, covered with a large towel, I can comfortably sit and allow the steam to penetrate my skin. As always, I caution the reader to use care and guard against being burned or scalded.

CULTIVATION

Yarrow is a perennial, winter-hardy plant that grows in bushy groups. It is a valuable and enduring bee attractor. Modest, it thrives in any soil but prefers a bright, sunny spot. Starter plants and seeds are available commercially although the latter maintain their ability to germinate for only a year. Sow the seeds outdoors in the open after mid-March in shallow furrows by pressing the seeds into the soil, later thinning seedlings to eight inches apart. Yarrow can also be sown into lawns because it can be trod upon without damage.

Like Chamomile, Yarrow belongs to the soil-healing plants who prevent diseases in their neighbors. For instance, when grown next to scented plants such as Rosemary, Hyssop, or Lavender, it intensifies their fragrance.

Besides the medicinally used Common Yarrow (*Achillea millefolium*), garden varieties in various colors and fragrances are available from your local nurseries. These include low-growing specimens suitable for rock gardens. Greek Yarrow (*A. ageratifolia*), originally from the Balkan mountains, makes a white-flowered ground cover with felty, grey leaves and a sweet-acrid scent. (This endearing feature is why the English call it "Sweet Milfoil.") Silvery Yarrow with its ivory blooms (*A. clavenae*, often sold as *A. argentea*) and *A. spinulifolia* also remain small and make interesting additions to a rock garden.

Some of the colorful species are perfect in late-season dried flower arrangements. These include the yellow-flowering Fernleaf Yarrow (*A. fili-pendulina*) with horticultural varieties like 'Coronation Gold' and 'Gold Plate.' Some of the lovely red-flowering varieties of *A. millefolium* are 'Cerise Queen,' 'Rosea,' and the three-foot grower 'Fire Brand.'

BOTANICAL CHARACTERISTICS

Name: Achillea millefolium — Yarrow

Distribution: Europe, North America, northern Asia, and southern Australia

Habitat: Meadows, ridges, waysides, and banks between fields; prefers arid and sunny spots over wet areas.

Description: Grows erect, 8 to 30 inches tall; the stem is hard and marrowy, mostly hairy; leaves are pointed, lanceolate, finely divided, two to three times pinnate; flowers are arranged in corymbs; white or pink ray flowers. Flowering time is May to October.

Confusion with similar plants: None

Collecting season:

   In spring, for a course of treatment with the juice.
   In its midsummer flowering, for tea and tincture.

Active ingredients: Essential oil with azulene, bitter compounds, and tannins

Astrological association: Venus

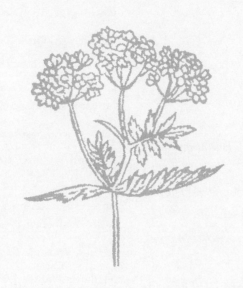

BIBLIOGRAPHY*

Aschner, Dr. Berhnard, *Paracelsus – Sämtliche Werke*, Jena 1932, Bd. I–X

Bach, Edward, *Blumen, die durch die Seele heilen*, München 1979

Bingen, Hildegard von, *Ursachen und Behandlung der Krankheiten*, Ulm 1955

dies., *Naturkunde*, Salzburg 1959

Bock, Hieronymus, *Kreuterbuch 1577*, Reprint Kölbl, München 1964

Bohn, W., *Die Heilwerte heimishcer Pflanzen*, Leipzig 1927

Buschheister-Ottersbach, G.A., *Handbuch der Drogistenpraxix*, Berlin 1919

Culpeper, Nicholas, *Culpetters complete Herbal*, Exeter

Dietrich, Dr. Karl, *Neues pharmazeutisches Manual*, Berlin 1919

Dinand, A.P., *Taschenbuch der Heilpflanzen*, Esslingen 1926

Eliade, Mircea, *Mythen, Träume und Mysterien*, Salzburg 1961

Fischer, Hermann, *Mittelalterliche Pflanzenkunde*, Hildesheim 1967

Fischer-Rizzi, Susanne, *Blätter von Bäumen*, München 1980

Fischer-Rizzi, Susanne, *Himmlische Düfte*, München 1989

dies., *Dufterlebnisse*, Isny 1989

dies., *Poesie der Düfte*, Isny 1989

Frater, Albertus, *Praktische Alchemie im zwanzigsten Jahrhundert*, Salt Lake City 1970

Frazer, James, *Der goldene Zweig*, Bd. I, II

Fritzsche, Helga, *Heilpflanzen biologisch ziehen*, München

Funke, Hans, *Die Welt der Heilpflanzen*, München 1979

Gessman, G.W., *Die Phlanzen im Zauberglauben*

Gessner, Dr. Otto, *Die Gift- und Arzneipflanzen von Mitteleuropa*, Heidelberg 1953

Grusche, Dr. H., *Heilpflanzen für dich und für mich*, Lerhrmeisterbücherei, Nr. 1325

Karl, Josef, *Phytotherapie*, München 1974

Künzle, Johann, *Chrut und Unchrut*, Locarno-Minusio 1962

Lonicerus, Adamus, *Krauterbuch*, 1679 / Reprint Kölbl, München 1962

Mabey, Richard, *Bei der Natur zu Gast*, Köln 1978

Madaus, Dr. Gerhard, *Lehrbuch der biologischen Heilmittel*, Band I–III, Leipzig 1938

Marzell, Dr. Heinrich, *Unsere Heilpflanzen*

ders., *Bayrische Volksbotanik*, Nürnberg

Müller, Ferdinand, *Das Große illustrierte Kräuterbuch*, Ulm 1874

Papyros Ebers, übersetzt von Dr. H. Joachim, Berlin 1973

Pelikan, Wilhelm, *Heilpflanzenkunde*, Bank I u. II, Dornach, 1958 / 62

Perger, von H. Ritter, *Deutsche Pflanzensagen* 1864 / Reprint, Leipzig 1980

Plenzat, Dr. Frider, *Duftende Pflanzen in Garten und Haus*, Frankfurt 1982

---

*This bibliographic listing is taken untranslated from the 1995 German edition of *Medicine of the Earth*. Rudra Press has not ascertained which, if any, of these works has been translated into English.

Pumpe, Heinrich, *Die 12 wichtigsten Heilkräuter in ihrer volkstümlichen Anwendung*, München 1957

Rademacher, Dr. Johann Gottfried, *Erfahrungsheillehre*, Bd. I u. II, Lorch 1939

Ranke-Graves, Robert von, *Die weiße Göttin*, Berlin 1981

Ripperger, Walther, *Grundlagen zur praktischen Pflanzenheilkunde*, Leipzig 1937

Schlegel, Emil, *Religion der Arznei*, Ulm 1960

Schloss, Lothar, *Comfrey – Wiedergeburt einer Heilpflanzen*, Bergen 1979

Schröder, Johann, *Höchstkostbarer Arzeney-Schatz*, Bd. I u. II 1685

Schott, Rolf, *Die Kunst sich gesund zu erhalten*, Regimen Sanitatis Salernitanum, Zürich 1964

Seifert, Alwin, *Gärtnern, Ackern – ohne Gift*, München 1971

Stoffler, Hans-Dieter, *Der Hotrulus des Walahfried Strabo*, Sigmaringen 1978

Tabernaemontanus, Jacobus Theodorus, *Neu vollkommen Kräuter-Buch*, 1731 / Reprint Kölbl, München 1975

Tisserand, Robert, *Aromatherapie*, Freiburg 1980

Waggerl, K.H., *Heiteres Herbarium*, Salzburg 1950

Weiss, Dr. R.F., *Lehrbuch der Phytotherapie*, Stuttgart 1974

Additional references
used in the English translation:

American Joint Committee on Horticultural Nomenclature, *Standardized Plant Names (SPN): A Revised and Enlarged Listing of Approved Scientific and Common Plants and Plant Products in American Commerce or Use*, 2nd Edition, Harrisburg PA, 1942

Bunney, Sarah, ed., *Illustrated Encyclopedia of Herbs*, New York: Barnes & Noble, 1994, (originally in Hungarian in 1984)

Editors of Sunset Magazine, *Western Garden Book*, Menlo Park: Lane Publishing Co., 1988

Fitter, R. & F. and Blamey, M., *Pareys Blumenbach: Wildblühende Pflanzen Deutschlands und Nordwesteuropas*, Hamburg, Berlin: Verlag Paul Parey, 1974. (Translated from the English *Wild Flowers of Britain and Northern Europe*.)

Hylton, William H., ed., *The Rodale Herbal Book*, Emmaus PA: Rodale Press, 1974

Lockie, Dr. Andrew and Geddes, Dr. Nicola, *Complete Guide to Homeopathy: Principles and Practices of Treatment*, London, New York, Stuttgart: Dorling-Kindersley, 1995

Lust, John, *The Herb Book*, Toronto, New York: Bantam Books, 1974

McIntyre, Anne, *The Complete Woman's Herbal*, New York: Henry Holt and Company, 1994

Mills, Simon Y., *The Essential Book of Herbal Medicine*, New York: Penguin Arkana, 1993

Moore, Michael, *Medicinal Plants of the Mountain West*, Santa Fe: Museum of New Mexico Press, 1979. Also *Medicinal Plants of the Pacific West*.

Pons Fachworterbuch Medizin Englisch / Deutsch, Deutsch / Englisch, Stuttgart, Dresden: Klett Verlag, 1992

Potterton, David, ed., *Culpeper's Color Herbal*, New York: Sterling Publishing Co., 1983

U. S. Department of Agriculture's Soil Conservation Service, *National List of Scientific Plant Names and Synonyms*, Washington DC, 1982 ed.

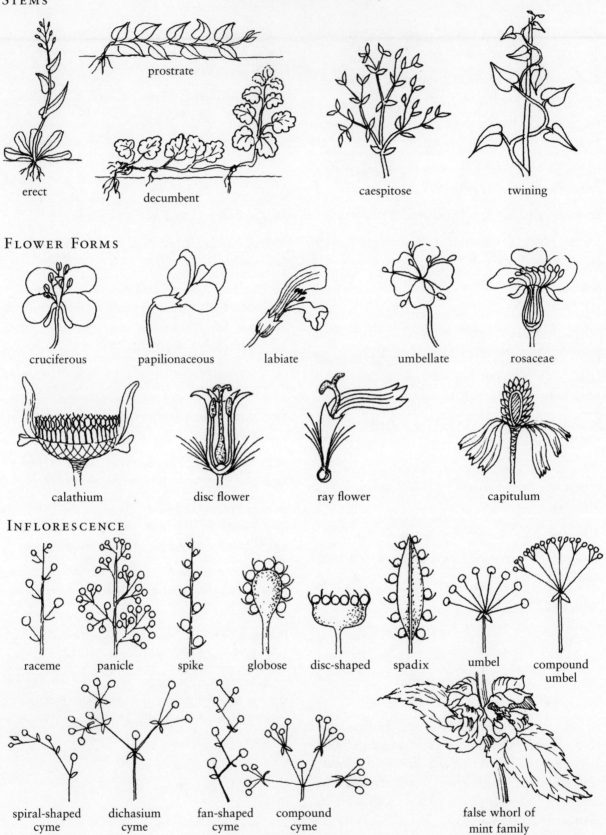

STEMS

erect

prostrate

decumbent

caespitose

twining

FLOWER FORMS

cruciferous

papilionaceous

labiate

umbellate

rosaceae

calathium

disc flower

ray flower

capitulum

INFLORESCENCE

raceme

panicle

spike

globose

disc-shaped

spadix

umbel

compound
umbel

spiral-shaped
cyme

dichasium
cyme

fan-shaped
cyme

compound
cyme

false whorl of
mint family

ARRANGEMENT OF LEAVES ON STEM

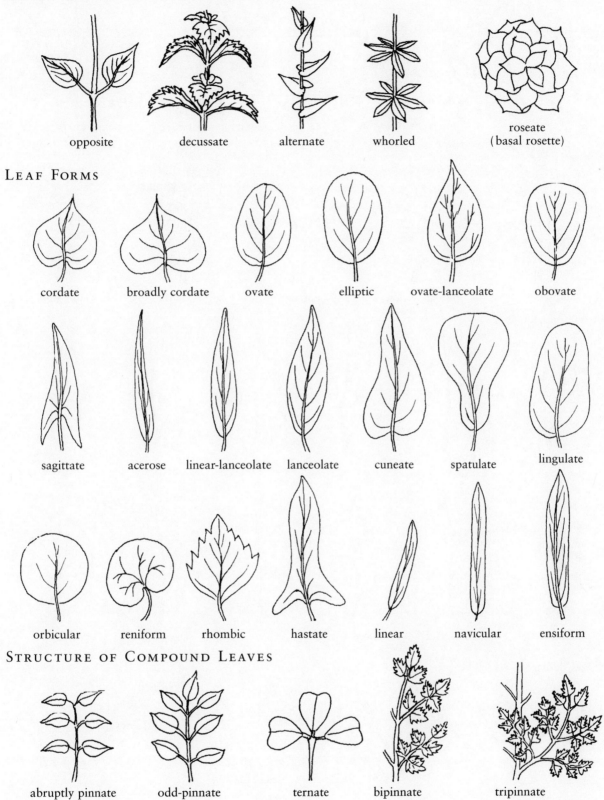

opposite   decussate   alternate   whorled   roseate (basal rosette)

LEAF FORMS

cordate   broadly cordate   ovate   elliptic   ovate-lanceolate   obovate

sagittate   acerose   linear-lanceolate   lanceolate   cuneate   spatulate   lingulate

orbicular   reniform   rhombic   hastate   linear   navicular   ensiform

STRUCTURE OF COMPOUND LEAVES

abruptly pinnate   odd-pinnate   ternate   bipinnate   tripinnate

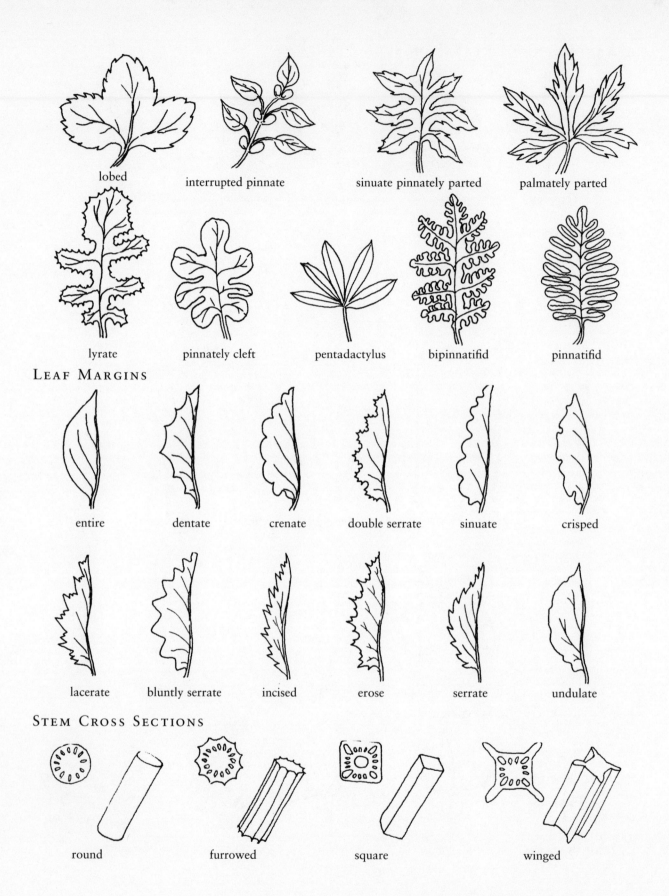

lobed   interrupted pinnate   sinuate pinnately parted   palmately parted

lyrate   pinnately cleft   pentadactylus   bipinnatifid   pinnatifid

LEAF MARGINS

entire   dentate   crenate   double serrate   sinuate   crisped

lacerate   bluntly serrate   incised   erose   serrate   undulate

STEM CROSS SECTIONS

round   furrowed   square   winged

INDEX

Toothed Wood Fern, 190
Tormentil, 78, 110, 281–87
 botanical characteristics of, 287
 cultivation of, 286
 healing properies of, 283–86
  powder, 285
  salve, 286
  schnapps, 285
  tea, 285
  tincture, 285
  toothpowder, 286
  wine, 285
 veterinary use of, 286
Tragopogon pratensis, 29
Treifolium pratense, 52
Trifolium repens, 52
Tumeric, 141
Tussilago farfara, 34, 49, 63, 64
Twoleaf Beadruby, 125

U
Umbelliferae, 9–10
Uric acid, 75
Ustilago equiseti, 174

V
Vaccinium myrtillus, 63
Valerian, 11, 213, 240, 266, 289–96
 botanical characteristics of, 296
 cultivation of, 294–95
 healing properties of, 292
  sleep pillow, 293
  tea, 292, 293
  tincture, 292
  wine, 293
 veterinary use of, 294
Valeriana mexicana, 291
Valeriana officinalis, 11, 213, 292
Verbascum bobmyciferum, 216
Verbascum longifolium, 216
Verbascum nigrum, 216
Verbascum olympicum, 216
Verbascum phoeniceum, 216
Verbascum thapsiforme, 108, 211
Verbascum thapsus, 216
Verbona, 56
Veronica officinalis, 63,108
Vervain, 204
von Bingen, Hildegard, 85, 164, 192, 200
von Crasinski, P. Cyrill, 191
von Goethe, J.W., 12
von Linné, Carl, 56, 125
von Mengenberg, Konrad, 202

W
Waggerl, Karl-Heinz, 47, 115
Wallflower, 39

Warts Herb, 165
Warts, remedy for, 142
Water Hemlock, 10
Water Hemp, 155
Water Marjoram, 155
Water Parsnip, 10
Weaning, tea for, 183
Weiss, Dr. R.F., 49
Wellbestow, 24
White Birch, 129
White Waterlilly, 57
Whortleleberry, 63
Wild Laurin, 48
Willowleaf Inula, 29
Winged Figwort, 107
Wolf's Eye, 23
Wolf's Herb, 31
Wolf's Thistles, 227
Wolf's Yellow, 23
Wolfberries, 227
Wolfman, 31
Wolfsgelega, 23
Women's Gratitude, 299
Women's Herb, 299
Women's Mountain, 40
Wood Avens, 49
Wood Tea, 33
Wood's Mother Herb, 273
Woodland Angelica, 10
Wormwood, 203, 213
Wort, definition of, 201
Woundherb, 24
Wounds, herbs for healing, 78–79

Y
Yarrow, 49, 147, 213, 299–306
 botanical characteristics of, 306
 in cosmetics, 304–305
 cultivation of, 305
 healing properties of, 302–304
  juice, 304
  tea, 304
  tincture, 304
  wine, 304
 veterinary use of, 304
Yellow Bedstraw, 141, 213
Yellow Gentian, 49
Yellow Sweet Clover, 63

Z
Zingiber officinale, 11, 49